RE-ENGINEERING CLINICAL TRIALS

RE–ENGINEERING CLINICAL TRIALS
Best Practices for Streamlining Drug Development

PETER SCHÜLER

BRENDAN BUCKLEY

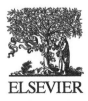

Amsterdam • Boston • Heidelberg • London
New York • Oxford • Paris • San Diego
San Francisco • Singapore • Sydney • Tokyo
Academic Press is an imprint of Elsevier

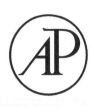

Academic Press is an imprint of Elsevier
32 Jamestown Road, London NW1 7BY, UK
525 B Street, Suite 1800, San Diego, CA 92101-4495, USA
225 Wyman Street, Waltham, MA 02451, USA
The Boulevard, Langford Lane, Kidlington, Oxford OX5 1GB, UK

ISBN: 978-0-12-420246-7

British Library Cataloguing-in-Publication Data
A catalogue record for this book is available from the British Library

Library of Congress Cataloging-in-Publication Data
A catalog record for this book is available from the Library of Congress

For information on all Academic Press publications
visit our website at http://store.elsevier.com/

Typeset by TNQ Books and Journals
www.tnq.co.in

Printed and bound in the United States of America

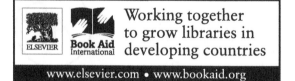

Working together
to grow libraries in
developing countries

www.elsevier.com • www.bookaid.org

CONTENTS

SECTION 2 What Does Our Industry and What Do Others Do

SECTION 3   Where to Start: The Protocol

SECTION 5   From Data to Decisions

SECTION 6   You Need Processes, Systems, and People

LIST OF CONTRIBUTORS

Urs-Vito Albrecht
Peter L. Reichertz Institute for Medical Informatics, Medical School, Hannover, Germany

Nicholas John Alp
ICON Clinical Research UK Ltd, Marlow, UK; Cardiovascular Medicine, Oxford University Hospitals NHS Trust, Oxford, UK

Pol Boudes
PFB Consulting, Pennington, NJ, USA

Brendan M. Buckley
ICON Clinical Research Ltd, Dublin, Ireland; School of Medicine and Health, University College Cork, Cork, Ireland

Malcolm Neil Burgess
ICON Clinical Research, Warrington, PA, USA

Martin Daumer
Sylvia Lawry Centre – The Human Motion Institute, Munich, Germany; TU Munich, LMU Munich and Trium Analysis Online GmbH

Simon Day
Clinical Trials Consulting & Training Limited, Buckingham, UK

Winfried Dietz
Unternehmensberatung Dietz, Wallenhorst, Germany

Patrick Frankham
Mcgill University, Quebec, Canada

Heather Fraser
Global Life Sciences & Healthcare Lead, Institute for Business Value, IBM, UK

Tatiana Gasperazzo
Lampe & Company, Berlin, Germany

Kenneth A. Getz
Tufts Center for the Study of Drug Development, Tufts University School of Medicine, Boston, MA, USA

Matthias Gottwald
Global Drug Discovery - Global External Innovation and Alliances, Bayer Pharma AG, Berlin, Berlin, Germany

Mike Hardman
Innovative Medicines, AstraZeneca, Macclesfield, UK

Clara Heering
Icon Plc, Medical & Safety Services, ICON, Langen, Germany

Liselotte Hyveled
Novo Nordisk A/S, Bagsvaerd, Denmark

Stan Kachnowski
Department of Management Studies, Indian Institute of Technology-New Delhi,
New Delhi, Delhi, India; Lasker Hall, CUMC Audubon Center, New York, NY, USA;
Overseas Unit, Royal Society of Medicine, London, England, UK; PI, Columbia
University Medical Center, New York, NY, USA

Kenneth I. Kaitin
Tufts Center for the Study of Drug Development, Tufts University School of Medicine,
Boston, MA, USA

Wayne Kubick
CDISC - Clinical Data Interchange Standards Consortium, N. Barrington, IL, USA

Johannes Lampe
Lampe & Company, Berlin, Germany

Christian Lederer
Sylvia Lawry Centre – The Human Motion Institute, Munich, Germany

P. Luisi
Mcgill University, Quebec, Canada

Michelle Marlborough
Medidata Solutions Inc., New York, NY, USA

Kevin McNulty
Product Marketing, Intralinks, Charlestown, MA, USA

Gareth Milborrow
ICON Clinical Research UK Ltd, Eastleigh, UK

Nick Milton
Knoco Ltd, Bath, UK

Andrew Mitchell
Intralinks, London, UK

Erich Mohr
MedGenesis Therapeutix Inc., Victoria, BC, Canada

Henrik Nakskov
Strandvejen, Charlottenlund, Denmark

Miguel Orri
InnovatOrri Pharma Consulting Ltd, Petaling Jaya, Malaysia

Oliver Pramann
Kanzlei 34 - Rechtsanwälte und Notare, Hannover, Germany

Johann Proeve
Global Data Management, Bayer Healthcare, Leverkusen, Germany

Wolfgang Renz
Boehringer-ingelheim, NY, USA

Martin Robinson
International Academy of Clinical Research (IAOCR), Maidenhead, UK

Andreas Hans Romberg
Lean Development & Innovation, Staufen AG, Köngen, Baden-Württemberg, Germany

Yuji Sato
Centre for Clinical Research, Keio University School of Medicine, Shinjuku, Tokyo, Japan

Peter Schüler
Medical & Safety Services, ICON, Langen, Germany

Linda B. Sullivan
Metrics Champion Consortium, Carmel, IN, USA

Jochen Tannemann
Life Science, Intralinks GmbH, Frankfurt am Main, Hessen, Germany

Chris Trizna
CSSi Clinical Site Services, Glen Burnie, MD, USA; Virginia Commonwealth University, Glen Burnie, MD, USA

INTRODUCTION

The pharmaceutical industry is experiencing a gap between investments in new medicines and the number of new drugs reaching the market. The return on investment is under increasing pressure because of global restrictions on reimbursement.

This book will outline a number of approaches that are readily applicable and are within the existing regulatory framework. Where we present more revolutionary ideas outside current regulations, this will be clearly detailed. The authors are subject-matter experts from within the drug development industry and from academia. They will assess a variety of new opportunities to apply new technologies to data acquisition and handling, and will also discuss the implementation in this industry of process improvement methodologies that are well established elsewhere. For instance, concepts such as Lean- and Shopfloor-Management could well be transferred to the program and protocol-development process. The regulatory authorities, such as FDA, EMA, and PMDA, appreciate the need for change and promote the adoption of new concepts such as adaptive/risk-based site monitoring. However, change in such a conservative industry needs to be managed by the people working in it, and accordingly new roles need to be developed with a consequent need for changes in qualifications as well.

The book is providing the readers a quick to read overview of all options to improve drug development. It covers all core aspects, such as systems, processes, people, by subject-matter experts. Regulatory authorities are open to innovation as long as it can be scientifically justified. However, the industry itself is reluctant to move away from established and conservative but often outdated and inefficient models. Nothing new needs to be invented to allow very significant improvement in drug development. However, it requires the combined application of technology integrated with fundamental process improvement and purpose-driven staff development to achieve the efficiencies in clinical trials that will allow more drugs to be developed more quickly (Figures 1 and 2).

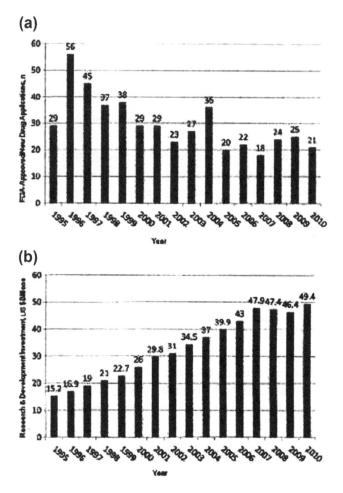

Figure 1 The number of newly approved drugs by FDA between 1995 and 2010 is rather stable, even though investment steadily increased until 2007, since when it has been stable, leaving a major productivity gap [1].

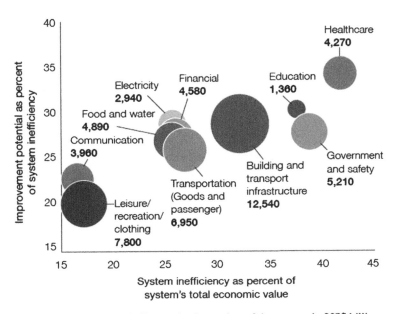

Note: Size of the bubble indicates absolute value of the system in US$ billions
Source: IBM Institute for Business Value analysis based on inefficiency
and improvement potential estimates reported during 2009 survey of 518
economists.

Figure 2 Of the US$15 trillion in inefficiencies within our global system, approximately US$4 trillion could be eliminated, with highest relative potential in the Healthcare sector [2].

REFERENCES

[1] Casty Frank E, Wieman Matthew S. Drug development in the 21st century: the synergy of public, private, and international collaboration. Ther Innovation Regul Sci May 2013;47(3):375–83.
[2] Korsten Peter, Seider Christian, IBM Institute for Business Value. The world's 4 trillion dollar challenge: using a system-of-systems approach to build a smarter planet. January 2010.

Why Does the Industry Need a Change?

CHAPTER 1

Why Is the Pharmaceutical and Biotechnology Industry Struggling?

Kenneth A. Getz, Kenneth I. Kaitin

Contents

1. INTRODUCTION

Industry insiders and observers would be hard pressed to find a macrolevel indicator showing that the drug development enterprise is *not* productive. Arguably the enterprise has been experiencing one of its most productive periods in recent history. The number of new molecular and biologic entities in the research and development (R&D) pipeline has been rising 7% annually and in 2014 exceeded 10,000 active drug candidates. And for each of the several years before that, productivity—as measured by the total number of new drugs and biologics approved by the U.S. Food and Drug Administration (FDA)—met or exceeded the average number of annual approvals over the preceding decade (see Figure 1.1) [1]. The number of new molecular entities (NMEs) approved by regulatory agencies in the European Union and Japan also increased steadily during that time [2].

A variety of discovery technologies have helped feed the drug development pipeline through more rapid and comprehensive target identification and optimization. To name but a few technologies: high-throughput screening has resulted in a 10-fold reduction in the cost of testing compound

Re-Engineering Clinical Trials
http://dx.doi.org/10.1016/B978-0-12-420246-7.00001-3

3

**Number of new drug
and biologics approvals**

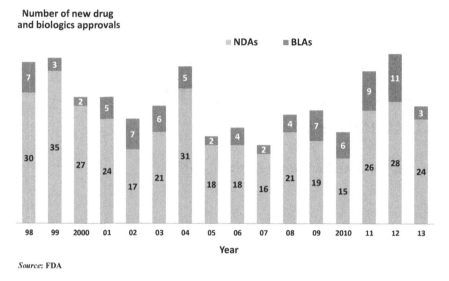

Source: FDA

Figure 1.1 New drugs and biologics approved annually.

libraries; combinatorial chemistry has increased 800-fold the number of new molecular entities to be potentially synthesized; the speed of DNA sequencing has rapidly accelerated since the first genome was sequenced in the 1970s [3].

But this snapshot of current productivity belies a crisis that is intensifying and threatening the long-term viability of the drug development enterprise. Pharmaceutical and biotechnology companies are struggling to bring candidates through R&D and to generate a sufficient return on investment. Inefficient processes, high uncertainty, complexity, and poor performance lie at the heart of the crisis that the drug development enterprise now faces.

This chapter provides an overview of critical factors that characterize a stifling and challenging operating landscape.

1.1 High Failure Rates

Despite efforts since the 1960s to improve drug development risk, the probability of successfully bringing a drug from discovery to commercialization is low—and is gradually getting worse [4]. According to the FDA, for every 10,000 new molecular entities discovered, only one will receive regulatory approval to be marketed. Tufts Center for the Study of Drug Development (CSDD) research indicates that within the

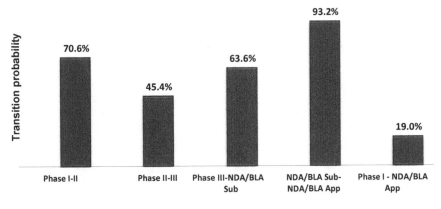

Source: **Tufts CSDD**

Figure 1.2 Phase transition probabilities for all drugs (1998–2008).

clinical development phase—the most expensive and last stage of R&D—only 19% of drugs that enter will be approved (see Figure 1.2) [5]. Success rates in the European Union are similar to those in the United States [6].

The transition from Phase II to Phase III has the highest attrition rate, with 55% of all compounds failing to advance to the final stage in clinical trials. Despite industry efforts over the years to improve success rates, current clinical approval rates are lower than that observed in the 1990s, when 21.5% of all drugs entering clinical testing were submitted to and approved by the FDA.

Overall clinical approval success rates and phase transition probabilities vary widely by therapeutic area. Oncology, immunology, and infectious diseases have the highest clinical approval success rates, ranging from 19.4% to 23.9%. Crowded drug classes targeting chronic diseases (e.g., central nervous system, cardiovascular and endocrine system disorders) have the lowest overall clinical approval success rates [7].

1.2 Long Development Timelines

Clinical phase durations currently are no shorter than they were in the early 1990s. Despite the implementation of a wide variety of new practices and technologies intended to accelerate clinical development cycle times, the opposite has occurred [8]. By 2010 the average clinical phase duration was 6.8 years, increasing 15% during the preceding decade (see Figure 1.3). Longer clinical phase durations are in large part a function of the therapeutic

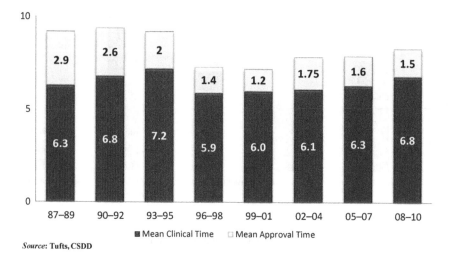

Source: **Tufts, CSDD**

Figure 1.3 Drug development timelines (cycle time in years from Investigational New Drug (IND) approval to New Drug Application (NDA) approval).

classes that dominate research activity (e.g., oncology and central nervous system). Drugs targeting diseases in these therapeutic areas have longer average development cycle times.

Although regulatory requirements have steadily increased since 2000, the average time from submission of a new drug or biologic application to regulatory approval is 1.5 years and has remained relatively flat over that time period. Whereas Western markets have the most stringent regulatory environments, companies in the United States and Western Europe typically outperform (e.g., time to market and number of simultaneous international market approvals) their peers in other geographic regions. One explanation for this finding is that requirements from mature market regulatory agencies have forced companies to be more selective in the compounds that they choose to develop and commercialize. Countries with more permissive regulations tend to produce drugs that may be successful domestically but are not sufficiently innovative to receive approval and gain market adoption elsewhere [6].

Operating inefficiencies are a major contributor to longer development cycle times. However, perhaps the largest contributor is poor study volunteer recruitment and retention rates. A Tufts CSDD study of several hundred global clinical trials found that sponsor companies must typically double the planned enrollment period to give investigative sites enough

Table 1.1 Study enrollment cycle times

	2012 screen to completion rates	Increase in planned study duration to reach target enrollment
Overall	56%	94%
Cardiovascular	59%	99%
Central nervous system	61%	116%
Endocrine/metabolic	41%	113%
Oncology	78%	71%
Respiratory	59%	95%

Source: Tufts CSDD (2012).

time to recruit study volunteers and complete a given clinical trial (see Table 1.1). Even when cycle times are extended, one of four (39%) investigative sites, on average, in any multicenter global clinical trial will underenroll, and one of every 10 (11%) will fail to enroll a single patient [1]. The other half of the sites in a given multicenter study eventually will either meet the enrollment target or exceed it.

It is estimated that one of every 200 people in the United States would need to participate in clinical trials at the present time if the clinical research portfolio were to be successfully completed. The failure of the drug development enterprise since the 1990s to elicit support and commitment from the public and patient communities and to engage them as partners in the clinical research process plays an instrumental role in challenging recruitment and retention effectiveness. National and international public opinion polls show that public confidence and trust in the clinical research enterprise has eroded during that time period. A more recent public poll conducted by the Kaiser Family Foundation, for example, has shown that the public has a strongly unfavorable view of pharmaceutical and biotechnology companies, with more than one-fourth of respondents saying that they do not trust pharmaceutical and biotechnology companies to offer reliable information about drug side effects and safety and nearly half saying that they do not trust research sponsors to inform the public quickly when safety concerns about a drug are discovered [1].

1.3 Steadily Rising Drug Development Costs

Total spending worldwide on pharmaceutical R&D will reach an estimated US$140 billion in 2014, representing a 4.9% compound annual growth rate

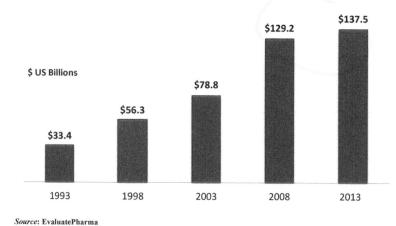

Figure 1.4 Total global research and development spending.

during the preceding 10 years (see Figure 1.4) [9]. Companies now report that they anticipate limiting growth in R&D investment to 2% annually for the foreseeable future to tie spending to expected increases in global industry revenue.

Enterprise wide, as overall drug development spending has risen, the number of new drugs introduced per year has been relatively flat. Between 2003 and 2013, the pharmaceutical industry spent a cumulative US$1.3 trillion on R&D, which resulted in 296 new drug and biologic approvals. This translates into US$4.4 billion average annual cost per approved molecule. In that same 10-year period alone, the average cost per new chemical and biologic entity during the second half of the decade increased 30% over the average during the first half (see Figure 1.5). Rising R&D investment generating less output is a long-standing trend. The number of new FDA-approved drugs per billion U.S. dollars of R&D spending by the drug development enterprise has halved approximately every nine years since the 1950s [10].

Annual development spending and its associated output tell only part of the story. High failure rates and long cycle times translate into very high levels of 12–15 years in capitalized investment required to develop a successful drug. The average capitalized cost to bring a single drug through R&D and into the marketplace now exceeds US$1.3 billion (see Table 1.2). Each successful drug must cover its own direct costs (30% of the total) plus all of the costs associated with failed drugs and the opportunity cost of capital amortized over the period of time that it takes to develop the successful drug candidate [5].

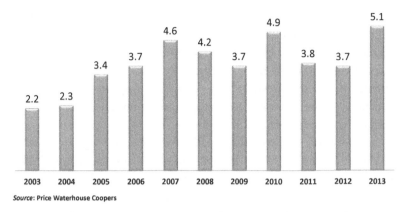

Source: Price Waterhouse Coopers

Figure 1.5 Cost per new molecular entity.

Table 1.2 Direct and capitalized development

	Direct costs		Capitalized costs	
Basic research through preclinical phase	$60 MM	17%	$186 MM	15%
Clinical phase through regulatory approval	$109 MM	34%	$189 MM	15%
Allocated failures	$166 MM	49%	$866 MM	70%
Total per approved drug	$335 MM		$1,241 MM	

Source: Tufts CSDD.

1.4 Rising Protocol Complexity

Several Tufts CSDD studies capture remarkable growth in protocol design scientific and operating complexity. In 2012, for example, to demonstrate safety and efficacy, a typical Phase III protocol had an average of 170 procedures performed on each study volunteer during the course of 11 visits across an average 230-day time span. Ten years previously, the typical Phase III protocol had an average of 106 procedures, 9 visits, and a 187-day time span. For the typical Phase III protocol conducted in 2012, study volunteers came from an average of 34 countries and 196 research centers, up from 11 countries and 124 research centers 10 years ago. Moreover, in 2012, to qualify to participate in a typical Phase III protocol, each volunteer had to meet 50 eligibility criteria—up from an average of 31 inclusion and exclusion criteria 10 years previously. And a typical Phase III study in 2012 collected nearly 1 million clinical data points, up from an estimated 500,000 a decade earlier (see Table 1.3) [11].

Rising study design complexity is inevitable. New scientific knowledge about the pathophysiology of many diseases, and new approaches to measuring disease progression and economic impact require collecting more data. Crowded classes of investigational therapies and the ongoing movement to develop stratified medicines are pushing research sponsors to collect more data and to target smaller patient subgroups to more effectively differentiate small- and large-molecule interventions. Research sponsors are collecting an ever-wider array of data, including biomarker, genetic, outcome, economic, and companion diagnostic, that may be analyzed as part of the study or stored and analyzed at a future date. And medical scientists and statisticians often add procedures to gather more contextual data to aid in their interpretation of the findings and to guide development decisions.

Rising study design complexity is also a function of risk management, risk avoidance, and outdated practices. Drug developers routinely add procedures guided by the notion that the marginal cost of doing so, relative to the entire clinical study budget, is small, whereas the risk of not doing so is high. Additional procedures are performed to hedge against the study failing to meet its primary and key secondary objectives. The data from these procedures may prove valuable in post hoc analyses that reveal new and useful information about the progression of disease and its treatment, as well as new directions for future development activity. Clinical research teams add procedures for fear that they may neglect to collect data requested by regulatory agencies and health authorities, purchasers, and payers. Failure to do so could potentially delay regulatory submission,

Table 1.3 Characterizing protocol complexity (a typical phase III protocol)

	2002	2012
Total number of end points	7	13
Total number of protocol procedures	106	167
Total number of eligibility criteria	31	50
Total number of countries	11	34
Total number of investigative sites	124	196
Total number of patients randomized	729	597
Total number of data points collected per patient[a]	500,000	929,203

[a]Medidata solutions.
Source: Tufts CSDD.

product launch, and product adoption. Medical writers and protocol authors also often permit outdated and unnecessary procedures into new study designs because they are routinely included in legacy protocol authoring templates and operating policies.

Phase II studies are the most complex and most burdensome to execute. An increasing number of research sponsors aspire to collect more data during Phase II clinical trials to avoid going into costly later stage studies. As a result, the growth in the number of new procedures performed during Phase II outpaces that observed in other phases. Several therapeutic areas, including anti-infectives, immunomodulation, central nervous system, and oncology, consistently have more complex protocols, as they represent areas in which it is more difficult to demonstrate clinical safety, efficacy, and economic benefit.

Most importantly, protocol complexity is correlated with higher development costs, longer study durations, and more protocol deviations and amendments [12].

1.5 Poorly Integrated and Fragmented Operating Models

Over the past two decades, the number of parties—from both internal and external sources—involved with an individual drug development program has grown dramatically. A wide variety of cross-functional areas now support clinical development programs, including clinical, clinical operations, patient recruitment, statistics, medical writing, regulatory affairs, clinical supplies, procurement, external alliance management, capacity planning and forecasting, and data management. Contract service providers support the drug development enterprise under a broad range of relationship models including integrated alliances, functional service providers, full-service, and specialty service provider arrangements.

Fragmentation in the drug development enterprise is the enemy of efficiency. Planning, communication, coordination, and collaboration are extremely difficult across such a highly fragmented collective of operating elements, particularly when they are—as is increasingly the case—more globally dispersed. Functional areas also tend to develop and execute strategies in an insular way without engaging and coordinating support across internal functions and among disparate external service providers. As a result, new solutions and practices are highly dependent on individuals championing change, and efficiency-boosting initiatives are typically implemented as uncoordinated point solutions, addressing only part of a larger systemic problem or challenge.

Silo-based execution of strategies and tactics is fraught with delays and disruptions. The current operating environment has prompted pharmaceutical companies to pursue collaborations to share risk and return. Joint development arrangements, in-licensing deals, and mergers and acquisitions (M&As) are examples of the most prevalent and pervasive shared innovation approaches utilized. Of late, the volume and scale of M&A activity has risen to such heights that even the largest companies can be takeover targets. Between 2008 and 2012, 5 of the top 10 largest pharmaceutical companies—as defined by global prescription drug sales—acquired and absorbed at least one major company (e.g., Merck acquired Schering-Plough; Pfizer acquired Wyeth; Sanofi acquired Genzyme). Tufts CSDD research shows that the fragmented and poorly integrated execution of shared innovation approaches consistently results in drug development durations that are significantly longer than the average, adding a median of 14.8 months of development time [13].

1.6 Tightening Sources of Capital

Capital to fund R&D innovation—from all sources, including global market consumption and the investment community—has become increasingly constrained. Economic conditions for pharmaceuticals are tightening. Internationally, countries are enforcing drug pricing and reimbursement limits. Worldwide, governments are cracking down on pharmaceutical detailing and promotional practices and requiring greater disclosure of interactions with health care purchasers and payers.

Health care reform—including the Affordable Care Act in the United States, which was enacted in 2010—seeks to reduce patients' out-of-pocket health care expenses, including drugs and medical interventions. Although the pharmaceutical industry is expected to see an additional 30 million U.S. citizens receiving health care coverage, the Affordable Care Act is projected to cost the industry US$12–15 billion annually in lost revenue during the coming decade [10].

Payers and other third-party providers, in their efforts to control rising health care costs, are increasingly demanding that research sponsors demonstrate that their products offer therapeutic or cost advantages over competitors' products and other medical interventions. Health technology assessment and comparative effectiveness movements in Western Europe and the United States are gaining momentum and challenging pharmaceutical and biotechnology companies to submit new drug applications demonstrating not only safety and efficacy but also economic and therapeutic value.

Blockbuster drugs that historically generated strong and highly profitable revenue streams are losing patent protection and seeing rapid erosion from generic equivalents. The "patent cliff"—between 2014 and 2018—represents approximately US$100 billion in lost sales due to generic competition (see Figure 1.6) [1]. From 2007 to 2014, the average revenue lost to patent expirations was 60% greater than the average for the prior five years, as a growing number of blockbuster drugs lost their market exclusivity.

Declining pharmaceutical company stock prices and market capitalizations indicate that the investment community expects its return on current and future R&D investments to be below the cost of capital and would prefer less R&D and higher dividends. A Tufts CSDD analysis of pharmaceutical company market capitalizations during the past 10 years indicates that more than half a trillion U.S. dollars in overall market value has disappeared as the investment community has shifted its attention to other more promising economic sectors [14]. The estimated internal rate of return (IRR) on small-molecule R&D between 2002 and 2007 was 7.5%, down from an IRR of 12% for a typical small molecule developed between 1997 and 2002 [15].

Yesterday's blockbuster drugs are today's generic offerings. Generic drug sales now capture nearly 80% of the total market for prescription

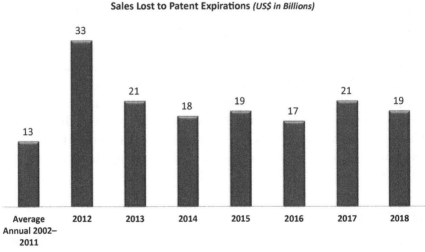

Sales Lost to Patent Expirations *(US$ in Billions)*

Source: **EvaluatePharma; Tufts CSDD**

Figure 1.6 The patent cliff.

medications annually. The growing number of generic drugs increases the complexity of the drug development process for new interventions and raises regulatory requirements and market hurdles for approval, adoption, and reimbursement. The large number of generic alternatives in certain therapeutic areas has served as an R&D deterrent within the research-based pharmaceutical industry for many diseases with significant morbidity and mortality. In response, many companies have refocused their R&D efforts on unmet and hard-to-treat medical needs and orphan indications, which often reduce the economic value of new drug innovations.

Economic and capital market conditions have contributed to high operating volatility. Only 10% of all drug development companies that existed 50 years ago are still operating today. The remaining 90% have failed, divested, merged, or been acquired [4]. As a result, it is difficult for new models of innovation to take hold and deliver sustainable change and impact.

1.7 Returning to a Viable R&D Innovation Model

The industry is struggling to innovate under the current operating conditions characterized in this chapter. These operating conditions are intractable, and they are getting worse. The R&D operating model, which served the drug development enterprise well during the past 50 years, is outdated and no longer viable.

Despite the dire current state of the R&D enterprise, there is much on the horizon that is cause for optimism. Demand for prescription drugs is expected to increase as Baby Boomers enter their retirement years and as emerging Eastern markets turn to Western medicine for treatment. New technologies including proteomics and platform technologies are expected to improve the predictability and accelerate discovery and nonclinical phase activity.

New models of collaboration, including open innovation platforms, the integration of big data systems that leverage structured and unstructured electronic health information, modification of legacy processes, the adoption of adaptive clinical trial designs and more patient centric clinical trials, are all emerging approaches that hold promise in transforming R&D process and performance.

REFERENCES

[1] Getz K. Transforming legacy R&D through open innovation. The Monitor 2011; 4(3):16–21.
[2] Dowden H, Jahn R, Catka T, Jonsson A, Michael E, Miwa Y, et al. Industry and regulatory performance in 2012: a year in review. Clin Pharmacol Ther 2013;94(3):359–66.

[3] Scannel J, Blanckley A, Boldon H, Warrington B. Diagnosing the decline in pharmaceutical R&D efficiency. Nat Rev Drug Discov 2012;11:191–200.

[4] Munos B. Lessons from 60 years of pharmaceutical innovation. Nat Rev Drug Discov 2009;8:959–68.

[5] Kaitin K, DiMasi J. Pharmaceutical innovation in the 21st century: new drug approvals in the first decade 2000–2009. Clin Pharmacol Ther 2011;89(2):183–8.

[6] Pammoli F, Magazzini L, Riccaboni M. The productivity crisis in pharmaceutical R&D. Nat Rev Drug Discov 2011;10:429–38.

[7] DiMasi J, Feldman L, Seckler A, Wilson A. Trends in risks associated with new drug development: success rates for investigational drugs. Clin Pharmacol Ther 2010; 87(3):272–7.

[8] Getz K, Kaitin K. Open innovation: the new face of pharmaceutical research and development. Expert Rev Clin Pharmacol 2012;5(5):481–3.

[9] EvaluatePharma. World Preview 2016.

[10] Arlington S. From vision to decision: pharma 2020. Price Waterhouse Coopers.

[11] Getz K, Stergiopoulos S, Marlborough M, Whitehall J, Curran M, Kaitin K. Quantifying the magnitude and cost of collecting extraneous protocol data. Am J Ther 2013. Published ahead of print. April 9, 2013.

[12] Getz KA, Stergiopoulos S. Therapeutic area variability in the collection of data supporting protocol end points and objectives. Clin Invest 2014;4(2):125–30.

[13] DiMasi JA, Kim J, Getz KA. The impact of collaborative and risk-sharing innovation approaches on clinical and regulatory cycle times. Ther Innov Regul Sci 2014; 48(4):482–7.

[14] Kaitin K, Honig P. Reinventing bioinnovation. Clin Pharmacol Ther 2013;94(3): 279–83.

[15] David E, Tramontin T, Zemmel R. Pharmaceutical R&D: the road to positive returns. Nat Rev Drug Discov 2009;8:609–12.

CHAPTER 2

What Are Current Main Obstacles to Reach Drug Approval?

Pol Boudes

Contents

1. THE NEED

Specific clinical requirements concerning the efficacy, the safety, and the risk–benefit of a drug have to be met for a new drug to be approved. These requirements are not always well understood and can constitute obstacles that are difficult to overcome [1]. A failure to demonstrate that a new drug brings a meaningful clinical benefit is a frequent issue encountered during the drug approval process. While a statistical significance on a primary outcome of efficacy is necessary, it is not sufficient for a drug approval. The nature of the outcome and the size of the effect have to be taken into account to demonstrate that data are clinically significant [2]. Another frequent underlying reason is related to the difficulty of selecting the appropriate dose and regimen [3].

In the European Union, contrary to the United States, the European Medicines Agency (EMA) has to disclose the reasons why drugs are withdrawn when their applications are refused. A recent study confirms the prominence of efficacy objections, notably because of a lack of clinical relevance, over any other issues such as safety or quality [4].

Concerning safety, the main question to address is not whether there is a safety signal or not, but rather whether any safety signal has been appropriately addressed. Safety signals should be characterized and quantified and, most importantly, addressed in the clinical practice context so, ideally, they can be managed [5].

Re-Engineering Clinical Trials
http://dx.doi.org/10.1016/B978-0-12-420246-7.00002-5

Ultimately, the analysis of efficacy and safety remains the cornerstone of drug development. A deficient or unfavorable risk–benefit analysis continues to be the main reason why drugs are not approved [1]. It is also important that regulators' feedback is taken into account. A recent European study indicated that a failure to follow the recommendations received during a scientific advice was ultimately associated with denial of approval [6].

At the same time, new obstacles arise and the drug approval process is becoming more complex and more expensive. Recent safety issues, such as the Cox-2 and glitazones controversies [7], have led regulators to accept less risk, especially for drugs that could be widely marketed. The toughening of regulatory guidelines, such as the need to demonstrate the cardiovascular safety of an antidiabetic compound, increases costs of drug development to such levels that investment is discouraged [8]. Other regulatory guidances, such as the biosimilar one [9], originally designed to facilitate access to biological drugs created confusion and led to the opposite result of their intent. Some other guidelines, intended to address specific situations, become the rule and create unnecessary complexity [10]. Sponsors might also have to develop new diagnostic assays as companion to a drug [11]. Such companion diagnostics help to better define treatment eligibility and the response to treatment. However, the development of an assay to support a drug approval brings complexity, time, and costs to the process.

Finally, a new reality emerges as some medical needs are now well addressed, and it is difficult to improve upon what is already approved [12]. For instance, the need for antihypertensive treatment, cholesterol-lowering drugs, and antiosteoporotic treatments are largely met for the general population. The bar for a new treatment approval is simply too high. Not surprisingly, over the past years, fewer drugs were approved [13].

2. THE SOLUTION

While an appropriate risk–benefit analysis remains the cornerstone for a drug approval (Table 2.1), sponsors have to change the way things are done. Instead of using a mass marketing strategy anchored on limited additional medical benefit, scientific progresses would allow the elucidation of diseases' pathophysiology and help to focus on unmet medical needs. Understanding and addressing new mechanisms of action shall pave the way to innovative new drugs [14].

Increases in development costs also mean that partnership, beyond academia and start-ups, is now essential between pharmaceutical companies [15].

Table 2.1 Recommendations to present risk–benefit analyses, based on an analysis of FDA advisory committee outcomes

Efficacy	Always explain and support clinical relevance
	Improve monitoring, increase sample size, include comparator (oncology trials)
	Support small sponsors with experienced ones (oncology trials)
	Use progression-free survival and biomarkers (oncology trials)
	Validate patient-reported outcomes
	Anchor symptomatic improvement to patients' satisfaction
	Explore data with multiple secondary analyses
	Document efficacy in key populations
	Rationalize dose regimen selection
Effectiveness	Avoid confusion with efficacy
	Summarize results over an entire database
	Explain results in the context of available treatments
Safety	Agree beforehand with regulators on size of database and extent of exposure. Reconsider status if a safety signal is identified.
	Identify all signals
	Explain to clinicians how to decrease and manage risk
	Build a consensus with experts to stand scrutiny during review
	Obtain a consensus with regulators on "potential" safety issues
Risk–benefit	Integrate previous recommendations
	Establish a risk–benefit profile for each indication or population

Source: Adapted from [1].

Regulators, for their part, have to realize that flexibility is essential to improve health [16]. A regulatory precedent exists: In the early 1990s, the flexibility demonstrated to tackle the AIDS epidemic led to the approval of many life-saving antivirals [17].

Today, innovations for the treatment of cancers and orphan diseases exemplify this new way of thinking. In cancers, a new patient–centric approach based on specific new mechanisms of action translates into remarkable drug efficacy and new drug approvals, albeit in a more targeted patient population [14]. Regulators' flexibility allows cancer clinical trials to break away from the dogma of clinical-trial designs. Trials for orphan cancer drugs that were approved are more likely to be smaller and use nonrandomized, unblinded designs and surrogate outcomes to assess efficacy [18]. For rare diseases, legislators have created the appropriate incentive to stimulate drug development and drug approvals [19]. In orphan diseases, few patients are available, and clinical trials to bring evidence of efficacy and safety are more imaginative (Table 2.2). Using natural history data comparisons to anchor efficacy instead of placebo comparisons, accepting

Table 2.2 Clinical study designs used in orphan diseases to support risk–benefit analysis

Small sample sizes require large effect size
Enrichment of study population (practical, prognostic, predictive)
Comparison with historical cohorts (life-saving drugs)
Comparison to baseline status (responder analysis)
Biochemical markers linked with disease pathophysiology
Composite endpoints
Extension phase
Registry

Source: Adapted from [20].

data from only one pivotal trial instead of two, and relying less on statistics and more on clinical significance have facilitated the approval of life-saving drugs [20]. In this context, it is noteworthy that orphan drugs have a better chance to get to a positive approval decision [6].

Finally, regulators and sponsors have to rely on patients and their organizations to understand where therapeutic needs are and which problems are the most important to address.

As a reminder of the benefit that was brought in by HIV-patient organizations to change the rules of drug development and to create the conditional approval, families and patients are now more involved in drug development [16]. Their contribution brings urgency to the drug approval process, helps to better define the medical needs, influences the design and recruitment of clinical trials, and, even, financially supports clinical research efforts [21].

3. SWOT

Strengths: Science driven, mechanism-of-action driven, large effect size, address medical needs.

Weaknesses: Innovation dependent, capital intensive, smaller patient populations.

Opportunities: New study design, new ways to address risk–benefits, patient involvement.

Threats: Regulatory flexibility, collaboration between sponsors.

4. APPLICABLE REGULATIONS

Draft guidance on biosimilars [9] and adaptive design [10], guidance on in vitro diagnostic [11], as well as FDA draft guidance on adaptive design and FDA guidance on bioanalytical validation.

Food and Drug Administration (FDA), Center for Drug Evaluation and Research (CDER), Center for Biologics Evaluation and Research (CBER), CVM. May 2001. BP.

5. TAKE HOME MESSAGE

As there is no precise way to calculate a risk–benefit profile, drug development and approval remain an art rather than a science. Beyond the strength of data, many other factors have to be taken into account. These include current medical needs, variable regulatory contexts, changing legislative and societal environments, tougher operational challenges, and higher costs of investment before any potential return. Breaking old dogmas, new study designs are attempted. Regulations, such as orphan drug designations, breakthrough therapy, or approval under exceptional circumstances stimulate investment and bring flexibility to the approval process.

The risk–benefit analysis remains the cornerstone for drug approval.

Recent scientific progresses help to better understand the pathophysiology of diseases and lead to the discovery of new mechanisms of actions and new drugs.

As demonstrated with cancers and orphan diseases, the approval of new drugs that bring important medical benefits is fueling the drug development engine.

Regulators will be flexible to approve drugs that bring important medical benefits.

REFERENCES

[1] Boudes PF. How to improve complex drug development a critical review at FDA advisory meetings. Drug Inf J 2007;41:673–83.
[2] Man-Son-Hing M, O'Rourke K, Molnart FJ, Mahon J, Chan KBY, Wells G. Determination of the clinical importance of study results. A review. J Gen Intern Med 2002;17:469–76.
[3] Sacks LV, Shamsuddin HH, Yasinskaya YI, Bouri K, Lanthier ML, Sherman RE. Scientific and regulatory reasons for delay and denial of FDA approval of initial applications for new drugs, 2000-2012. JAMA 2014;311:378–84.
[4] Tafuri G, Trotta F, Leufkens HGM, Pani L. Disclosure of grounds of European withdrawn and refused applications: a step forward on regulatory transparency. Br J Clin Pharmacol 2012;75:1149–51.
[5] Boudes PF. The challenges of new drug benefits and risks analysis. Lessons from the ximalagatran FDA advisory committee. Contemp Clin Trials 2006;27:432–40.
[6] Regnstrom J, Koenig F, Aronsson B, Reimer T, Svendsen K, Tsigkos S, et al. Factors associated with success of market authorization applications for pharmaceutical drugs submitted to the European Medicines Agency. Eur J Clin Pharmacol 2010;66:39–48.
[7] Hiatt WR, Kaul S, Smith RJ. The cardiovascular safety of diabetes drugs. Insights from the rosiglitazone experience. N Engl J Med 2013;369:1285–7.

[8] Viereck C, Boudes P. An analysis of the impact of FDA's guidelines for addressing cardiovascular risk of drugs for type 2 diabetes on clinical development. Contemp Clin Trials 2011;32:324–32.

[9] Guidance for Industry. Biosimilars: questions and answers regarding implementation of the biologics price competition and innovation act of 2009. Draft guidance. US department of Health and Human Services. FDA. CDER. CBER. February 2012. Biosimilarity; 2012.

[10] Guidance for industry. E14 Clinical evaluation of QT/QTc interval prolongation and proarrythmic potential for non anti-arrythmic drugs. Questions and answers. US department of HHS, FDA, CDER, CBER, November 2008 ICH; 2008.

[11] Guidance for industry and Food and Drug Administration staff – in vitro companion diagnostic devices. (2011). US department of HHS, FDA, CDER, CBER; July 14, 2011.

[12] Anonymous. Where will new drugs come from? Editor Lancet 2011;377:97.

[13] Scannell JW, Blanckley A, Boldon H, Warrington B. Diagnosing the decline of pharmaceutical R&D efficiency. Nat Rev Drug Disc 2012;11:191–200.

[14] Hamburg MA, Coliins FS. The path to personalized medicine. N Engl J Med 2010;363:301–4.

[15] Mullard A. Partnering between pharma peers on the rise. Nat Rev Drug Disc 2011;10:561–2.

[16] Sasinovski FJ. Quantum of effectiveness evidence in FDA's approval of orphan drugs. Washington DC: National Organization for rare disorders; 2011. Available at: http://raredoseases.org/docs/policy/NORDstudyof FDAapporvaloforphandrugs.pdf.

[17] Breckenridge A, Feldschreiber P, Gregor S, Raine J, Mulcahy L-A. Evolution of regulatory frameworks. Nat Rev Drug Disc 2011;10:3–4.

[18] Kesselheim AS, Myers JA, Avorn J. Characteristics of clinical trials to support approval of orphan vs nonorphan drugs for cancer. JAMA 2011;305:2320–6.

[19] Seone-Vasquez E, Rodrigues-Monguio R, Szeinbach SL, Visaria J. Incentives for orphan drug research and development in the United States. Orphanet J Rare Dis 2008;3:33–40.

[20] Boudes PF. Clinical studies in lysosomal storage diseases. Past, present and futures. Rare Dis 2013;1:e26690.

[21] Gallin EK, Bond E, Califf RM, Crowley WF, Davis P, Galbraith R, et al. Forging stronger partnerships between academic health centers and patient-driven organization. Acad Med 2013;88:1220–4.

CHAPTER 3

Japan: An Opportunity to Learn?

Yuji Sato

Contents

1. THE NEED

1.1 General Background

Multinational multisite clinical trials are regarded as a crucial method of addressing essential clinical questions from within academia, e.g., how to establish the comparative effectiveness among several treatment options [1], and from within the pharmaceutical industry, which seeks to efficiently pursue new drug development for international regulatory approval with as little delay as possible across countries. In addition to the scientific and regulatory standards required for such global trials, including sound study protocols and compliance with relevant regulations, operational coordination across participating countries has become increasingly critical in the day-to-day conduct of trials at investigational sites: even given the best possible protocols and complete regulatory compliance, the quality of clinical data can be compromised, sometimes irretrievably, if the trial operation fails. Arguably, high scientific standards, regulatory and ethical compliance, and operational excellence are the three indispensable prerequisites for high-quality clinical trials, but attention seems hitherto to have focused mostly on the former two prerequisites, with the latter prerequisite regarded as somewhat less crucial.

Among the several noteworthy limitations inherent in double-blind controlled trials [2], which are touted as one of the major cornerstones of evidence-based medicine today, an important limitation is the increasing

Re-Engineering Clinical Trials
http://dx.doi.org/10.1016/B978-0-12-420246-7.00003-7

23

costs of ever larger trials involving many countries and thousands of patients. As neither the scientific rigorousness of trials (e.g., sample size calculation) nor regulatory requirements (e.g., data quality assurance by on-site monitoring) can be sacrificed to control skyrocketing budgets, the operational component alone ends up being scrutinized for elements that can be curtailed or economized. Attempts in this regard include identifying investigational sites in locations where operational costs, mostly personnel expenses, are seen as comparatively low, and outsourcing trial-related operations to commercial contract research organizations (CROs).

However, the unfortunate failures of global trials that not infrequently occur indicate the many problems and challenges involved in clinical trial operations, many of which reflect the immense difficulty of striking a sensible balance between minimizing costs and maintaining, let alone improving, the quality of trials. This chapter attempts to illustrate some of the major operational issues affecting international clinical research operations. It also presents some perspectives on how Japan, as a participant in multinational large-scale trials, can effectively manage these issues.

1.2 Operational Challenges in Multinational Large-scale Clinical Trials

As clinical trials globalize, they involve more and more players. Figure 3.1 illustrates an example of a global pharmaceutical company sponsoring a global multisite trial involving Japanese investigational sites. Normally, global companies operating in Japan have their own domestic subsidiaries with varying degrees of clinical developmental capacity in place locally. It has become common for the headquarters to have a master agreement with an international CRO that then assigns the required local clinical research operations to its own subsidiary. If the project happens to involve codevelopment with a domestic pharmaceutical company, the domestic company contractually plays some part in clinical trial operations along with the subsidiary of the global pharma, the patent holder of the novel compound, and the subsidiary of the global CRO. As a result, three different organizations on the sponsoring side are simultaneously involved in one single trial. Having these multiple organizational layers leads at times to situations where, should some issue arise at a site, e.g., how certain procedures defined in the protocol should be interpreted, clarification can only be made after time-consuming toing and froing involving many e-mail communications, teleconferences, misunderstandings, and misplaced concerns between the site, the three local organizations and the two headquarters. All these

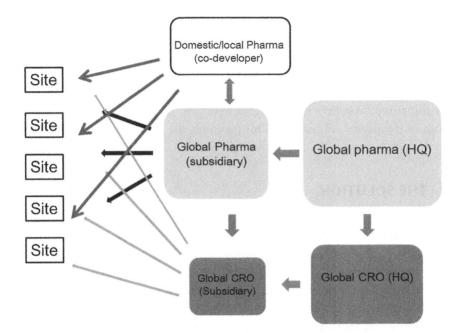

Figure 3.1 Current operational scheme of multinational trials. As more trial operations are outsourced to contract research organizations, more interactions and communications among related professionals are required, increasing the risks of communication gaps, misinterpretations, and misinformed decision-making. The large numbers of arrows pointing toward the investigational sites imply conflicting instructions and explanations coming from different parties, often with delays involved. HQ, headquarters.

interactions cause significant delays in the conduct of the trial and may negatively affect the quality of the trial itself.

Teamwork and communication may seem too banal and commonplace to be mentioned in business administration, and when globalized clinical trial operations are discussed, the ostensibly banal issue of communication among multiple trial-related professionals and organizations is seldom taken up as a potential stumbling block in clinical development that can be as serious as that of budget constraints. Ramifying and sophisticated trial designs with novel exploratory endpoints, sensitive but sometimes unstable biomarker evaluations, and updated electronic data-capturing systems—all recent examples of conscientious efforts to further improve trial quality—need to be understood and properly addressed by all of the multiple players in the complicated reporting lines. It should be borne in mind that the anticipated added value of these novel measures cannot be fully achieved if the eventualities arising from them cannot be dealt within actual daily operations. It is also frequently the case that the introduction of new information technology that is supposed to decrease operational workload, increase accuracy and efficiency, and thereby minimize trial costs, is in the end quite counterproductive, because it complicates trial execution due to malfunctions, updating requirements, and lack of familiarity with it on the part of the personnel using it. This prolongs the trial period and prevents trials from being conducted within the planned developmental budget.

2. THE SOLUTION

In terms of cost-effectiveness, Japan has not been widely regarded as an ideal country for large-scale multinational trials. Perceived drawbacks [3] have included local regulations and business practices that used to look somewhat different from those of other developed countries [4], language differences, limited motivation for patients to participate in trials, high trial costs, and insufficient availability of clinical research support at investigational sites. However, the past 10 years have seen drastic improvements in the clinical research infrastructure under the aegis of the Japanese MHLW to boost clinical trials, together with painstaking efforts by both the pharmaceutical industry and investigational sites in modernizing trial operations, partly to address the so-called drug lag issue Japan has been facing [5]. Therefore, apart from the remaining issue of trial costs, which are still relatively high by international standards, it is fair to say that the other posited obstacles have been largely overcome. Furthermore, the operational excellence common to Japanese manufacturing industry at large, and particularly to the automobile industry, as seen in attention to detail, conscientious adherence to regulations and standards, and constant efforts to improve quality [6], is equally to be found in clinical trial operations, which leads to high-quality trial results and outstanding operational metrics.

Detailed cross-national comparisons of operational quality in clinical trials are scarce. This is understandable to some extent, because in industry-sponsored trials the main objective is to publish the final major results on efficacy and safety, and not such operational data (a recent comparative analysis of GCP compliance at American and Chinese investigational sites [7] is an exceptional publication in this regard). Thus, there is little published evidence to support the above-mentioned claims about the excellence of clinical trial operations in Japan. However, the analysis presented below of three recent multinational trials in two different therapeutic areas shows that the inter-rater reliability of the Japanese data exceeded that of the United States and European countries.

In complex diseases where diagnosis and evaluation of treatment response require specialist expertise and sophisticated clinical judgment, the establishment and maintenance of high inter-rater reliability, which are critical in large-scale trials involving multiple sites and investigators, are always a challenge. One innovative way to ensure high inter-rater reliability is to establish a dual process of eligibility assessment under central coordination [8–11] (Figure 3.2). Patients considered by an investigator to meet the inclusion criteria and no exclusion criteria can be deemed inappropriate and excluded from the trial in cases where the central assessor at the central coordinating center double-checks the eligibility and finds that the inclusion criteria are not fully met; this is termed screening failure. In one study of acute and severe disorders in intensive care units (unpublished), the

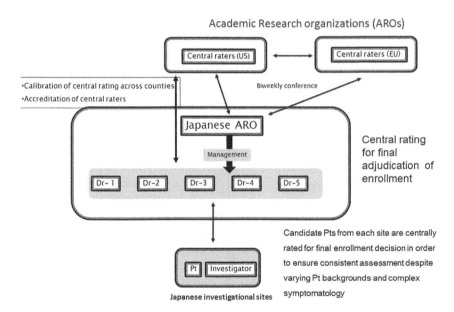

Figure 3.2 A recent example of central coordination by collaborative trial management through what are often called AROs in the United States. In this case, inter-rater reliability was dually ensured: first by central raters in each country to adjudicate case identification and enrollment, and second by having the central raters themselves regularly "calibrated" across three areas with respect to their patient identification process. This model has been successfully implemented in three global trials across different therapeutic areas, and screening failure, i.e., enrollment of patients (Pts) who do not squarely meet the inclusion criteria, was minimized.

screening failure rate was lowest in Japan, followed by the European Union (EU) and the United States (10%, 30%, and 50%, respectively), whereas the enrollment efficiency (finally enrolled patients per investigational site per month) was highest in the United States, followed by the EU and Japan (0.33, 0.19, and 0.07, respectively). This example highlights the difficult balance between enrollment efficiency, an important factor affecting trial period and costs, and the appropriate screening of criteria fulfillment, a critical point in ensuring high data quality.

These experiences suggest that, even with the financial and time constraints prevailing in the current competitive research and development (R&D) environment, Japan is a reasonable investigational location for trials with complex trial designs involving diseases that require particular attention and expertise for diagnosis and evaluation. Without such attention and expertise, successful clinical development is likely to fail in establishing safety and efficacy.

3. SWOT

Strength	Weakness
• Enhances probability of success in clinical trials in terms of efficiency, appropriate case identification, and smooth trial conduct • Allows close and timely collaboration among related professional groups to achieve teamwork excellence	• Attention to detail and preconceived procedures can at times impede swift and flexible adaptability in the face of unexpected challenges • Individual variability in communication adeptness can lead to miscommunication detrimental to whole trial implementation
Opportunities	**Threats**
• Conducive to difficult trials that involve operational hurdles, diagnostic challenges, and complicated endpoint evaluations	• Rapid enrollment at reasonable price for relatively simple trials can be better handled in other emerging locations

4. APPLICABLE REGULATIONS

The International Conference on Harmonization (ICH) Good Clinical Practice (GCP) and all applicable US, EU, and Japanese regulations (Japanese Ministry of Health, Labor and Welfare (MHLW): The Pharmaceutical affairs law, The MHLW ethics guideline for clinical research).

5. TAKE HOME MESSAGE

- Japan should play a larger role in multinational clinical trials, particularly in those requiring evaluation of subtle endpoints in complex and severe diseases.
- Increased expenditure can be compensated for by data quality and smooth trial conduct in therapeutic areas where subtle diagnostic and outcome evaluations are critical.
- Timely and smooth communication is the sine qua non of multinational trials, but it is too often given little serious attention in trial management. The unexpected flaws and problems that crop up in trial designs and operational procedures and manuals can be resolved with good communication and teamwork, but not without such communication.

6. CONCLUDING REMARKS

A recent analysis by Chakma et al. [12] suggests a decline in US financial competitiveness in biomedical R&D with an industrial trend to reallocate its funding to Asia–Oceania, where the costs of conducting R&D are lower, thanks to cheaper labor and the availability of greater government subsidies. This shift is only encouraged by the increase in development expenditure required for Food and Drug Administration drug approval. However, if a trial conducted cheaply ends up being a failure due to operational mishaps and the drug in question, whose efficacy and safety might have been successfully established if the trial was conducted properly, cannot be marketed, this is a complete waste both scientifically and financially.

The ideal environment for a clinical trial must be identified in strict accordance with the specific requirements of the trial in question, as governed by its therapeutic area, the targeted disease, endpoints, patient population, operational readiness, and cost structure. Good infrastructures for clinical research, including medical and operational expertise, do not come cheaply, so although selecting a location primarily on the basis of financial factors may look cost-effective and rational in the short term, it can be a fatal choice in the long term. As clinical development of a novel compound is always a time-consuming long-term enterprise, the greatest challenge we all face now may be how to juggle short-term business needs with long-term scientific integrity.

REFERENCES

[1] Martin DF, Maguire MG, Fine SL. Identifying and eliminating the roadblocks to comparative-effectiveness research. New Eng J Med 2010;363:105–7.

[2] Rawlins M. De testimonio: on the evidence for decisions about the use of therapeutic interventions. Lancet 2008;372:2152–61.

[3] Sato Y, Kouyama K. Clinical research in Japan: past, present and future. Keio J Med 2010;59(3):104–9.

[4] Colby MA, Birt MP. Negotiating the Gray Maze – the business of medicine in Japan. Connecticut: Floating World; 1998.

[5] Hirai Y, Kinoshita H, Kusama M, Yasuda K, Sugiyama Y, Ono S. Delays in new drug applications in Japan and industrial R&D strategies. Clin Pharmacol Ther 2009;87:212–8.

[6] Liker J, Franz JK. The Toyota Way to continuous improvement: linking strategy and operational excellence to achieve superior performance. New York: McGraw-Hill Professional; 2011.

[7] Chang JJ, Xu J, Fan D. A comparative method of evaluating quality of international clinical studies in China: analysis of site visit reports of the Clinical Research Operations and Monitoring Center. Contemp Clin Trials 2008;29:654–62.

[8] Targum SD, Pollack MH, Fava M. Redefining affective disorders: relevance for drug development. CNS Neurosci Ther 2008;14:2–9.

[9] Targum SD, Nakagawa A, Sato Y. A cross-cultural comparison study of depression assessments conducted in Japan. Ann Gen Psychiatry 2013;12:9–15.

[10] Opal SM, Laterre P-F, Francois B, LaRosa SP, Angus DC, Mira J-P, for the ACCESS Study Group, et al. Effect of eritoran, an antagonist of MD2-TLR4, on mortality in patients with severe sepsis – the ACCESS randomized trial. JAMA 2013;309(11):1154–62.

[11] Aikawa N, Takahashi T, Fujimi S, Yokoyama T, Yoshihara K, Ikeda T, et al. A Phase II study of polyclonal anti-TNF-a (AZD9773) in Japanese patients with severe sepsis and/or septic shock. J Infect Chemother 2013;19:931–40.

[12] Chakma J, Sun GH, Steinberg JD, Sammut SM, Jagsi R. Asia's ascent—global trends in biomedical R&D expenditures. N Engl J Med 2014;370:3–6.

CHAPTER 4

The "Clinical Trial App"

Urs-Vito Albrecht, Oliver Pramann

Contents

1. THE NEED

In highly specialized medicine, conducting research close to patients to retain a complete and unbiased set of individual data is a methodological and economical challenge. Inherent to the use of personal mobile technology in the form of smart devices is the capability to bridge possible gaps, specifically differences in know-how and understanding between all parties. This technology is ubiquitously available, user friendly, and offers many features that make it attractive for research and a valuable resource to count on in conducting clinical trials in the future. Developing mechanisms and strategies to assure mobile data quality, validity, and reliability is crucial.

2. THE SOLUTION

Patient-oriented data collection might provide benefits to the conventional researcher-focused method as it provides additional valuable (individual) information. The population-based research (field-work) aspect is also of interest when researching long-term effects of approved pharmaceuticals and medical products in post-marketing trials or for gathering additional data on product safety. Considered as personal, but nevertheless powerful, communication devices, smart devices, and trial applications running on them have the potential to provide considerable support for clinical research as they are widely available and broadly accepted by the general public.

Re-Engineering Clinical Trials
http://dx.doi.org/10.1016/B978-0-12-420246-7.00004-9

Smartphones and Tablet PCs are ubiquitously available and are an integral part of our daily lives. According to IDC market research, 1 billion devices were sold in 2013, and expectations are that this number will rise to 2.3 billion per year by 2017 [1]. Other smart devices, some of them wearable, e.g., glasses, watches, or necklaces, will join the market. Small, downloadable software applications (apps) can be run on such devices and make use of their integrated functionalities and sensors, many of them having been manufactured according to high industrial standards. Some of the functionalities include built-in accelerometers, gyroscopes, cameras, microphones, touch screens, GPS, as well as communication features: audio, video, and textual information. However, the real strength of these devices ensues from the fact that they allow their users physical and, more importantly, psychological proximity resulting in their broad acceptance.

This makes them interesting for research as they have the capability to track a persons' activities and to combine this information with other related data to profile the user—without any additional effort or perceived discomfort for that user. The opposite is in fact the case. With integrated comfort functions for the purpose of simplifying a user's life and adding comfort, users willingly consent to participate in data sharing that has the stated intent to allow improving the necessary services for them. Naturally, a responsible and trustworthy policy on data acquisition, data sharing, and data protection is essential to avoid breaching the personal rights of users and to develop a technology that does not add pitfalls or threats for them, be it in the present or the future. With smart devices, users become both receivers and senders of information. As we all are social beings, spreading and receiving information in a swift and comfortable way is the aspect that fuels the flame of innovation of that technology. Personalization of devices makes them even more attractive to the users. A pleasing design and high usability level make them a perfect technical extension to our needs. Enriched with web technology and various social media aspects, the technology is tailored to the individual.

The above-mentioned aspects make smart devices attractive for research as well. As of 2014, several studies relating to smart devices exist, mainly concerning smartphones. In medicine, the focus is mostly on epidemiology, and lies, for example, in identification of the prevalence of smoking in cars [2], in performing tests with psychological background [3], and also in a pharmacovigilance [4]. The authors mainly praise the efficient and low-cost recruitment as well as the large numbers of cases they were able to collect for their studies. This is certainly an important aspect, but certainly not the only one making this trial-app-based approach interesting for clinical trials [5].

3. SWOT

1. Strengths

Clearly, large cohorts may be recruited from all over the world with relatively little effort by using the synergistic effects triggered by trends that are accompanying the boom in smart devices, specifically mobile internet and social media usage. Another strength of the mobile data sharing approach that becomes possible with trial apps is the chance to investigate cohorts independent of constraints due to time or space. By using smart devices and apps, the individual data are constantly collected, managed, and comfortably sent to the data pool.

2. Weaknesses

The main weakness goes hand in hand with the strengths of the approach. The smart devices and apps are not deployed in a standardized clinical setting, such as in a laboratory of a study center, but rather in the private environment of the user. Thus, not all environmental factors can be accounted for while planning an app. Therefore, uncertainty remains as to the quality of the results delivered, some of this being due to unknown hardware specifications of user's devices as well as other software that may run on these devices and may have an influence on the study app, or other unforeseen events. Provoked as well as nonprovoked breaches of the protocol by the study participants may be easy to track, but are often hard to interpret, as the information needed for detecting them may not be readily available along with the recorded data.

3. Opportunities

Adherence to the protocol by the study participants may be improved by comfort functions of the app, such as providing reminders to take a drug or for appointments at the study center. The individual progress of participants on the trial time line, as well as their physical progress, may be visualized to give feedback. Communication among the study participants and between the participants and the conductors of the study may be enhanced by using social media components and the improving information flow. Information material and updates on the study may be delivered directly, without any media break (i.e., switching to an additional device or method of delivery) and without time delay [5,6]. Table 4.1 presents the strengths of the approach.

Table 4.1 Possible fields of application and features of the clinical trial app

Field of application	Examples
Recruitment	• Worldwide, via social media and the Internet
Study documentation	• Study documentation by questionnaires answered on the smart devices
	• Patient diaries documented on the device
Study-related tests	• Trial-related tests performed on the device
	• Sensor-based data collection of the patient for trial reasons
Adherence	• Continually available information on the trial
	• Information and orientation on the trial time line
	• Reminders for drug intake or appointments
	• Study-related communication
	• From study participant to study center (and vice versa), example: scheduling study visits via the app
	• Within the study (participants exchange experiences)

Cost and time savings in recruitment, data acquisition and management are to be expected, depending on the setting in which the smart device and the app is deployed.

4. Threats

Strategies for improving the quality of mobile data collection with respect to validity and reliability and that allow judging the relevance remain to be developed and implemented. Also, gathering highly sensitive individual and personalized data goes hand in hand with the necessity for study participants to carry higher responsibility and become more involved in data collection than is the case in conventional studies. From the technical point of view, data protection is of extreme importance and the highest levels of encrypting technologies are to be ascertained [5,6].

Depending on the intended use of the app and smart device by the manufacturer, it is likely that the device—and in such cases the app is defined as a medical device as well—underlies regulatory oversight as a medical device according to national law. The consequences lie within the fulfillment of the regulatory demands, as for example, applying for premarket approval in the United States and conformity assessment procedures needed to gain a CE label, which is necessary to market an app within the European Union.

Furthermore, ethical aspects with respect to that kind of research need to be discussed, e.g., the necessity of providing adequate information to cover all aspects that may serve to improve trust in the app, the trial, and its sponsor. This has already been discussed for apps intended for the consumer market [7].

4. APPLICABLE REGULATIONS

Depending on the intended use of the application or the smart device, it may be classified as a medical device. In this case, the manufacturer has to make sure that he observes all applicable regulations for medical devices. For the European Market, the European Commission provides the manufacturer with information on whether an application is classified as a medical device or not. The MEDDEV Guideline 2.1.1/6 of January 2012 is legally not binding but very helpful for interpreting the appropriate European regulation.

A software application is defined as standalone software. If the application is intended for diagnosis or therapy, it will become a medical device in the legal sense. Examples could be software applications for the presentation of a patient's heart rate or other physiological parameters during routine checkups or for intensive care, monitoring in general, or software for measuring interpedicular distance or sagittal diameter of the spinal canal.

The consequences of the previously raised issues underline the necessity of obtaining a CE label for an app that is rated as a medical device before the manufacturer is allowed to put the application on the market. The CE mark may only be assigned after the appropriate conformity assessment procedures. The details of the procedures depend on the potential risk of the medical device.

For the US market, the FDA defines a medical device as "an instrument, apparatus, implement, machine, contrivance, implant, in vitro reagent, or other similar or related article, including a component part, or accessory which is recognized in the official National Formulary, or the United States Pharmacopoeia, or any supplement to them, intended for use in the diagnosis of disease or other conditions, or in the cure, mitigation, treatment, or prevention of disease, in man or other animals, or intended to affect the structure or any function of the body of man or other animals, and which does not achieve its primary intended purposes through chemical action within or on the body of man or other animals and which is not dependent upon being metabolized for the achievement of any of its primary intended purposes" [8].

The manufacturers need a premarket notification if the device underlies the regulation. A letter of substantial equivalence from the FDA is necessary.

Without obtaining this, manufacturers are not allowed to commercially distribute their devices.

On September 25, 2013, the FDA published a guideline for developers of mobile medical apps. Its intent is comparable to the MEDDEV guideline in the European Regulation, provided by the European Commission.

If apps are used in clinical studies, their use has to comply with the fundamental rules for clinical research, e.g., the Declaration of Helsinki or the ICH-GCP.

5. DATA PROTECTION

Personal-health-related data are of key importance when doing research following this clinical trial App approach. For participants providing their data for research, it is even more important, as they share sensitive and highly personal information related not only to their health, but also about their daily living routines as well as information about their environment and interactions. From the ethical perspective, this results in the responsibility of the beneficiaries, namely the researchers, to establish the best possible measures for data protection to avoid unintended and unwanted data sharing with third parties. Policies for data security and privacy differ between countries but recently, the European Union proposed a General Data Protection Regulation to harmonize rules on data protection within the 28 member states and their national laws on data protection [9]. It is meant to replace the Data Protection Directive 94/46/EC from 1995 with the intention to strengthen the digital privacy rights of EU citizens, improve the EU's online economy, and strengthen the free market [10]. The draft regulation prohibits the processing of sensitive personal data including "data concerning health" that comprise "[…] any information which relates to the physical or mental health of an individual, or to the provision of health services to the individual" (Article 4, No. 12). The draft also allows exceptions for data processing for research and statistics "[…] where grounds of public interest so justify" (No. 42). The Article 81 on "processing of personal data concerning health" gives a detailed description that is in line with the current directive.

Besides other changes, the key element of the planned regulation is that individuals must give explicit consent for data to be processed [10]. Also, individuals will be granted easier access to their data and with the "right to data portability," they will be enabled to more easily transfer their data from one service provider to another [10].

It is expected that the regulation will take effect within the next two years. A sponsor has to make sure that the appropriate laws are observed but should keep track of the new aspects of the forthcoming regulation for future studies making use of personal health data.

6. TAKE HOME MESSAGE

- The implementation of smart devices and (clinical trial) apps inherits great potential for improvement of data acquisition and study participant adherence in clinical trials.
- Trial planning needs to consider new methodological aspects adapted to the deployment of the new technology.
- *Clinical trial apps allow for better* integration of study participants in trials since media breaks are avoided but also give them new responsibilities as they might perform clinical tests with the devices and apps.
- *Clinical trial apps* must follow the highest possible standards in development in all relevant areas (data acquisition and management, data protection). It is also important to provide a transparent and detailed standardized description of the app's functionality and to specify the rationale for the trial.
- *Regulatory oversight* is highly likely as clinical trial apps are a medical product.
- One should keep track of new aspects of the forthcoming General Data Protection Regulation that will affect the clinical trial app approach.

REFERENCES

[1] Llamas RT, Stofega W. Worldwide smartphone 2013–2017 forecast update: September 2013. IDC Corporate USA; 2013.
[2] Patel V, Nowostawski M, Thomson G, Wilson N, Medlin H. Developing a smartphone 'app' for public health research: the example of measuring observed smoking in vehicles. J Epidemiol Community Health May 2013;67(5):446–52. http://dx.doi.org/10.1136/jech-2012–201774. Epub 2013 Feb 26.
[3] Dufau S, Duñabeitia JA, Moret-Tatay C, McGonigal A, Peeters D, Alario F-X. Smart phone, smart science: how the use of smartphones can revolutionize research in cognitive science. PLoS ONE 2013;6(9):e24974. Epub 2011 Sep 28.
[4] Baron S, Goutard F, Nguon K, Tarantola A. Use of a text message-based pharmacovigilance tool in Cambodia: pilot study. J Med Internet Res 2013;15(4):e68. http://dx.doi.org/10.2196/jmir.2477. URL: www.jmir.org/2013/4/e68. PMID: 23591700.
[5] Albrecht U-V, von Jan U, Pramann O. Mobile Labore für Feldversuche. Dtsch Arztebl 2013;110(31–32):A-1478/B-1301/C-1285.
[6] Pramann O, Albrecht UV. Smartphones und Software Applikationen (Apps) in klinischen Studien. Pharmind, in press.

[7] Albrecht UV. Transparency of health-apps for trust and decision making. J Med Internet Res 2013;15(12):e277. http://dx.doi.org/10.2196/jmir.2981. URL: http://www.jmir.org/2013/12/e277/.

[8] FDA, Federal Food, Drug, and Cosmetics Act, Chapter II – Definitions, sec.201. [21U.S.C.321].

[9] European Commission. Parliament and of the Council on the protection of individuals with regard to the processing of personal data by competent authorities for the purposes of prevention, investigation, detection or prosecution of criminal offences or the execution of criminal penalties, and the free movement of such data 2012. /* COM/2012/010 final – 2012/0010 (COD) */. URL: http://eur-lex.europa.eu/LexUriServ/LexUriServ.do?uri=CELEX:52012PC0010:en:NOT.

[10] European Commission. Commission proposes a comprehensive reform of data protection rules to increase users' control of their data and to cut costs for businesses 2014. URL: http://europa.eu/rapid/press-release_IP-12-46_en.htm?locale=en (press release). European commission (2012). Proposal for a Directive of the European.

What Does Our Industry and What Do Others Do

CHAPTER 5

Re-Engineering Clinical Trials: Best Practices for Streamlining the Development Process

P. Luisi, Wolfgang Renz, Patrick Frankham, Stan Kachnowski

Contents

With the globalization of healthcare research, current clinical trials are technical, time-consuming, costly, and to a degree misunderstood by the public. Barriers to clinical trials may include access, awareness, and general understanding of what they entail for participants. With the convergence of mobile and electronic health, social media, and big data, the current model for developing novel medicines will see important changes. For clinical trials to innovate anew, they must (1) reduce time to market and (2) provide a better match of promising new therapies to the patient population and thus better individualized treatment, among others. Although clinical trials are only one phase of the research and development process, as the industry faces challenges across drug development, a re-engineering is required to more readily meet the needs stakeholders. To re-engineer clinical trials,

Re-Engineering Clinical Trials
http://dx.doi.org/10.1016/B978-0-12-420246-7.00005-0

adjacencies, such as point-of-care devices, telemedicine, and portable and wearable technologies will enable manufacturers to accelerate the development of innovative medicines.

1. THE NEED

The advent of high-cost, high-risk clinical trials has already arrived, and all stakeholders in the drug development field face the imperative to innovate or absorb these increasing costs and risks. The current approach to bring a drug to market includes 6–9 years of clinical development and additional costs related to increased regulatory requirements, cost-effectiveness studies, high recruitment costs, and accounting for subpopulation needs in study design [1,2]. To continue to deliver cutting-edge pharmacotherapies, a whole scale re-engineering of the clinical trial is required. The phase III randomized control trial must be contextualized in the framework of real-world medication outcomes and thus must leverage from existing investments health technologies, including social media, health informatics, telemedicine, biomedical innovations, mobile applications, and wearable monitors.

2. THE SOLUTION

With the conversion of mobile and electronic health technologies, pharmaceutical manufacturers are aiming to incorporate "smart" devices into clinical development. New technologies and innovations will provide the ability to screen, monitor, and communicate with study participants on an ongoing basis, abilities that will, in practice, decrease cycle times and reduce recruitment sizes if participants are more likely to stay engaged. Telemedicine will be used to conduct virtual trial visits, allowing for a more centralized approach to patient and participant engagement and follow up. Collection of a new set of patient reported outcomes using accelerometer technologies that can assess calorie expenditure, sleep duration and quality, and activity will be leveraged by trial sponsors and healthcare providers alike in their search for tools to analyze patient health and improvement. Innovative technologies using video, short messaging services (SMSs) or text, wearable monitors, and simple application programming interfaces to allow databases to speak to one another have already been pioneered in the consumer health sphere and are now poised to impact and drastically change the ways in which clinical trials are planned, conducted, evaluated, and sponsored.

3. RE-ENGINEER TRIALS WITH NEW TECHNOLOGIES AND INNOVATIONS

The repurposing of new software and hardware technologies toward healthcare as well as the discrete design of electronic health (ehealth) and mobile health (mhealth) technologies for healthcare has provided for a new framework to envision more efficient clinical trials. These technologies (Table 1) and their actual or potential impact on re-engineering the clinical trial are examined here as are other nontechnology innovations and more distant future space for visionary clinical trials.

Table 2.1 Construct of new technologies for clinical trial reengineering

Technology/innovation	Exists in consumer space	Current use in clinical trials
Social media	Yes	Low
Telehealth	Yes	Moderate
Wearable technologies and activity monitors	Yes	Low
Biomedical technologies	No	Moderate

4. NEW TECHNOLOGIES

4.1 Social Media

The ubiquitous nature of social media via Twitter, Facebook, and patient platforms has already begun to transform how current patients interact with the brand and manufacturer of their prescription drug [3]. With the recent first draft commentary from the Food and Drug Administration (FDA) on the acceptable uses of pharmaceutical advertising and interaction with current and potential patients, this stands to continue growing [4]. In the clinical trials space, social media has been used and has the potential being used as a patient recruitment tool. Platforms, especially disease-specific community sites (e.g., PatientsLikeMe) and disease management applications, may reduce cycle time for recruitment of patients away from traditional healthcare trial enrollment points. Although the U.S. government's clinicaltrials.gov has long served as a database and access point for clinical trials recruitment, Acurian was a pioneer in this area through launch of its clinical trial awareness and patient recruitment social networking application in 2008 [5].

A year after its introduction, Acurian announced Click it Forward, and their Recruitment Manager™ generated 50% of their clinical trials patient referrals through social medial platforms and networks [6].

Acurian and other recruitment firms have forged ahead with innovative recruitment strategies even without specific FDA guidance on the topic. Other innovative trials by major pharmaceutical players have included Pfizer's virtual clinical trial [7]. Pfizer forged new concepts for involving patients at each point in the clinical trial but was not without the challenges, including low recruitment and slow-down issues related to regulatory compliance. Still, within the trial, there are lessons that social media platforms have the potential to serve as future touch points for both recruitment and evaluation of add-on technologies that may improve medication-based adherence and outcomes in real-world settings.

4.2 Health Informatics and Electronic Records

Algorithms and computer-assisted culling of electronic medical platforms and other hubs of patient data can provide more accurate prediction of clinical trial recruitment. Recent research has demonstrated the feasibility of using health plan and registry databases to select the fewest feasible recruitment sites [8]. Simple algorithms based on inclusion and exclusion criteria can provide trial sponsors with identification of the most populous sites with the most number of eligible patients [8]. Preliminary research has also suggested that electronic health records (EHRs) patient indices may be predictive of a trial's ability to fulfill sample size and should be included as a preliminary check in trial assessment planning [9].

Clinical trial managers seeking patients may use EHRs platforms to perform data capture after using it for matching of clinical trials. Cooperation among data capture systems and clinical trial stakeholders will be essential to improving efficiency and reliability of these processes. The Clinical Data Interchange Standards Consortium is one example of a successful consortium that seeks to enable higher levels of interoperability among data capture and clinical trial stakeholders. Joint partnerships between data scientists, electronic record providers, and the pharmaceutical research industry will further develop the efficiency of clinical trial matching and recruitment, thus reducing cycle times and outreach costs.

Affordable home-based DNA testing provided by companies (e.g., 23andMe) have increased access to genetic profiles and disease risk information while also providing a social community for learning and exchanging familiar disease and genealogical experience. Based on a recent FDA warning letter to 23andMe for misrepresentation of their services and the lack of integration in standard healthcare provider and patient relationships, home DNA services have yet to prove that affordable technologies will positively affect healthcare. Future use of such tests, however, remains plausible for inclusion into pre- and post-marketing development for pharmaceutical companies. For example, the innovative marketing of such health and genetic kits that require provision of DNA materials for health or genealogical materials demonstrates that there is a high threshold for provision of such data into consumer databases. Pharmaceutical stakeholders may be able to leverage that threshold into alterative provision of biological data from patients in its clinical and postmarket studies.

4.3 Telehealth for Patient Management

Telehealth was defined by the Institute of Medicine in 1996 as the "use of electronic information and communications technologies to provide and support healthcare when distance separates participants [10]." Almost two decades later, telehealth, or telemedicine, still holds tremendous potential for achieving value across healthcare and more specifically in clinical trials. Telehealth, in its multiple channels including mobile applications, video-conferencing, telephone, and SMSs or text, has applications for patient recording, visits, and monitoring adherence.

As trial sponsors look to innovate collection of patient reported outcomes, investment by sponsors into customized, password-protected mobile applications to collect data are both reliable and potentially cost-effective. Although some of these systems have only been evaluated in consumer and posttrial market settings, they hold high likelihood for potential integration into clinical trials [11]. In addition, social media applications through web and mobile-based platforms are also suitable for collection of views of patients in the trial setting on perceived effectiveness, health status, and quality of measures [12]. A strength of this approach is regulatory approval for patient-reported collection instruments is suggestive of a causal, pragmatic pathway.

Patient reported outcomes and all other study data collected through electronic data capture, through such systems such as Phase Forward and Medidata, hold a key perspective for understanding how systems have been adopted by pharmaceutical and life sciences partners and have actually generated revenue [13]. Electronic data systems and their historical demonstrated value add through shareholder revenue generated by public offerings and large buyouts will provide an analog for other clinical trial innovations. The sustainability of these companies and inclusion of their technologies over the long term may be predictive of the large-scale buy-in required to support companies offering innovations in clinical trials. Furthermore, new electronic data collection systems will continue grow and be expanded with the advent of other major changes related to re-engineering of clinical trials.

Study visits, often requiring study reimbursement, clinician and study personnel time, and other overhead costs related to location servicing, may be mitigated through the inclusion of remote and electronic visits. Although the FDA has voiced preference for in-person study visits, telemedicine has been accepted across a number of specific disease areas for traditional healthcare; thus, the Pfizer trial paved the way for alternate frameworks that allow for appropriate protocols to be modified for telehealth visits [7,14].

Clinical trials require high levels of patient adherence to oftentimes complex medication regimens that may be further confounded by environmental and socioeconomic factors. There are high levels of evidence that technology, from SMSs to behavioral modification applications, have the potential to improve adherence [15–17]. As higher levels of adherence during the trial have the potential to reduce patient enrollment needs and execute studies more expeditiously, interventions including behavioral modification software and hardware should be explored. Beyond text messaging, physical reminders for medication adherence, including robots and wireless pill bottles (e.g., AdhereTech), may hold promise based on prototypes currently being evaluated in medication adherence studies [18,19].

Smart blister pack technologies, such as those offered by Qolpac, Mevia, Medic, and Cypak, all use a combination of subscriber identification module, radiofrequency identification, packaging technologies, integrated circuitry, and ehealth interfaces to improve adherence in both clinical trial settings and traditional standard care settings. There has been some evidence of the products' ability to improve adherence and outcomes, although it is not yet consistently demonstrated across all disease states [20]. If successfully demonstrated, these smart pill devices or systems may not only increase adherence but also provide a more accurate reading of medication possession ratios for pharmacy benefits managers, providers, and researchers, thus further elucidating the hazy world of medication compliance and patient outcomes. The potential to leverage success in postmarket adherence studies with clinical trials is worthy of attention by industry trial sponsors.

4.4 Wearable Technologies and Activity Monitors

The new advent of wearable fitness monitors powered by triaxial accelerometers has tremendous application for adding value to clinical trials. Consumer-facing devices available at major retailers such as the UP by Jawbone, Fitbit, and Nike Fuel are forging a discussion about the inclusion of activity as a measure for analysis by healthcare professionals and study personnel alike. Laboratory-validated accelerometers are largely accepted for providing reliable activity and sleep data, although the validation of consumer-facing monitors is largely still in development [21,22]. Add on technologies for the current wearable triaxial accelerometers will soon include heartbeat monitoring and pulse oximetry, improving upon the field of wearable devices. Companies such as iRhythm Technologies Inc. have paved the way for easier access to long-term continuous cardiac monitoring with the latest addition of accelerometry. The combination of multiple technologies or sensors may enable earlier disease diagnosis, overall healthcare savings, and better clinical outcomes.

Future FDA validation of these devices will be dependent upon consumer health companies expanding into medical device classification. In the interim, postmarket drug studies and other health economics outcomes research should be carefully exploring ways to integrate activity monitoring into protocols across a wide range of therapeutic areas, including diabetes, diseases of the nervous system, and all other disease states that may have improved patient outcomes when the patients on medication can use wearable monitors to improve their physical activity and sleep outputs [23,24].

Wearable monitors on the consumer market offer the ability to use application programming interfaces to collect customized data from the monitors. These interfaces will require private development customized to research needs and data points available for the monitor; thus, the space has still to grow to meet the needs of clinical trial sponsors [25]. As the space develops, the interfaces should explore inclusion of new analytic and algorithm measures that will provide new, potentially compelling evidence about the effect of medications in real time. Adherence to medications, as well as the daily changes in activity measures such as caloric burn and step count, could be included today in postmarket drug studies and in future phase II and phase III trials. Health literacy is variable across demographic subgroups as is technology literacy [26,27].

Future clinical trial sponsors integrating wearable technologies should carefully assess the population readiness to use such wearable devices, what kind of system will be required to collect and transport the data (e.g., wireless, cellular, location-based docking stations), and other barriers. Real-time monitoring of patients using wearable devices may produce unease about constant monitoring, especially if nonadherence to the device prompts an intervention from the study personnel to the patient. Still, if wearable monitors are able to reduce study dropout as a product of future algorithms created around continued use and trial adherence, the monitors may in the end reduce the number of patients needed for a study. Another yet-to-be-addressed issue is the acceptability of activity as an independent measure for health improvement. Activity, when tied to improved quality of life or reduced body mass index, may be acceptable to healthcare professionals, but the current steps, sleep, and sleep-quality data produced by consumer facing wearable monitors has yet to fully integrated in healthcare professional viewpoints. As the field in this area grows and more patients access these devices on their own, clinical trial sponsors and healthcare professionals alike will be pressed to define the meaningfulness of wearable monitor measures for clinical care.

The diffusion rate of wearable monitors continue to grow, and more households in the United States report knowledge of such devices; thus, the knowledge and acceptance rate of monitors may be a critical level [28]. Importantly, comfort and familiarity of the devices may serve to strengthen recruitment tactics if the devices are available for full reimbursement or through other subsidized models. Validity of the data is still of question as participants in trials may not wear the device 24 h a day or may deal with technical failures that distort the data. These opportunities and challenges should be studied further in postmarket clinical trials and in within health populations to understand the real-world change capable from consumer wearable devices.

4.5 Biomedical Technologies

Handheld palm and mobile devices are on the cusp of revolutionizing patient and clinical data in the field. Both low- and high-resource areas have high potential value add from devices that can collect biological data (e.g., sputum, blood). Investors in technologies from venture capital and pharmaceutical alike should investigate applicable innovations across the United States and global biotechnology start-up. Competitions, such as the Healthcare Innovation World Cup and the Pilot Health Tech NYC, are highlighting these technologies and providing an opportunity for clinical trial stakeholders to invest in companies before they are bought by larger ventures. Healthcare technology incubators such as Rock Health and Blueprint Health aim to support and fund start-up technologies that will diffuse at an increasing rate if the technology proves robust. This is a highly valuable area for re-engineering clinical trial decision-making.

4.6 New Models for Innovation

The clinical trials field is also ripe for integrating lessons learned from nontraditional stakeholders. Product development partnerships such as the Global Alliance for TB Drug Development and Drugs for Neglected Diseases Initiative are using government and private grant funds to develop robust drug pipelines for largely nonrevenue-generating treatments. Because these groups are nonprofit and are beholden to grant makers, they are forced to spend clinical trial dollars more wisely and thus have using outsourced models in low-resource areas to expedite time to market for new regimens. In looking to alternative clinical trial methods, the pharmaceutical industry may find innovations that suit their current needs and deliver cost savings.

5. EXISTING AND UNSEEN CHALLENGES

The evolution of technology in domestic and international settings requires diversity, necessity, and technology innovation [29]. To deliver true, sustainable innovation to clinical trials, these three elements should be assessed across the field of burgeoning products and processes. More specific elements to pharmaceutical research and development should also be included in the assessment to prepare and meet the challenges ahead.

The plethora of new ideas and technologies in clinical trials is evidence of the diversity of thought being flourished by health-focused start-ups, corporations, and investors. Still, the diversity of ideas will only lead to successful technologies if these idea makers and supporters include the perspective of future patients. If sponsors ask participants to include a technology model into their everyday life a framework for acceptance of the technology model will be required to be understood by the process designers of the trial. Low health and electronic literacy issues will continue to pose challenges if the technologies are designed with the user experience at front of mind. Additional failure rates, variable use case scenarios, and infrastructure needs will eliminate potential participants in trials unless the introduction of the technology is done with appropriate research on the population's diversity.

Although there is necessity for the development of the technologies from the part of the pharmaceutical industry stakeholders as well as patients seeking medication, regulatory agencies have not voiced their concern over the necessity to innovate clinical trials. Thus, the industry sponsor and their advocates will have to continue in the face of nonexistent or unclear regulatory guidance in low-risk settings such as postmarket studies until clarity is achieved. A further challenge is that consumer technology companies may not see the need to seek medical device classification if their product is successful outside of the realm of research. Thus, investors should seek technology development partners who are committed to seeking appropriate classification for their device that meets current FDA or other regulatory standards. The acceptability of the data provided by new devices must also be of necessity to clinical trial investigators, healthcare providers, patients, and regulatory bodies. Without necessity for additional data, decision makers will be reticent to invest in technologies even if they have the potential to improve the patient experience. Acceptability of the data and high potential for cost savings will be the most important necessities for including a re-engineering technology in a clinical trial.

Technological evolution in clinical trials has been limited in the past two decades, thus slowing the growth of an area of research and development that should have continued to evolve. Patient privacy concerns have certainly contributed to the stunted growth in the field. The newest Cloud and health technology platforms in the consumer face have worked to overcome these challenges. Leveraging the device- and consumer-facing companies in health, clinical trial sponsors should be able take lessons from their success combined with the latest in health information protection systems to overcome these challenges. Still, as technology evolution is organic and also dependent on the acceptance of human users, trust, acceptability, and usability are of utmost importance for meeting the call to re-engineer clinical trials.

Successful use of technology in the consumer health sphere should enlighten clinical trial planners and sponsors that their current speed and cost of research is too high to be sustainable and that there are existing concepts that should be seriously considered for inclusion. The new ecosystem of technology innovation provides an exciting space for evaluating new devices or tools in a pilot or low-risk postmarket setting. With those learnings, especially if accomplished in a rigorous, statistically significant study, conscientious regulators and pharmaceutical compliance and medical stakeholders will be more willing to move forward with new methods for trials. Thus, the clinical trials industry and its stakeholders should champion these innovations through early stage investment, pilot testing, sharing results when successful and unsuccessful, and collectively advocating their potential to improve medicines and diagnostics to regulators and future patients.

6. SWOT

Why is the new concept better (**S**trength) than established method, what are potential **W**eaknesses, such as outstanding buy-in from stakeholders, **O**pportunities (cost- or time savings), and **T**hreats (e.g., regulatory limitations)

Strengths	Weaknesses
• More connected trial • Faster cycle times • More data collection • Fewer in clinic visits (e.g., completed from home setting) • Sourcing patients through social media increases recruitment times	• Patient confidentiality • Cloud-based data storage • Data validation issues
Opportunities	**Threats**
• Following participants in real-world setting • Potential decrease in clinical trial development costs	• Regulatory acceptance of data • Good clinical practice guidance, site monitoring visits, unclear deviations • Big reliance on technology, multiple technology platforms to be sourced and integrated into database

7. APPLICABLE REGULATIONS

- Policy and regulation will have to be adapted to include real-time data collections.
- Classification of existing consumer devices and technologies for the clinical trial markets.
- Validation and patient protection are key barriers.
- The danger of collecting too much data since trials are already data intense.

8. TAKE HOME MESSAGE

- Convergence of mobile and electronic health (e.g., EHR) will enable the next wave of innovation in clinical trials.
- Clinical trials need to be adapted for health-seekers, or information-seekers that will have considerable information about their disease and treatment options.
- Policy and regulatory concerns, namely around exchange of confidential information.
- New entrants into the clinical trial space (e.g., technology companies, AdhereTech, FitBit) who will have considerable data expertise with customers.

REFERENCES

[1] Kaitlin K. Deconstructing the drug development process: the new face of innovation. Clin Pharmacol Ther 2010;87(3).

[2] Getz KA, Wenger J, Campo RA, Seguine ES, Kaitin KI. Assessing the impact of protocol design changes on clinical trial performance. Am J Ther 2008;15:450–7.

[3] Steele R. In: Mukhopadhyay SC, Postolache OA, editors. Utilizing social media, mobile devices and sensors for consumer health communication: a framework for categorizing emerging technologies and techniques, vol. 2. Springer Berlin Heidelberg; 2013. pp. 233–49. http://dx.doi.org/10.1007/978-3-642-32538-0_11.

[4] U.S. Department of Health and Human Services, Food and Drug Administration. Guidance for industry: fulfilling regulatory requirements for postmarketing submissions of interactive promotional media for prescription human and animal drugs and biologics; 2014.

[5] Acurian. Click it forward; 2014. Click it Forward Web site. https://ols15.acuriantrials.com/jsp/facebook/default.html. Updated 2008. accessed 2/9.

[6] Connor S. Acurian generates over 50% of clinical trial patient referrals from proprietary relationships with online health networks & social media platforms; 2014. Acurian Generates over 50% of Clinical Trial Patient Referrals from Proprietary Relationships with Online Health Networks & Social Media Platforms Web site. http://www.businesswire.com/news/home/20100304006150/en/Acurian-Generates-50-Clinical-Trial-Patient-Referrals#.Uvgv7D84EQk. Updated 2010. accessed 2/9.

[7] Pfizer tests a concept that could modernize drug studies. NJ.com; 2014. http://www.nj.com/business/index.ssf/2012/01/pfizer_tests_a_concept_that_co.html. [accessed 2/9/2014].

[8] Curtis JR, Wright NC, Xie F, et al. Use of health plan combined with registry data to predict clinical trial recruitment. Clin Trials 2014;11(1):96–101.

[9] Sumi E, Teramukai S, Yamamoto K, Satoh M, Yamanaka K, Yokode M. The correlation between the number of eligible patients in routine clinical practice and the low recruitment level in clinical trials: a retrospective study using electronic medical records. Trials 2013;14:426–6215.

[10] Schwamm LH. Telehealth: Seven strategies to successfully implement disruptive technology and transform health care. Health Aff (Millwood) 2014;33(2):200–6.

[11] Schapranow M, Plattner H, Tosun C, Regenbrecht C. Mobile real-time analysis of patient data for advanced decision support in personalized medicine. In: The fifth international conference on eHealth, telemedicine, and social medicine; 2013. pp. 129–36.

[12] Baldwin M, Spong A, Doward L, Gnanasakthy A. Patient-reported outcomes, patient-reported information. Patient: Patient-Centered Outcomes Res 2011;4(1):11–7.

[13] Akami. Case study – phase forward; 2014. http://www.akamai.com/html/customers/case_study_phase_forward.html. Updated 2013. [accessed 2/11].

[14] Roehr B. Pfizer launches virtual clinical trial. BMJ 2011;342:d3722.

[15] Hou MY, Hurwitz S, Kavanagh E, Fortin J, Goldberg AB. Using daily text-message reminders to improve adherence with oral contraceptives: a randomized controlled trial. Obstet Gynecol 2010;116(3):633–40.

[16] Linn AJ, Vervloet M, van Dijk L, Smit EG, Van Weert J. Effects of eHealth interventions on medication adherence: a systematic review of the literature. J Med Internet Res 2011;(4):13.

[17] Mbuagbaw L, van der Kop ML, Lester RT, et al. Mobile phone text messages for improving adherence to antiretroviral therapy (ART): a protocol for an individual patient data meta-analysis of randomised trials. BMJ Open 2013;3(5):10. 1136/bmjopen-2013-002954.

[18] Takacs B, Hanak D. A prototype home robot with an ambient facial interface to improve drug compliance. J Telemed Telecare 2008;14(7):393–5.

[19] AdhereTech | home http://adheretech.com/; 2014 [accessed 2.09.2014].

[20] Mahtani KR, Heneghan CJ, Glasziou PP, Perera R. Reminder packaging for improving adherence to self-administered long-term medications. Cochrane Database Syst Rev 2011:9.

[21] Bassett Jr DR, Rowlands A, Trost SG. Calibration and validation of wearable monitors. Med Sci Sports Exerc 2012;44(Suppl. 1):S32–8.

[22] Plasqui G, Bonomi A, Westerterp K. Daily physical activity assessment with accelerometers: new insights and validation studies. Obes Rev 2013;14(6):451–62.

[23] O'Driscoll DM, Turton AR, Copland JM, Strauss BJ, Hamilton GS. Energy expenditure in obstructive sleep apnea: validation of a multiple physiological sensor for determination of sleep and wake. Sleep Breath 2013;17(1):139–46.

[24] Machac S, Prochazka M, Radvansky J, Slaby K. Validation of physical activity monitors in individuals with diabetes: energy expenditure estimation by the multisensor Sense-Wear armband Pro3 and the step counter omron HJ-720 against indirect calorimetry during walking. Diabetes Technol Ther 2013;15(5):413–8.

[25] Postolache O, GirÃ£o P, Postolache G. In: Mukhopadhyay SC, Postolache OA, editors. Pervasive sensing and M-health: vital signs and daily activity monitoring, vol. 2. Springer Berlin Heidelberg; 2013. pp. 1–49. http://dx.doi.org/10.1007/978-3-642-32538-0_1. 10.1007/978-3-642-32538-0_1.

[26] Jensen JD, King AJ, Davis LA, Guntzviller LM. Utilization of internet technology by low-income adults: the role of health literacy, health numeracy, and computer assistance. J Aging Health 2010;22(6):804–26.

[27] Gazmararian JA, Yang B, Elon L, Graham M, Parker R. Successful enrollment in Text4Baby more likely with higher health literacy. J Health Commun 2012;17 (Suppl. 3):303–11.

[28] MobiHealth News. Consumer health apps by the numbers; 2013.

[29] Basalla G. The evolution of technology. Cambridge: Cambridge University Press; 1989.

CHAPTER 6

How Can the Innovative Medicines Initiative Help to Make Medicines Development More Efficient?

Matthias Gottwald

Contents

1. THE NEED

Despite continuously increasing efforts, attrition rate, even in later phases of clinical development, is still high, leading to an overall unsatisfyingly low success rate in medicines development. At the same time, the nature of healthcare is changing with an aging population and increasing burden of chronic diseases. Science offers great opportunities, but it is also becoming more complex and its integration in the innovation cycle more difficult. Resulting from a deeper molecular analysis of disease mechanisms and the availability of first stratification markers in a few indications, the demand for generally more targeted therapies is increasing. Nevertheless, current research and regulatory and healthcare delivery models are not yet adapted to this changing environment and are unsustainable in light of these advances, putting the entire healthcare value chain at risk [1]. None of these challenges can be solved by any single company or institution alone.

Re-Engineering Clinical Trials
http://dx.doi.org/10.1016/B978-0-12-420246-7.00006-2

2. SOLUTION

2.1 What Is the Innovative Medicines Initiative?

In 2008, the pharmaceutical companies, organized in the European Federation of Pharmaceutical Industries and Associations (EFPIA) and the European Commission (EC), jointly started the Innovative Medicines Initiative (IMI) (www.imi.europa.eu). This biggest public–private partnership in healthcare research aims at making medicines research and development (R&D) processes more efficient and effective, addressing major challenges in society and healthcare (Figure 6.1). Experts from small and big industries, academia, regulatory authorities, patient organizations, and payers work together in critical mass consortia on a broad range of topics all along the value chain. The topics are defined by the participating pharmaceutical companies thereby ensuring that topics of high relevance for the development of innovative medicines are addressed. The EC provides 1 billion Euros as funding for public partners in collaborative projects while the EFPIA companies contribute another billion Euro "in-kind," e.g., by participation of their experts in projects. The overall philosophy of IMI is to

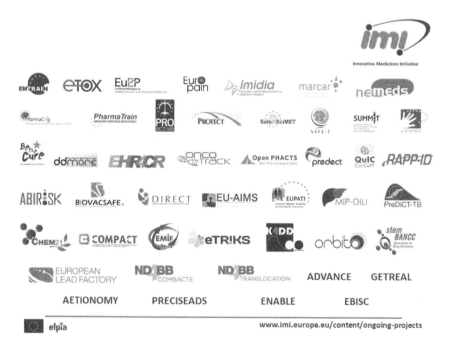

Figure 6.1 IMI's ongoing projects.

make the results as broadly as possible available to all parties working in the area of medicines R&D; this is reflected by a specific Intellectual Property (IP) policy that strives for a balance between a reasonable protection of results and broad publication and distribution. All relevant results will be published; more standardized processes will create a more reliable environment for everybody working in medicines development, and IP protected outcomes will be made available to interested third parties under fair and reasonable terms [2].

2.2 Achievements Made So Far

In the meantime, 59 projects have been initiated, using the complete budget of 2 billion Euro; 46 of these projects finished their negotiation and planning phase and have started work (Figure 6.2). The results from the first projects show that this new model of collaboration works successfully. The projects cover important aspects of the whole value chain from early research and preclinical development up to clinical trial design, pharmacovigilance, and relative effectiveness measurement [3,4]. Of particular interest in IMI are organizations involved in clinical research, since they can contribute specifically with their access to patient samples and their experience in running clinical trials (Table 6.1).

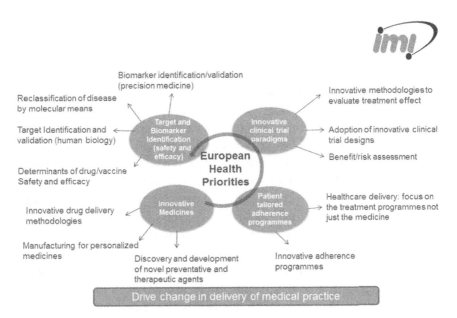

Figure 6.2 IMI2 is expected to start Q2 2014: major planned research areas.

Table 6.1 Examples of achievements from current IMI projects

Area	Examples of achievements
Establishment of robust, validated models for drug development	Touchscreen rat model for schizophrenia and Alzheimer's (NewMeds [5]), animal model mimicking nonsyndromic autism disorder (EU-AIMS)
Development of biomarkers and tools predictive of clinical outcomes (efficacy and safety)	Novel biomarkers in Schizophrenia and depression (NewMeds), diabetes (Imidia), colon cancer (OncoTrack), kidney-, liver-, and CV-safety (SAFE-T, eTOX)
Identification of new drug targets	Potential novel targets in autism (EU-AIMS), diabetes (SUMMIT), and pain (EUPAIN)
Clinical trials—improved design and process	Improved trial design, e.g., in schizophrenia (NEWMEDS), pain (EUPAIN), and asthma (U-BIOPRED)
	New business model for electronic health records data reuse for research (EHR4CR)
"Big Data"—solutions to leverage knowledge	Improved IT infrastructure and data collection processes (ETRIKS, EMIF)
Education and training for new-generation R&D professionals	Biggest course catalog in biomedicine (on-course®, EMTRAIN), modular master programs in safety sciences (SafeSciMET), pharmacovigilance (EU2P), and along the whole R&D process (PharmaTrain)

In the following, a few of the projects are described in some more detail to give a perspective of the approaches taken.

Jointly developed, reliable, clinically validated systems for prediction of safety and efficacy of new compounds help to select the most promising development compounds before entering clinical trials. This has, for instance, been approached in the project NEWMEDS (www.newmeds-europe.com), where a new touchscreen rat model has been developed which is expected to have a much higher predictive value for the clinical situation than former models [5]. Biomarkers help to stratify patients for clinical trials and to monitor disease progression and treatment effects. One example in this field is the project ONCOTRACK (www.oncotrack.eu), which aims at a better understanding of the heterogeneity of colon cancer patients via a systems medicine approach. A comprehensive molecular analysis of tumor samples from more than 200 colon cancer patients is performed, including whole genome analysis and the analysis of the methylome and other relevant molecular data. These data—more than one terabyte per patient—then undergo a simulation model to identify novel patterns of biomarkers allowing a more precise patient stratification in the future.

Of high relevance in this context is the close interaction with and often direct participation of the regulators in the project permitting the new tools and processes to become regulatory-approved standards in industrial and academic clinical development. One example is the project SAFE-T (www.imi-safe-t.eu), in which the evaluation of 153 biomarkers for drug-induced injury of the kidney, liver, and vascular system has been completed, and 79 have been selected for further assessment in exploratory qualification studies. The qualification processes have been adapted and aligned across agencies (EMA and FDA [6,7]).

Sharing of data and knowledge from many stakeholders is another important approach to improve processes in clinical development. For example, in the project NEWMEDS, five major companies reanalyzed data from 34 clinical trials with 11,670 schizophrenia patients, resulting in the recommendation to reduce the number of patients per trial from 79 to 46 and the duration from 6 to 4 weeks without a significant loss of statistical power (unpublished information).

The e-TOX project (www.e-tox.net) has gathered an unprecedented amount of data from preclinical toxicity trials which now, together with the simultaneously developed new simulation approaches, allows a better safety prediction for novel compounds [8,9]. ETRIKS (www.etriks.org) is on the way to devise and implement a novel IT platform for translational research which has the potential to become a standard platform for preclinical and clinical data management, thereby offering the opportunity for a better comparison and sharing of data beyond the current silos. This platform is already used by several other IMI projects. The European Medical Information Framework (EMIF) project (www.emif.eu) aims to build an integrated, efficient framework for consistent reuse and exploitation of currently available patient-level data to support novel research. First indication areas are Alzheimer disease and metabolic diseases. And, in the PROTECT project, coordinated by the EMA, new approaches in pharmacovigilance and pharmacoepidemiology are established and implemented. This includes a comparison of the existing adverse event repositories and the development of novel methods for earlier signal detection (www.imi-protect.eu). The link to "real-world" data plays an important role in this project and is also addressed in a new project called GET REAL, in which regulators and payers jointly work in a multistakeholder consortium on the optimization of the development processes needed for an early proof of the socioeconomic value of new medicines (unpublished information).

Another area addressed by several IMI projects is education and training (E&T). Operational excellence is important along the whole value chain of medicine R&D, and in a rapidly changing world, it is of utmost importance that up-to-date training opportunities exist for everybody working in this field or entering it. SafeSciMET (www.safescimet.eu) has developed a modular master program on preclinical and clinical safety sciences; EU2P (www.eu2p.org) is a modular master and PhD program on pharmacovigilance and pharmacoepidemiology. PharmaTrain (www.pharmatrain.eu) has established a standardized European diploma and master program on medicines R&D, covering the whole process from target identification up to the market. The program is now delivered at 12 universities in different European countries and is currently also taken up by universities in Asia and the Americas. This is complemented by a program for training clinical investigators and an additional master program for regulatory affairs professionals. Finally, the project EMTRAIN (www.emtrain.eu) generated LifeTrain, a framework for continuous professional development/life-long learning for professionals in biomedicine in Europe [10], and the course portal on-course®. With more than 5000 courses, it is now the biggest database with course information in this area [11].

Reaching out beyond the professionals working in medicines R&D, the most recently launched E&T project (February 2012) is the European Patients' Academy on Therapeutic Innovation (EUPATI, www.patientsacademy.eu). It consists of a consortium of patient organizations, academia, NGOs, and industries—30 organizations in total. The project sets out to develop and disseminate objective, credible, correct, and up-to-date public information about medicines R&D for the lay public by administering a certificate training program, by creating an educational toolbox which can be used by patient advocates, and by creating a public library on medicines R&D on the Internet translated into seven languages, published under "creative commons license" for reuse by the public. This is also intended to foster a better and earlier involvement of patients in the development of novel medicines.

The fact that the EMA is leading an IMI project and is in an advisory role in several other IMI projects shows that this new "neutral" platform is ideal to foster dialogue across stakeholder boundaries and to define common priorities and standards jointly. The projects which have already taken up their work currently bring together more than 6000 scientists from academia, SMEs, pharmaceutical companies, regulators, payers, and patients all across Europe. Moreover, regulatory authorities outside Europe have already started to liaise with IMI projects, e.g., via project advisory boards.

2.3 Plans for the Future

Based on the positive experiences with IMI, the EU Commission and EFPIA decided to develop a successor program (IMI2) under the EU Research Framework Program HORIZON 2020. IMI2 will draw on the experiences from IMI1 but with an expanded scope and budget. The overarching topic for IMI2 will be to support the transition toward a more targeted medicine, allowing the development and delivery of the right prevention and treatment for the right patient at the right point of time (Figure 6.3). It starts with critical mass research projects to get a better molecular understanding of complex diseases and to identify and validate novel targets and biomarkers for safety and efficacy. The second pillar is dedicated to the development of innovative clinical trial paradigms, leading to clinical trial designs or benefit–risk approaches better fit to a more stratified approach, e.g., including companion diagnostics. This is closely related to the third pillar, which deals with patient adherence programs and the

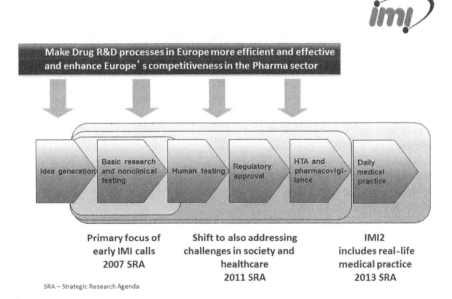

Figure 6.3 The scope of IMI and the road to IMI2.

understanding of the real-world situation in an aging population. Potential projects here could be worked on devices that allow a better remote monitoring of a patient's physical situation. And last, but not least, IMI2 will look into improving targeted delivery and manufacturing methods and the clinical development of products in areas with a high societal need, but limited incentives for industry, like in antibiotics.

Starting 2014 and until 2020, groups of pharmaceutical companies will publish ideas for projects in these topic areas. Consortia formed by experts from academia, hospitals, SMEs, regulatory authorities, or patient organizations in Europe and associated countries are invited to formulate proposals for addressing these topics and apply for funding. The best applicant consortium—selected in a peer review process—will, together with the involved pharmaceutical companies, develop the detailed work plan and both will jointly execute the project. Interested parties may use the partnering tool on the IMI JU Website (www.imi.europa.eu) to identify potential partners to form an applicant consortium.

3. SWOT

Strength	Weakness
Public–private partnership approach of IMI proven to be ideally suited for addressing overarching challenges in healthcare	Continuous support by pharmaceutical companies in competition to proprietary company projects with a shorter and easier measurable return on investment
Early involvement of regulators allowing faster development of the regulatory framework for clinical development toward the needs of a more targeted ("personalized") medicine	Global scope of the drug development process has to be taken up more actively in the framework for IMI2
Neutral platform attractive for dialogue with all stakeholders including patients and payers	

4. APPLICABLE REGULATIONS

Applicable regulations (e.g., EMA) apply to clinical trials, pharmacovigilance, advanced therapies, antimicrobial resistance, and scientific guidelines.

5. TAKE HOME MESSAGE

Many challenges in healthcare, and especially the development of innovative preventive and therapeutic approaches, are too big to be addressed by one institution alone. The Innovative Medicines Initiative (IMI) has proven that this model of public–private partnership works to address major challenges and is an unprecedented example of knowledge sharing across stakeholders and competitors. A neutral platform like IMI is ideal for the dialogue of pharmaceutical companies with regulators, payers, patients, academia, and SMEs to define common priorities and standards.

Looking at the achievements from the first IMI projects approaching their project end after five years, it can be expected that IMI2 will also significantly contribute to the development of a more robust environment for medicines development with a better understanding of many complex diseases and tools and processes to conduct targeted clinical research in a more efficient and effective way.

REFERENCES

[1] Munos B. Lessons from 60 years of pharmaceutical innovation. Nat Rev Drug Discov 2009;12:959–68.
[2] Goldman M. Reflections on the innovative medicines initiative. Nat Rev Drug Discov 2011;10:321–2.
[3] Laverty H, Gunn M, Goldman M. Improving R&D productivity of pharmaceutical companies through public–private partnership: experiences from the Innovative Medicines Initiative. Expert Rev Pharmacoecon Outcomes Res 2012;12(5):545–8.
[4] Vaudano E. The innovative medicines initiative: a public private partnership model to foster drug discovery. Comput Struct Biotechnol J 2013;6(7):e201303017.
[5] Talpos A, Fletcher JC, Circelli C, Tricklebank MD, Dix A. The pharmacological sensitivity of a touchscreen-based visual discrimination task in the rat using simple and perceptually challenging stimuli. J Psychopharmacol 2012;221(3):437–49.
[6] Matheis K, Laurie D, Andriamandroso C, Arber N, Badimon L, Benain X, et al. A generic operational strategy to qualify translational safety biomarkers. Drug Discov Today 2011;16(13–14):600–8.
[7] Dieterle F, Schuppe-Koistinen I, Prats N, Brown L, Cacoub P, Poynard T, et al. The European IMI SAFE-T Consortium: qualification of translational safety biomarkers. Toxicol Lett 2009;189(Suppl. 1):S157.
[8] Briggs K, Cases M, Heard DJ, Pastor M, Pognan F, Sanz F, et al. Inroads to predict in vivo toxicology – an introduction to the eTOX project. Int J Mol Sci 2012;13(3):3820–46.
[9] Obiol-Pardo C, Gomis-Tena J, Sanz F, Saiz J, Pastor M. A multiscale simulation system for the prediction of drug-induced cardiotoxicity. J Chem Inf Model 2011;51(2):483–92.
[10] Hardman M, Brooksbank C, Johnson C, Janko C, See W, Lafolie P, et al. LifeTrain: towards a European framework for continuing professional development in biomedical sciences. Nat Rev Drug Discov 2013;12:407–8.
[11] Payton A, Janko C, Renn O, Hardman M. on-course® portal: a tool for in-service training and career development for biomedical scientists. Drug Discov Today 2013;18(17–18):803–6.

CHAPTER 7

2E: Experiences with Lean and Shop Floor Management in R&D in Other Non-Pharmaceutical Branches

Andreas Hans Romberg

Contents

1. THE NEED

In almost every industry, there is a tremendous need and sometimes already a pressure for streamlining processes and increasing effectiveness—which means "Do the right things!"—as well as to increase efficiency—which means "Do the right things right!"

Lean and shop floor management approaches, as the management and leadership part of good lean management systems implementations, have already generated notable achievements. Most of the lean approaches started with lean in production. Around five years ago, lean management implementations had arrived in administrative areas—especially in Research and Development (R&D).

Re-Engineering Clinical Trials
http://dx.doi.org/10.1016/B978-0-12-420246-7.00007-4

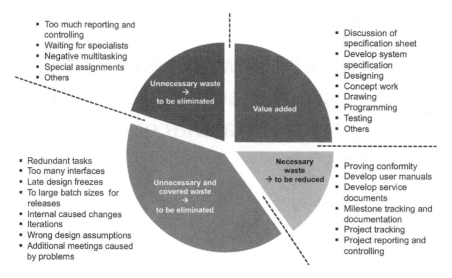

- Too much reporting and controlling
- Waiting for specialists
- Negative multitasking
- Special assignments
- Others

- Discussion of specification sheet
- Develop system specification
- Designing
- Concept work
- Drawing
- Programming
- Testing
- Others

Unnecessary waste → to be eliminated

Value added

- Redundant tasks
- Too many interfaces
- Late design freezes
- To large batch sizes for releases
- Internal caused changes
- Iterations
- Wrong design assumptions
- Additional meetings caused by problems

Unnecessary and covered waste → to be eliminated

Necessary waste → to be reduced

- Proving conformity
- Develop user manuals
- Develop service documents
- Milestone tracking and documentation
- Project tracking
- Project reporting and controlling

Figure 7.1 Value adding and waste in product development [1].

The idea behind lean management can be described best by the following metaphor: "Imagine you are an idea or a drawing or a component within a development project or process! What would be your favorite path of life? I am sure you would aspire to a condition of continuous flow from one place of adding value to the next. That would be the guarantee for shortest lead time without any boring waiting time."

One continuous process chain without any interface, without any waste, is the ideal state. That's the rational ergonomic target of lean management: to maximize "customer value" while minimizing waste. It can also be stated as creating more value for customers with fewer resources. Waste concludes everything which has no contribution to adding value (Figure 7.1). Eliminating waste along the entire value stream helps to create processes that need less human effort, less space, less capital, and less time to make products and services at far fewer costs and with much fewer defects, compared with traditional business systems.

2. THE SOLUTION

2.1 Benefits of Lean Management in Other Non-Pharmaceutical Branches

Many branches such as mechanical engineering, white goods, brown goods, and automotive have already started with lean management implementations within indirect areas.

Substantial key performance indicators (KPIs) to measure improvements and benefits of those implementations, especially in R&D and Development and Engineering (D&E) areas, are:

- **Hit rate** or **reliability factor** shows the adherence to delivery dates and schedules of teams working on projects in R&D and D&E to reduce disturbances, the target for this KPI is 100%.
- **Lead-time reduction** describes the least time needed for the same kind of projects/processes/activities after implementation of lean management/shop floor management.
- **Efficiency improvement** describes the ratio of reduced resource capacity needed after improvement to the resource capacity that is needed before improvement for same tasks and activities.
- **Project throughput** describes the increased number of projects an organization can handle with the same resources in the same span of time.
- **Increase of innovation rate**—this KPI describes the turnover of products younger than half of the average product life cycle time.

Typical results of lean development implementations in aforementioned branches are:

- Increase of hit rate: >90–95% (coming from 40 to 45%)
- Reduction of lead time: 30–60% (with same resources)
- Efficiency improvement: 20–40%
- Increase of project throughput: 20–30% (with same resources)
- Increase of innovation rate: >25%

However, not every single approach of lean in production can be transferred one-by-one to lean in R&D. But solutions for successful lean management implementations within R&D areas will also refer to well-known lean vocabulary like takt time, work in progress (WIP), process standards, and product standards.

2.2 Negative Multitasking is One Major Source of Waste to be Eliminated

R&D and D&E are involved in different value streams; that is the reason for disturbances, resulting in a major source of waste (Figure 7.2). Out of each process there is a permanent stream of tasks to be worked on by the resources. Some of the tasks are coming in constantly, others are coming in batchwise, and some of them also permanently change priorities. The higher the WIP,

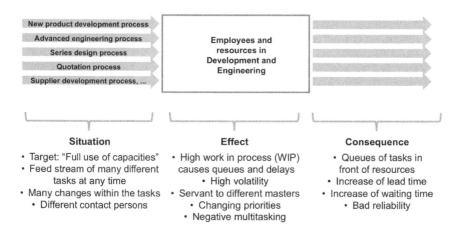

Situation	Effect	Consequence
• Target: "Full use of capacities" • Feed stream of many different tasks at any time • Many changes within the tasks • Different contact persons	• High work in process (WIP) causes queues and delays • High volatility • Servant to different masters • Changing priorities • Negative multitasking	• Queues of tasks in front of resources • Increase of lead time • Increase of waiting time • Bad reliability

Figure 7.2 Dealing with different value streams causes disturbances and waste within development teams.

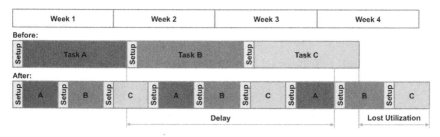

Figure 7.3 Negative multitasking—a major source of waste.

the more all the competing tasks in front of a resource cause "negative multitasking" (Figure 7.3).

Negative multitasking is the most common and important originator of waste especially within administrative areas such as R&D and D&E [1].

Reducing negative multitasking is possible by the following lean management methods, rules, and tools:

• Organizing multiproject environments to **prioritize and stagger projects** and to respect a maximum capacity load of resources of 80% (Figure 7.4).
• Try to separate the responsibility for the different value streams by **segmentation of the organizational structure**.
• **Reduction of work in process** (WIP) for each resource by a maximum of at least one work-week package in advance.

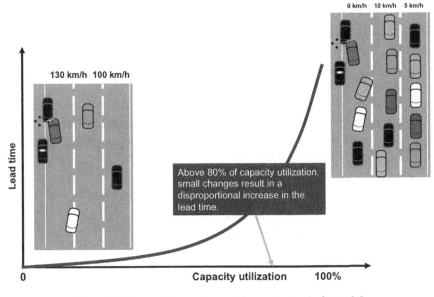

Figure 7.4 Respect a maximum of capacity load of 80% [2].

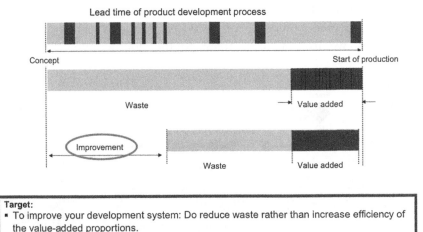

Figure 7.5 Waste indicator: Lead time ≫ value-adding time [3].

- Every single resource should work continuously on one task as long as needed and possible; disruptions should be reduced as much as possible.

Product development processes in traditional and not lean environments show a lot of waste. The value-added proportion is only about 25–30%—that means there is much room for improvement (Figure 7.5).

2.3 Some Aspects of Lean Management in R&D and D&E

To improve the lead time, as well as the efficient and effective use of capacity in R&D and D&E, it is better to reduce waste rather than making the value-adding part more efficient. To do so, lean companies are normally working on:

- Increasing effectiveness ("Do the right things!") by implementing, for example, interdisciplinary "frontloading" at the beginning of each R&D or D&E project using a set-based concurrent engineering (SBCE) approach.
- Increasing efficiency ("Doing the right things right!") by implementing a process-oriented shop floor management (SFM), for example, for multiproject environments. SFM helps to reduce disturbances within the processes using fast feedback loops by enforcing a takt time for R&D as well as E&D activities (takt time is a maximum of one week).

2.4 Frontloading

Frontloading follows a five-stage process with different steps of concretion (Figure 7.6) and enforces effectiveness.

Frontloading is a high-grade interdisciplinary approach. People from different functional departments are working together to create a robust and customer-oriented product or service. Through multidisciplinary approaches, we have an easy access to the holistic knowledge about

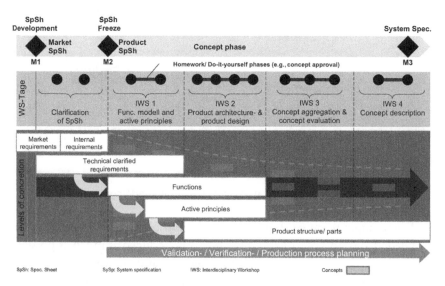

Figure 7.6 Frontloading is the key success factor for effectiveness—doing things right!

developing, producing, and servicing products in a very early stage of a project. This helps to assume risks before they appear—that means front-loading actively avoids risks in the late stages of a project and the product's life cycle. Avoiding/reducing risks stands for reducing costs. And, by the way, multidisciplinary working together in this case is a synonym for highly parallel working without interfaces, compared to working in time-consuming sequences and loops, which is a daily occurrence in many traditional engineering environments.

Another benefit of frontloading is the application of set-based concurrent engineering (SBCE). Traditional design practices, whether concurrent or not, tend to quickly converge on a solution, a point in the solution space, and then modify that solution until it meets the design objectives. This seems to be an effective approach, unless one picks the wrong starting point; subsequent iterations to refine that solution can be very time-consuming, expensive, and lead to a suboptimal design. By contrast, SBCE begins by broadly considering sets of possible solutions and gradually narrowing the set of possibilities to converge on a final solution. A wide net from the start and gradual elimination of weaker solutions makes finding the best or better solutions more likely [4].

2.5 Shop Floor Management

Shop floor management (SFM) in multiproject environments applies agile project management methods to control volatile situations (Figure 7.7).

SFM uses visual management for transparency to show deviations within processes and projects. A weekly (takted) and cascaded regular communication, based on transparency, enables the teams to organize a real-time control and to plan processes and projects (Figure 7.8).

Problems behind deviations will be prioritized and solved one-by-one. Systematic problem solving has to be supported by GENBA-visits to get a deep understanding of correlations where and when a problem occurs. GENBA (→Japanese) are all places in our daily working environment where problems and disturbances can happen. After problem solving, the improvement has to be approved by the team to make sure that the problem will never occur again. That is real day-by-day continuous improvement, which helps to create sustainable, robust processes, and process environments. That means SFM, applied in the right way, causes a change of management and leadership culture as well as a change of business culture, for example, how to deal with errors and mistakes in the daily business.

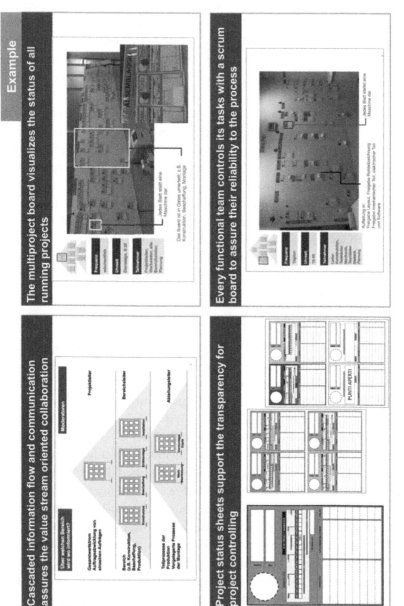

Figure 7.7 Example for a "paper-based" multiproject shop floor management.

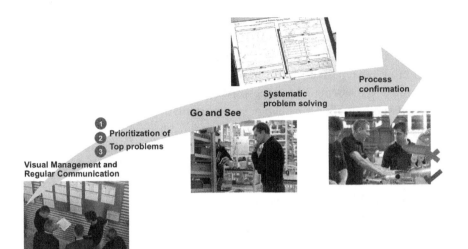

Figure 7.8 Shop floor management: process and methods.

	Step 1 Basis	Step 2 Insight	Step 3 Commitment	Step 4 Pilot projects	Step 5 Ideal state	Step 6 Roll-out
See	Awareness	Best practice visits/ sensitivation		Project communication and project marketing	Assessment of pilot projects/planning roll out	
Learn		Qualification of internal lean practitioners		Qualification of Lean Practitioners "on the project"	Further qualification on demand	
Act		Quick check and selection of pilot projects		Implementation of pilot projects within dedicated process and functional areas	"Do-it-yourself" roll out; coaching by consultant	
Live				Training/Coaching of shop floor management → performance improvement	Selective coaching by consultant	

Lead-time: round about 24 months

Involvement of cnsultants / *Involvement of employees*

Figure 7.9 Sustainable lean transformations respect necessary cultural changes.

From different points of view, the implementation of lean management is a multilayer procedure. First of all, lean management is not an installation of some different methods and tools. Lean management is a systems approach that respects and combines strategically, process-related, and structural as well as managerial aspects. Successful and sustainable lean development transformations follow a proven and stringent approach (Figure 7.9). A successful transformation is effective on four different levels:

- **Level 1—See**: Fully convinced people (management and concerned employees) will easily support a change or transformation process such as the implementation of lean management. Major issues are the creation of awareness at the beginning of and the continuous information about a transformation process. Also, the evaluation of the achieved improvements after the change is important.
- **Level 2—Learn**: A successful and sustainable transformation process should be carried out with the participation of internal qualified people (internal multipliers). Theoretical training, followed by pragmatic on-the-job-training, helps to get a good basis for the later "do-it-yourself" roll out and further improvement.
- **Level 3—Act**: Nothing is more successful than success, especially within their own company/organization. Hence the recommendation is to carry out a "lighthouse project" within a pilot area to show what kind and how much improvement is possible.
- **Level 4—Live**: Certain management behavior and leadership methods, which are different from the traditional ones, are very important to learn and adopt for a sustainable, lean approach. This "learning and coaching phase" will be carried out in parallel with the lighthouse project. Management acts as a role model and is the permanent driver of the improvement process. Management is striving for excellence in everything the company is doing.

The lean management approach in R&D and D&E is aiming at a maximum of throughput, a minimum of lead time, and customer orientation through waste reduction instead of only watching on a maximum of utilization of resources. This leads to tremendous lead-time reductions, cost savings through the increase of efficiency and effectiveness, as well as increase of project throughput with the same resources. Waste reduction, in general, starts at the personal desk and, with self-management, is followed by a value-stream orientation within the teams and departments. These are experiences out of many projects in different branches. Experiences, on the other hand, are also something that lean management needs for an outstanding buy-in and commitment from management. A sustainable management commitment guarantees sustainable transformations. During transformation and after, in the running system, management has to act as a role model. That necessitates a change of management behavior. Besides speeding up the development process through waste reduction, we need value-stream and lead-time orientation within our management skills. Reliability in collaborative systems (such as multiproject environments within product development) and customer orientation is as important as high-quality content work. Lean and agile development/project management is the only way to face volatile multiproject environments. Better and detailed planning will never be able to replace agile development/project management. Detailed planning only provides security through a kind of pseudo-accuracy.

We also learned from our project experiences that existing norms, standard procedures, and regulatory standards in the different branches sometimes influence or reduce parts of the benefit coming from lean management approaches; for example, some homologation procedures and requirements induce waste and inefficiency through non-essential specifications. Nevertheless lean management in R&D is worth being followed in every branch.

3. SWOT

1. **Strength:** Lean management, used as a holistic approach to increase efficiency, is in common use in many different non-pharmaceutical branches.
2. **Weaknesses:** Sustainability of lean management is very dependent on the awareness and buy-in of top management. Management has to act as a role model. Limitations for the reduction in lead time may be affected by physical lead times or official channels and regulations.
3. **Opportunity:** The pharmaceutical branch could transfer that knowledge and learn and earn from that experience. The increase of productivity when applying lean management is enormous (>50%), for example, by reduction of project lead times, increase of throughput by the same resources, etc. Permanent efficiency improvement has no limits.

4. APPLICABLE REGULATIONS

Start the reduction of waste by reducing **disturbances** in daily work. This is the only way to create **flow** within your business. Flow is the basis for minimizing waste and increasing value creation.

5. TAKE HOME MESSAGE

- Waste reduction in general starts at the personal desk and with self-management followed by a value-stream orientation within the teams and departments.
- Reliability in collaborative systems (such as multiproject environments within R&D and D&E) and customer orientation is as important as high-quality content work.

- Speed up the development process through waste reduction, value-stream, and lead-time orientation within management skills.
- Sustainable lean transformations need management attention and management commitment.
- Lean and agile development/project management is the only way to face volatile multiproject environments; better and detailed planning will never be able to replace agile development/project management. Detailed planning only provides security through a kind of pseudo-accuracy.

Substantial KPIs to measure improvements of lean management implementations in R&D areas and their results in mechanical engineering, white goods, brown goods, and automotive are:

- Hit rate or reliability factor: >95% (coming up from 40%)
- Project lead-time reduction: 60% (with same resources)
- Efficiency improvement: 40%
- Project throughput increase: 30% (with same resources)
- Increase of innovation rate: >25%

REFERENCES

[1] Romberg A. Schlank entwickeln, schnell am Markt - Wettbewerbsvorteile durch Lean Development. Log-x-Verlag; 2010.
[2] Reinertsen DG. The principles of product development flow: second generation lean product development. Celeritas Publishing; 2009.
[3] Liker JK, Morgan JM. Toyota product development system. Taylor & Francis Inc; 2006.
[4] Sobek DK, Ward AC, Liker JK. Toyota's principles of set-based concurrent engineering. MIT Sloan Management Review; 1999.

CHAPTER 8

Failure Mode and Effects Analysis (FMEA): Well-Known Methodologies, But Not in Our World

Winfried Dietz

Contents

1. THE NEED

Increasing globalization over the past decades has significantly increased the pressure on products, service offers, and design and production processes. Fierce competition from emerging countries, increasingly stricter standards and regulations, changing habits and needs on the part of consumers, a growing diversity of needs, and enormous price pressure are just a few of the challenges faced by companies. The effective and efficient anticipation of possible malfunctions during the product development process has, therefore, become imperative for survival.

The historical development of the quality management techniques in the context of industrial production can be outlined in three phases.

Re-Engineering Clinical Trials
http://dx.doi.org/10.1016/B978-0-12-420246-7.00008-6

1.1 Quality Inspections

Tests and inspections of products after manufacturing operations to identify existing defects were developed around 150 years ago in the wake of the development of mass production. These procedures were necessary due to the extreme division of labor in industrial manufacture in the early days of mass production. However, quality controls exacerbated the problems of forms of organization involving a division of labor and responsibilities. This was aggravated by the fact that this is the most expensive way of achieving quality objectives and that these processes, like all other processes, are subject to error. Consequently, quality inspections are not suitable to achieve zero-defect targets and cost objectives.

1.2 Quality Assurance

In the 1960s, many industries started to develop preventive methods to achieve quality objectives in the various fields of production. Examples include statistical control methods for product and process characteristics, continuous improvement processes, systematic instruction and training methods, and systematic and adaptive approaches for preventive maintenance and repair.

1.3 Quality Management

In the 1980s, the idea of a preventive approach toward achieving quality objectives was extended to all domains of organization. A very strong impetus was given in this respect by the first normative standards for quality management. In particular, the standard series ISO 9000 to ISO 9004 proposed many approaches as to how preventive quality management should be implemented. Specifically, the ISO 9001 norm called for risk analyses from the outset of product development. It is now apparent that the current major revision of this standard will demand a risk-based approach for all processes from 2015 onwards.

2. THE SOLUTION

In the domain of product and process development, the technique of failure mode, effects and criticality analysis (FMEA) provides us with a capable tool to learn the "developmental" or "development-concomitant" anticipation of:
- potential malfunctions and their effects, and can learn to:
- evaluate future risks, and
- conduct preventive and detection measures during the product development process.

The method was first described by the US armed forces in 1949 in the military procedures document MIL-P-1629 (*Procedures for Performing a Failure Mode, Effects and Criticality Analysis*). The objective was to evaluate the reliability and the repercussions of malfunctions of technical systems and equipment. The procedure model has been continuously developed since the first deployment of the method, and the application of FMEA has constantly spread throughout many sectors of industry. Historically, the technique represents the first "method-based" approach to achieve a transition from a "remedial and reactive" quality control methodology toward a preventive quality assurance procedure. Such a proactive approach to quality will also benefit the pharmaceutical industry, where a wide variety of complex, but somewhat regulated and thus standardized, processes need to be followed to develop a new medicinal product. The European Medicines Agency (EMA) guidance recommends FMEA for better study designs.

2.1 The Historical Development and Milestones of FMEA in Overview

1949: Description of FMEA in the military instruction procedures MIL-P-1629

1955: Development of the "Analysis of Potential Problems (APP)" by Kepner-Tregoe

1963: Application of FMEA by NASA for the Apollo project

1971: FMEA application in the food industry

1975: FMEA application in nuclear technology

1977: Beginning of FMEA application in the automotive industry (Ford; Q1)

1990: FMEA use in medical technology, communications engineering, and mechanical engineering

1995: FMEA application in software development

1996: Optimization of the FMEA methodology by the VDA (German Automotive Industry Association) (VDA Volume 4.2)

2015: Introduction of FMEA in Drug Development processes?

The black line in Figure 8.1 shows the progress and the effort of "change management" in a conventional product development process. The greatest expenses lie closely before and after the start of series production (SOP). At this late stage, the costs for any changes or modifications are extremely high since any changes have complex repercussions due to the existing level of production maturity. And, they also mostly affect the "hardware" (manufacturing facilities).

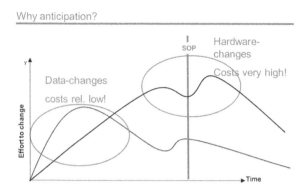

Figure 8.1 Why is anticipation necessary?

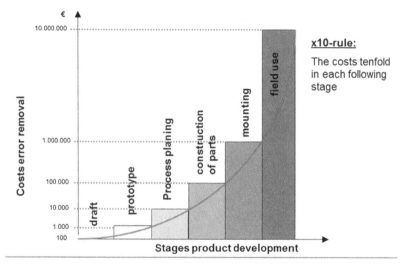

Figure 8.2 Exponential cost increases in the product development process.

The blue curve shows a development process characterized by anticipatory processes. The lion's share of the change management, and therefore the adaptive learning process, takes place well before the SOP. The costs are significantly lower as a result (see also Figure 8.2).

2.2 The FMEA Method: Success Factors and Pitfalls

FMEA is a tool to detect possible errors and defects at an early stage parallel to development and planning and to prevent their occurrence in products and processes.

The following FMEA models are deployed.

2.3 System FMEA

System FMEA analyzes proposed solution concepts. It is based on the following:

- System concepts
- Functional descriptions
- Requirement specifications

2.4 Design FMEA (e.g., Clinical Development Plans or Study Protocols)

The Design FMEA analyzes the planned development solutions. It is based on the following:

- System concepts
- Function analyses
- Requirement specifications
- Performance specifications
- Design drawings
- Formulations and compositions
- Circuit diagrams
- Norms and standards
- Directives

2.5 Process FMEA

The process FMEA analyzes the planned manufacturing process (e.g., of medicines or devices). It is based on the following:

- Design construction drawings
- Process plans
- Assembly concepts
- Production plans
- Inspection schedules
  The methodological approach.
  FMEA essentially always establishes a relationship between:

1. Cause
2. Failure mode
3. Effects

Figure 8.3 shows an example of such a chain of events. This representation is relevant for design FMEA.

Until 1996, the method was focused on working through standardized forms. These exist in various industry-specific variants. In the English-speaking realm, the processing of forms remains the usual method today for the development of FMEA.

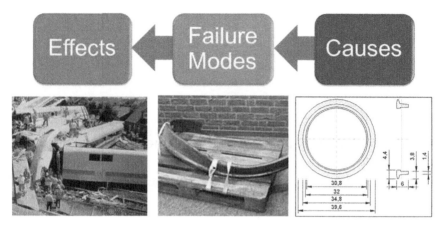

Figure 8.3 Basic principle of FMEA (cause, failure mode, effects): inappropriate design of the wheels of a German high-speed train, ICE, (cause) led to the breakage of one of the wheels at top speed, with the effect of a disastrous accident with 101 deaths in 1998.

In the respective columns, for example, the following information has to be entered:

1. Item
2. Function
3. Requirements
4. Potential failure mode
5. Potential effects
6. Severity
7. Potential causes
8. Design control
9. Occurrences of the cause
10. Detection actions

The processing of the specified information in the form frequently led to inconsistent analyses. The levels of causes, failure modes, and effects are not demarcated in a homogeneous manner. In the case of causes and failure consequences, in particular, this leads to an inappropriate generation of measures and incorrect risk assessments (Figure 8.4).

The FMEA process model of the VDA shows one possible solution. Its steps involve:

1. System structure (analysis/definition of system boundaries)
2. Function analysis
3. Malfunction analysis

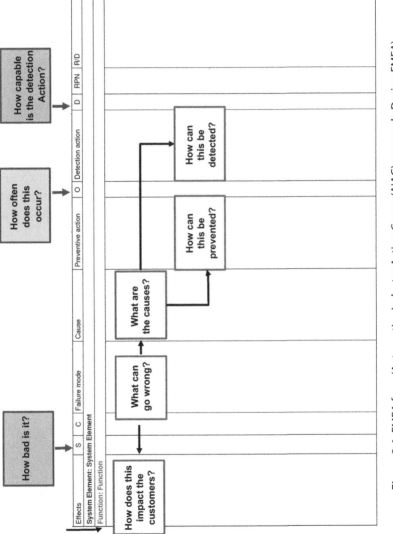

Figure 8.4 FMEA form (Automotive Industry Action Group (AIAG) approach; Design FMEA).

4. Measures analysis (risk analysis)

5. System optimization (through additional prevention and detection measures)

The system structure for a design defines the system boundaries of the components and their logical connections.

Which level in a complex structure is defined as a "focal plane" and, therefore, later defines a form-sheet view is determined by the position of the design responsibility of the respective organization (Figures 8.5 and 8.6).

In the functional analysis, the interactions between the functions of assemblies, components, parts, and their design features are depicted (Figure 8.7).

In the failure analysis, the interactions of the failures of assemblies, components, parts, and their design features are presented (Figure 8.8).

In the action analysis, the development-related preventive and detection measures are documented and evaluated as to their effectiveness. These results represent the risk assessment of the object of analysis (Figure 8.9).

In the system optimization, additional preventive and detection measures are developed and implemented for all causes, error, and effect combinations with a high-risk assessment (Figure 8.10).

With the aid of software, this information can also be displayed in the familiar form views. In the VDA approach, the form has been reduced to a presentation view of analysis results (Figure 8.12).

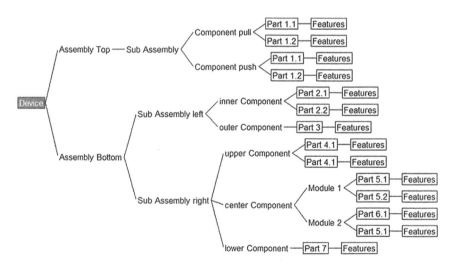

Figure 8.5 Design system structure.

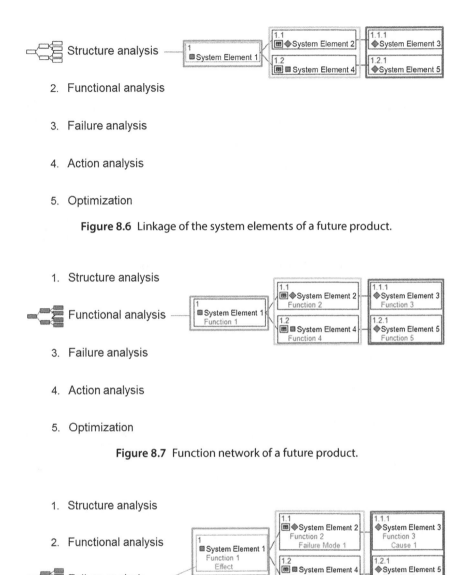

Structure analysis

2. Functional analysis

3. Failure analysis

4. Action analysis

5. Optimization

Figure 8.6 Linkage of the system elements of a future product.

1. Structure analysis

Functional analysis

3. Failure analysis

4. Action analysis

5. Optimization

Figure 8.7 Function network of a future product.

1. Structure analysis

2. Functional analysis

Failure analysis

4. Action analysis

5. Optimization

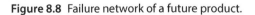

Figure 8.8 Failure network of a future product.

1. Structure analysis

2. Functional analysis

3. Failure analysis

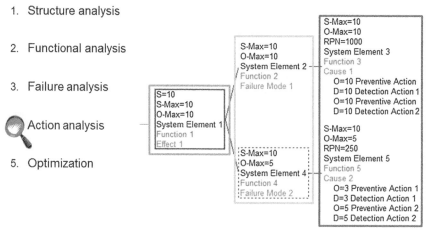

Action analysis

5. Optimization

Figure 8.9 Action analysis of a future product.

1. Structure analysis

2. Functional analysis

3. Failure analysis

4. Action analysis

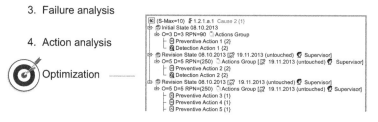

Optimization

Figure 8.10 System optimization of a future product.

2.6 Factors for FMEA Success

Among other aspects, the following decide the success or failure of an FMEA procedure (Figure 8.11):

1. Early and development-parallel use of FMEA in the production development process

2. Availability and substantive leadership on the part of the experts for the object of analysis

3. Methodological reliability of the moderator (Figures 8.12 and 8.13)

Effects	S	C	Failure Mode	Causes	Preventive Action	O	Detection Action	D	RPN	R/D
1.3.a.1 non continuous or invalid control/ no control brake system {1}	2		1.3.2.b.1 no or wrong monitoring of brakesys- tem {1}	unknown degree of validity of sensor signal post processing/ pressure sensors	ment preparation input signal values {1} Green, Amadou develop signal processing algorithm for environmental disturbunce exclusion {1} verify that there is no missinterpretation of sensor signal (sample rate is around 2 times the frequency of pumping, the shannon-nyquist theorem says more than 2 times will be needed) Copper, Andrew	4	signal values {1} Green, Amadou review of model to verify correct implementation of preparation input signal values {1} Green, Amadou	2	(56)	07.10.2013 Milestone 04 in revision
			1.3.2.2.b.1 don't define or defines wrong output states for actuator control (airpump, adblue pump, switchover value) {1} simple technical verification if values became set - must be caught by standard HIL (hardware in the loop) test procedure	Initial State: 18.10.2012					
					develop requirements specification to set output states for actuator control (airpump, adblue pump, switchover valve) {1} Green, Amadou develop test requirements specification to verify correct settings of output states for actuator control (airpump, adblue pump, switchover valve) {1}	4	apply automated HIL-tests based on test requirements specification to verify correct settings of output states for actuator control (air-pump, adblue pump, switchover valve) {1} Green, Amadou perform hydraulic and engine test bench operation to verify correct setting of output states for actuator	6	(168)	Copper, Andrew; Green, Amadou 07.10.2013 Milestone 04 in revision

Figure 8.11 FMEA form view of a future product.

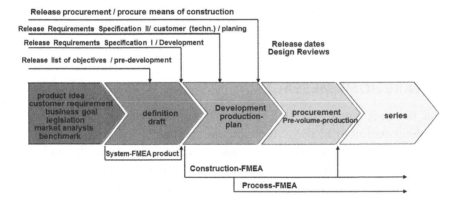

Figure 8.12 Development-concomitant deployment of FMEA in line with the VDA.

3. SWOT

S: FMEA is a well–established and powerful tool to proactively manage quality, also used for design and development processes.

W: It is mainly understood as a tool applicable to production, although it is also useful for service industry and process design. It is a complex method that is not easy to implement the first time.

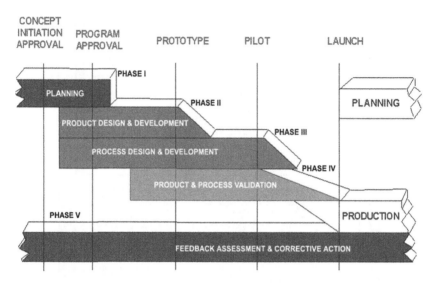

Figure 8.13 Development-concomitant deployment of FMEA in line with the Automotive Industry Action Group (AIAG).

O: The clinical development process may create more quality output (leading to better designed studies) with a more standard cycle time.

T: Inappropriate implementation and use of FMEA may create suboptimal results.

4. TAKE HOME MESSAGE

For the next few years, other sectors of industry will be involved in the implementation of FMEA. Much like the food and packaging industry, for example, the textile sector will be making adaptations within that industry and applying FMEA techniques. Moreover, strong development impulses are being generated by requirements imposed by standards in the field of functional safety. Quality assurance will become another driving force along with cost control. This also relates to the development and production processes in the pharmaceutical industry. In this context, the Fault Tree Analysis will grow together with FMEA as a deductive method through the development of software tools for FMEA applications.

5. APPLICABLE REGULATIONS

EMA/269011/2013, November 18, 2013, Reflection paper on risk-based quality management in clinical trials.

Where to Start: The Protocol

CHAPTER 9

No Patients—No Data: Patient Recruitment in the Twenty-first Century

Chris Trizna

Contents

1. THE NEED

As a patient recruitment leader with more than 20 years in this business, I have been witness to many "silver bullets" that claim to be the best tactics for recruiting patients. These tactics started with broadcast advertising on television and radio in the 1990s and moved to direct mail through targeted "opt-in" databases. Today, we use the new technologies such as Web site search engine optimization (SEO), search engine advertising, social media, and SMS texting. The truth is, there is no single solution that fits every recruitment need, but there is a better process to developing a solid recruitment and enrollment plan.

Is it any wonder that upwards of 80% of clinical trials fail to meet their enrollment timelines? Today's protocols are more complex, there are more studies competing for the same patients, and the overall perception of clinical trials is negative. In a CISCRP survey of general public

Re-Engineering Clinical Trials
http://dx.doi.org/10.1016/B978-0-12-420246-7.00009-8

and patient perceptions about clinical research, respondents reported on safety in clinical studies.

- *36% said that they generally believed clinical research studies are very safe*
- *58% said that they believed them to be somewhat safe*
- *5% said they did not believe them to be very safe*
- *1% said they did not believe them to be safe at all [1]*

In the twenty-first century, we need to do a better job of educating the patient population about conditions, promote more awareness about clinical trials, and finally we need to rethink our process of patient recruitment to meet our enrollment timelines.

2. THE SOLUTION

Every patient for every trial will be "recruited" into the trial. Whether it is a stage four metastatic breast cancer study or an osteoarthritis pain study, some basic steps need to be taken every time. First, there is awareness that comes from advertising, community outreach, from a medical professional, or from the doctor on the study. Patients need to understand their treatment options (including a clinical trial) as it relates to their condition. Moreover, patients should understand what a clinical trial is and what is involved with the study they are being presented with.

3. SWOT: STRENGTHS—PLANNING

The development and execution of an enrollment plan by each site will significantly increase the rate of enrollment over historic rates. The basics of patient recruitment are not complex, but simple steps are rarely (and consistently) taken to ensure successful enrollment within timelines.

This chapter will discuss fundamental steps necessary to develop successful enrollment plans and tools to maximize your enrollment.

4. SWOT: WEAKNESSES—SITE PERFORMANCE

We hear and see it on nearly every study: "10–20% of your sites are enrolling most of your study, and 10–20% of sites don't enroll a single patient." Site performance is a major issue with meeting enrollment timelines. But is it solely the responsibility of the sites to develop effective enrollment plans, or can we do more to set up each site for successful enrollment? When we leave enrollment planning up to the sites, we will continue to see substandard results.

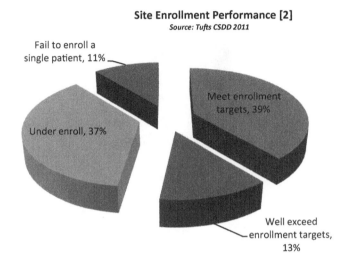

Site Enrollment Performance [2]
Source: Tufts CSDD 2011

Fail to enroll a single patient, 11%

Meet enrollment targets, 39%

Under enroll, 37%

Well exceed enrollment targets, 13%

5. SWOT: OPPORTUNITIES—THE ENROLLMENT PLAN

Who is our ideal patient? We need to determine the best ways to identify our target audience—where they will be found during their everyday routine and what motivates them. For example, while the protocol calls for people 18+, where is the greatest prevalence? Who is most likely to have the particular condition? Narrow your target audience to the closest age range and gender.

Remember, your target may not be the patient. You need to identify the people that will make and/or influence the decision for someone to participate in the clinical trial. For example, for a pediatric asthma study, we obviously would not target children with asthma; we would target their mothers, women aged 30–45. For a moderate to severe Alzheimer's study, we would target the children or caregivers of these patients: adults aged 45–64. These target audiences can vary in different countries around the world based on the culture and health care systems.

Once the target audience or audiences are identified (and there can be more than one), we need to determine how to reach them during their everyday lives to get information in their hands about the study. This step is what we call *defining the patient pathway*.

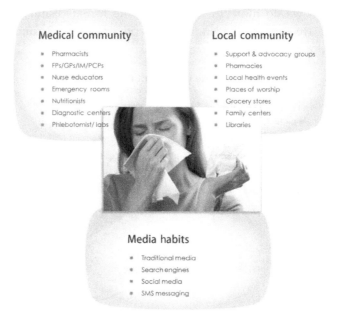

Medical community

- Pharmacists
- FPs/GPs/IM/PCPs
- Nurse educators
- Emergency rooms
- Nutritionists
- Diagnostic centers
- Phlebotomist/labs

Local community

- Support & advocacy groups
- Pharmacies
- Local health events
- Places of worship
- Grocery stores
- Family centers
- Libraries

Media habits

- Traditional media
- Search engines
- Social media
- SMS messaging

To define the pathway, we look at three areas to reach people in their everyday lives. The first is the *medical community* (primary care physicians, specialists, diagnostic, pharmacists, urgent care, nutritionists, physical therapists, etc.); second is in the *local community* where they might be found during a regular weekly routine (family centers, grocery stores, day care, local events, health fairs, support and advocacy groups, etc.); and finally, we use *media vehicles* (television, radio, print, mail, Internet, transit, etc.).

Once your target audience is defined and you know where the target audience can be found, you can now start developing the creative messaging strategy (advertisements) and tactics to recruit them.

Your message and/or advertisement is one of the most important aspects of recruitment that is often overlooked. Your message needs to quickly capture your target audiences' attention, and provide them with information so that they can make an informed decision regarding potential participation in the clinical trial. Once they have this information, you need to make sure there is a call to action—whether it is speaking to their physician, filling out an online screener, or picking up the telephone.

When working on a global study, you may not be able to use the same approach for all countries. There are cultural nuances to take into consideration. For example, in some parts of the world you cannot show feet in an advertisement, and you must match the race/ethnic look of the region. Colors can also be very important, as they have different meanings in different countries. For example, yellow represents mourning in Egypt, but in Japan it means courage. In India, red stands for purity while in South Africa, it is the color of mourning. White represents clean, pure, and angels in North America, but quite the opposite in China, where it means death and mourning. Utilizing the appropriate colors in each country is key.

5.1 Recruitment Tactics

The most compliant and most cost-efficient patient comes from within the site's patient population itself. When developing an enrollment plan, start with tactics that focus on the site's patient population in and around the site. Sites typically already have a relationship with the patient, and there is a level of trust between the doctor and patient. When thinking about recruitment at the site, there are proactive tactics and reactive tactics.

Tactics in the office often include:

1. Chart reviews of upcoming patient visits (proactive; site to patient)
2. Doctor letters to patients within the database (proactive; site to patient)
3. Fliers, brochures, and other materials in the waiting or exam rooms (reactive; patient asks site)
4. Patient referrals (reactive; patient asks site)

Once we have identified a patient for the study, how effective is the site in presenting the study through the informed consent? I have heard too many times of study coordinators mailing the informed consent to the patient, never to hear from them again. Sadly, I am not surprised by the lack of interest after receiving a consent by mail. Pretend you are the potential participant; going over the informed consent can be very intimidating to the patient and family members (who will influence the decision to participate). This is a time where training and support tools can increase the enrollment rate on many studies. More training should be done with this process at the site or during the investigator meeting. There are many tools that can be developed to help in the process:

- Flip charts: Clearly define and illustrate the study to the patient in a well thought-out process
- Videos: Similar to the flip chart, the video makes it easy for people to comprehend all the medical terms and processes in which the patient will be asked to participate
- Electronic informed consent: Typically done on a computer or tablet, this system will help the patient better understand the informed consent through

videos, images, and charts. The system can also ask periodic questions of the patient to ensure that they understand the informed consent.

As we discussed earlier, there are other medical patient pathways to consider. After looking for patients at your site, think about where else your target patients would go to manage their condition or conditions. There may be other specialists or therapists that could interact with the patient. Are there other conditions that may affect this patient and different physicians treating them? For example, if you are working on a hypertension study, the target audience you are focused on is men 45–64 years of age. This patient population may also be treated for diabetes and under the care of an endocrinologist or nutritionist.

The *medical community* includes physicians, pharmacists, nurses, nutritionists, physical therapists, and other medical professionals. These are people whom the patient can trust to provide medical advice. Working with the medical community typically is based on professional relationships. Once a network is established, you will want to keep your network aware of your studies and potential medical options for their patients. The more informed your referral network is, the more likely they will refer patients to you for your studies. Tools for this tactic include: Doctor-to-doctor letters, brochures, inclusion/exclusion criteria cards, and study fliers.

Example: Medical Pathway of a Psoriasis Arthritis Patient

Family Practitioner diagnoses a patient with psoriasis.

Refers patient to a **Dermatologist** for further evaluation and topical treatment (**Pharmacist**).

Patient is referred to a **Rheumatologist** when arthritis symptoms present.

A **Physical Therapist** is recommended as well as a **Nutritionist**.

Nurse educators follow up with the patient for additional care.

In some instances, **social workers** intervene to support the patient's treatment.

In this example, eight different medical professionals were identified and targeted for recruitment.

Reaching out to the *local community* is not as difficult or time-consuming as most people think. It is a process that has to be tended to and expanded every week. The most important part of community outreach is education and awareness. Once you establish a network of organizations in the community, you will want to stay in touch with them on a regular basis, providing them with information about your practice and clinical trials. People want information and don't always know where to find it. This educational outreach also helps reduce people's fears about clinical trials, removing a major barrier to participation. Some of the high-traffic community organizations include community centers, senior centers, fitness centers, grocery stores, pharmacists, day care, places of worship, etc. Tools that you will need include brochures, fliers, videos, and general clinical trial information. Refer back to your target audience to help determine the best organizations to target.

The third area of a recruitment campaign is to reach out to the local population through *advertising*. Advertising offers the greatest reach to people with the condition. Advertising is not always the most efficient method, but at times necessary to identify additional patients for your study. Advertising is not an easy process, and many facets of planning media are best performed by a professional media planner and buyer. *Knowing your target population is critical* with this phase. With radio, your stations have very different audiences based on the format: top 40, pop, oldies, sports/talk radio, country, urban, etc. Each of these formats draws a unique audience. Similarly, when buying television, each show will draw a different audience. Your media buyer will know what questions to ask to ensure your media plan is focused on your target audience. The lowest cost for a spot (advertisement) is not always the best spot to buy. Costs are based on the number of people watching the show. Newspaper, while not as popular as it was 20 years ago, is still useful with different target audiences and can be effective. These three traditional media options will reach the largest population of people. Cable television is more segmented (more options through an expanded offering of networks) and can be used to focus on a very narrow audience, especially with specific cultural/ethnic backgrounds. Not only can a media planner put your message in the best possible location, but can negotiate the lowest cost for those purchases.

Online media have served as a very effective venue for recruitment, and, most importantly, they provide a measurable way of determining who is being reached. The Internet has become an important part of our everyday lives. It is not just young people searching the Web, but people of all ages. Internet users are active consumers of online wellness information. According to Pew Research, 72% of Internet users say they looked for health information online within the past year [3]. There are a few online platforms to recruit; here are the most frequently used initiatives:

1. Search engine paid key words
2. Social media paid advertising
3. Banner advertising

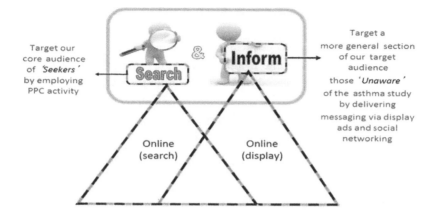

At CSSi, we use online media in most of the recruitment campaigns we launch. Depending on your target audience, the strengths of online recruitment are endless. One of the biggest benefits of online recruitment is the ability to both demographically and geographically target your audience. If you employed online advertising in the past, it went out to the entire World Wide Web. Today, you can customize your plan to specific genders, ages, and locations—all the way down to a zip code. Unlike traditional media buys, online tactics are highly measureable and you do not have to commit a large budget to the tactics. If it is working well, you can easily add additional budget or quickly end the campaign.

Unlike traditional media, where your message is sent out quickly and to hundreds of thousands of people, online tactics take a little more time and effort to get your message out to a large population. You may have to use multiple online tactics to distribute your message. Online media buying is not as simple as one might think; daily monitoring and adjusting is necessary to maximize the benefit of this tactic.

An online campaign provides a great opportunity when you are trying to reach a very small target population or if you are in a very large media market, like Los Angeles or New York City, where people are less likely to travel great distances to participate in your study. Traditional media's "reach" can be too large—most people hearing or seeing your ad won't consider your study because of the travel distance. Online recruitment enables you to effectively place ads geographically where people will be more willing to travel. Overall, it is a very efficient recruitment tactic.

The biggest challenge with online recruitment is the ever-changing environment of Web sites and applications. Something that is popular today will be old school the next year. Keeping up with the trends is a challenge.

When running global online campaigns, you must check with the local Ethics Committee (EC) to see what is allowable.

5.2 Search Engines

When looking for specific information, people will use search engines. They type in their key word or phrase and the search engine will identify Web sites that are relative to their search. You can pay to have your message appear on the first pages of those search results. In Google, these are typically the top three results or the results on the right side of the page. Advertisers will pay a little extra to appear at the top of the list. You only pay the fee (typically $3.00–$6.00) when someone clicks on your advertisement. When they click on your ad, typically it will take them to a study announcement or study Web site.

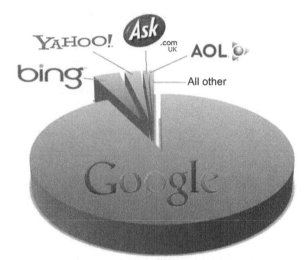

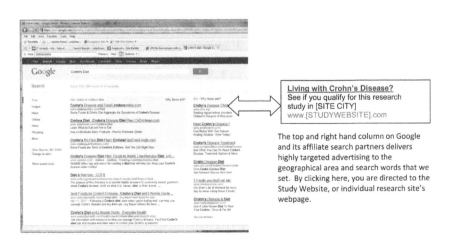

Living with Crohn's Disease?
See if you qualify for this research study in [SITE CITY]
www.[STUDYWEBSITE].com

The top and right hand column on Google and its affiliate search partners delivers highly targeted advertising to the geographical area and search words that we set. By clicking here, you are directed to the Study Website, or individual research site's webpage.

5.3 Social Media

Facebook.com is the largest social media Web site with over a billion users worldwide. Social media Web sites include Twitter, LinkedIn, Pinterest, Google Plus, Tumblr, and Instagram, just to name a few. There are hundreds of social media Web sites and the number grows weekly. Let's focus on the most popular social media site: Facebook. Like Google advertising, Facebook has a similar model. Users tell Facebook all about themselves and advertisers use this information to target their audiences. When someone clicks the "like" feature to indicate, for example, support of something they have read, a person, or an organization, Facebook can direct ads to that party. Similar to Google, ads appear on the side of the page. There are also a myriad of geographic and demographic targeting options available. When people click on the ad, you are charged a fee.

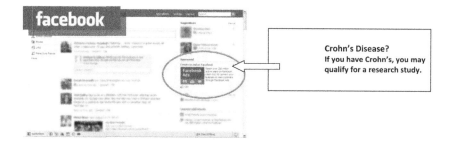

When considering global regions, one should look beyond Facebook to market-specific social networks such as Tuenti in Spain and Nasza-Klasa in Poland. The popularity of these sites will change on an annual basis!

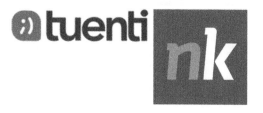

5.4 Display Advertising

Online display advertising is useful when you have a Web site that your audience is visiting on a regular basis. Your "message" would appear within the site in a variety of locations and/or sizes. Display advertising fees can be charged by the number of impressions it gets or visitors to that page, or by the number of clicks.

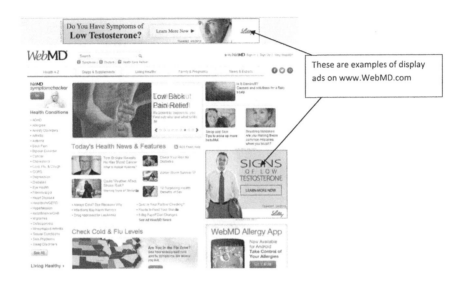

These are examples of display ads on www.WebMD.com

5.5 Enrollment Planning

Once you have done your research on the study population, it is time to develop the enrollment plan. A plan should be built for each country where you have sites. Developing a plan for each country is necessary, as there are restrictions on EC-approved recruitment tactics, and creative concepts will vary based on cultural differences. The enrollment plan is based on how you will reach the target audiences as described earlier; it is important to identify the best tactics and tools for each country. These will be the tools and tactics the sites will use to customize their unique enrollment plan. By developing the right tools and determining the best tactics to reach your target audiences, you set up the sites for successful enrollment planning.

Each site is unique and has different enrollment needs and challenges. For this reason, each site will need an individualized enrollment plan. The challenge with today's recruitment services is that recruitment companies focus on a single solution, when the sites want a solution unique to their individual needs. When each site has its enrollment plan built based on its needs, the site is more compliant and enrollment performance increases. The enrollment plan should contain specific strategies and tactics to be implemented on a specific timeline. Each tactic should have some type of measurable response or result to quantitatively determine success and failure. Areas to track include:

1. Budget spent
2. Number of responses (calls, inquiries, clicks on your Web site, etc.)
3. Number of responses that resulted in a screening
4. The screen failure (SF) rate with each tactic

Here is an example of an individual site enrollment plan timeline.

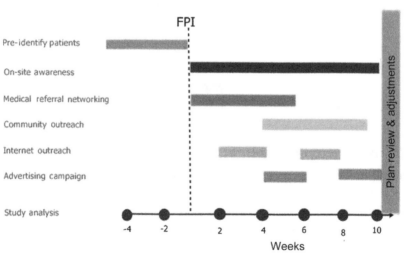

Sample site enrollment plan

6. SWOT: THREATS—SITES AND REGULATIONS

We have always let the sites run their own recruitment/enrollment plans without any accountability, and enrollment timelines are consistently missed. The site should be held accountable for implementing the plan and providing results. If sites make a commitment and are held accountable to the plan, sponsors will see more patients enrolled at each site and, thus, more well-performing sites.

7. APPLICABLE REGULATIONS

Any recruitment tactics that involve interface directly with patients will require approval by the agencies that regulate that application. The agencies that are referenced in this chapter include the Institutional Review Board (IRB), EC, and Ministries of Health. IRB includes both the local and national IRB governing boards. For example, the tools that CSSi provides to site coordinators to help a participant understand the informed consent process, such as flip charts and videos, all need to be approved by the applicable national and local IRB agencies. All advertising, whether through traditional media or online campaigns, must be approved by the appropriate regulations agency. When running a global online campaign for a study, approval must be granted from the local ECs to make sure that the material is allowable.

Every country needs to have a specific enrollment plan developed for them, because EC-approved recruitment tactics and creative concepts will be varied due to cultural differences; what is acceptable in Australia may not be culturally appropriate for Germany. When developing a recruitment and enrollment plan for your study, it is critical to make sure that all your materials have been reviewed and approved by the appropriate regulatory committee to avoid delays once the enrollment timeline begins and recruitment is underway.

8. TAKE HOME MESSAGE

In our world of well though-out clinical trials and collection of measureable data, our approach to recruiting patients for clinical studies should be no different. Take the time to follow these simple steps:
1. Pinpoint your target population
2. Identify the patient pathway
3. Develop tactics to raise awareness about your study
4. Create recruitment tools to educate, inform, and motivate people to inquire
5. Construct unique enrollment plans for each site
6. Measure your results and make adjustments based on recruitment metrics

Planning for recruitment is a simple and necessary step that will increase the likelihood of successful enrollment. While simple, this process takes patience, experience, and due diligence to develop an effective enrollment plan; it is not always easy. Setting your sites up for successful enrollment through this process will keep your study on schedule—and maybe even enable early completion.

REFERENCES

[1] CISCRP. Perceptions and Insights Study: Public and Patient Perceptions of Clinical Research; 2013. Retrieved from: https://www.ciscrp.org/wp-content/uploads/2014/01/2013-CISCRP-Study-General-Perceptions.pdf.
[2] Getz K. Director, Sponsored Research Programs. Industry Update. SCRS Site Solutions Summit 2012 - Typical Enrollment Performance. Retrieved from: http://myscrs.org/wp-content/uploads/2012/10/SSS-October-2012-Ken-Getz.pdf.
[3] Pew Research Center. Health Fact Sheet: Highlights of the Pew Internet Project's research related to health and health care; 2014. Retrieved from: http://www.pewinternet.org/fact-sheets/health-fact-sheet/.

CHAPTER 10

The Impact of Bad Protocols

Kenneth A. Getz, Kenneth I. Kaitin

Contents

1. A CRITICAL NEED TO ADDRESS RISING PROTOCOL DESIGN COMPLEXITY

Under an ideal resource-rich research and development operating environment, the regulatory approval of safe and effective medical products would be the ultimate test for whether study designs are good or bad. In the current resource-constrained operating environment, however, bad study design is defined as one that wastes resources, gathers extraneous data, and exposes study subjects to unnecessary risk. Ten years of research on protocol design practice at the Tufts Center for the Study of Drug Development (Tufts CSDD) shows that a high proportion of study designs today include elements that lead to inefficiency and waste. But the studies also suggest that there are numerous opportunities for improvement.

This chapter summarizes studies conducted by Tufts CSDD and others examining the impact of protocol design practices on drug development performance and cost. The chapter concludes with a discussion of how the growing awareness of and concern about bad protocol design are affecting change within the pharmaceutical industry and leading to new and compelling approaches to study design.

Re-Engineering Clinical Trials
http://dx.doi.org/10.1016/B978-0-12-420246-7.00010-4

2. IMPACT OF BAD DESIGN ON DIRECT PROCEDURE COSTS

In a 2012 study, Tufts CSDD found that sponsors were spending US$4 to $6 billion annually in direct costs to administer protocol procedures that were not tied to primary or key secondary end points and regulatory requirements. The incidence of these less essential or extraneous procedures had nearly doubled during the decade before that [1].

Noncore procedures are added to protocols for a variety of reasons: for example, clinical scientists and statisticians may want to collect more contextual data to help interpret study findings and guide development decisions. Context-setting variables may not appear in any statistical plan but they may provide clinical validation and explanation for unusual and unexpected results that may be observed during a clinical trial. Clinical scientists may also collect additional study data with the hope that, should the study fail to meet its original objectives, post hoc analyses will reveal useful new insights into the characteristics and treatment of disease. Most companies can point to incidences in which exploratory data in fact led to the discovery of a novel therapy. Nonetheless, this is a relatively rare phenomenon.

The presence of noncore protocol procedures may also be a function of authoring processes and practices and an insurance policy against risk. Medical and protocol writing professionals may incorporate outdated and unnecessary procedures into new protocols because those procedures are included in legacy authoring templates and policies.

Clinical teams may also collect additional data in cautious anticipation of requests from regulatory agencies, purchasers, and payers. Past experiences with unplanned and unexpected data requests from these parties have resulted in delayed submissions, later-than-planned product launches, and slower product adoption rates. They have also resulted in stalled career advancement and, in some cases, company restructuring and downsizing.

Fifteen midsized and large pharmaceutical and biotechnology companies provided data for the Tufts CSDD study on 116 Phase II and III protocols targeting diseases across multiple therapeutic areas and executed by investigative sites dispersed globally since 2009. Medidata Solutions provided direct procedure cost data to supplement those provided by participating companies. To minimize atypical and unusual designs, pediatric, medical device, orphan drug, and extension studies were excluded from the analysis.

Participating companies classified each protocol procedure according to the objective and end point it supported as defined by the clinical study report (CSR) and the study's specific statistical analysis plan (SAP). In total,

25,103 procedures were reviewed, and half of the total were classified as "core" to the study. These procedures supported primary or key secondary end points. More than one of every five procedures (22.3%), however, were "noncore," as they supported supplemental secondary, tertiary, and exploratory end points. One of every four (24.7%) procedures performed per Phase III protocol and 17.9% of all Phase II procedures were classified as noncore. Core procedures made up approximately half of all procedures by phase—47.9% of Phase III and 54.3% of Phase II studies (see Table 10.1).

Each study had an average of $2.9 million in total direct procedure costs. Nearly half (47.9%) was spent to administer core procedures. An average of $1.1 million per protocol (17.9%) was spent to cover the direct cost of performing noncore procedures. The direct cost of administering "required" and "standard" procedures for Phase II and III protocols was an average of $1.3 million (21.7%) and $0.8 million (12.5%), respectively.

For Phase III protocols, the average total direct cost to administer all procedures was $9.4 million. Approximately half of the total direct cost (46.0%, or $4.3 million on average) was spent on administering core procedures; 18.5%, or $1.7 million, was spent on administering noncore procedures. The direct cost of administering procedures supporting screening requirements and regulatory compliance was $2.2 million, or 24% of the total. Noncore procedure administration costs were on average $0.3 million, or 13.1%, of the total direct costs for Phase II protocols.

Wide variability in the incidence of procedures supporting end-point classifications was observed across therapeutic areas. Protocols targeting endocrine and central nervous system (CNS) disorders contained a higher relative average number of procedures supporting supplementary, tertiary, and exploratory procedures (e.g., noncore) end points. Oncology protocols had the highest relative proportion of procedures supporting core end points and objectives and the lowest relative proportion supporting noncore end points [2].

The proportion of direct costs of administering endocrine protocol procedures supporting noncore end points and objectives was significantly higher than that observed in oncology and CNS studies. The results of the Tufts CSDD study highlight the need to evaluate the feasibility of each protocol individually based on the end points and objectives as defined by the CSR and SAP.

Tufts CSDD studies looking at the direct cost of administering extraneous procedures do not include any of the indirect costs associated with personnel capturing, monitoring, cleaning, analyzing, managing, and storing the data. These costs are many multiples higher than the direct costs

Table 10.1 Distribution of procedures and direct procedure costs by end point type

End point type	Definition	Phase II procedures	Phase III procedures	Phase II direct procedure costs	Phase III direct procedure costs
Core	Supporting primary and key secondary end points	54.4%	47.7%	55.2%	46.7%
Required	Supporting compliance-related requirements	8.0%	10.0%	16.3%	22.7%
Standard	Supporting baseline and routine volunteer visit assessments	19.7%	17.6%	15.4%	12.0%
Noncore	Supporting supplementary, tertiary, and exploratory end points	17.9%	24.7%	13.1%	18.6%

Source: Tufts CSDD (2012).

measured. Tufts CSDD also did not attempt to estimate the ethical costs of exposing study volunteers to unnecessary risks associated with conducting noncore procedures.

3. IMPACT OF BAD DESIGN ON STUDY PERFORMANCE

Research published in the peer-reviewed and trade literature shows a very clear inverse relationship between study design scope and study performance and quality. Study designs that include a relatively large number of eligibility requirements and unique procedures conducted frequently have poorer study volunteer recruitment and retention rates, take longer, and generate lower quality clinical data than designs without such features.

Friedman and colleagues found, for example, that the high volume of data now collected in clinical trials distracts research scientists, compromises the data analysis process, and ultimately harms data quality [3]. Nahm, Pieper, and Cunningham found that as more data are collected during protocol administration, error rates increase [4]. And Barrett showed that the more procedures included per protocol, the higher the incidence of unused data in new drug application submissions [5].

Higher levels of study design complexity are also associated with longer cycle times and lower patient recruitment and retention rates. Clark found, not surprisingly, that the collection of excessive and unnecessary clinical data drives longer study durations, and he suggested that longer durations may delay regulatory agency submission and ultimately reduce the likelihood of approval [6].

Ross and colleagues conducted a comprehensive analysis of peer-reviewed academic studies and found that health professionals were less likely to refer patients to, and patients were less likely to participate in, more complex clinical trials [7]. Madsen showed that patients are significantly less likely to sign the informed consent form when facing a more demanding protocol design [8].

In a study conducted by Boericke and Gwinn, it was shown that the higher the number of study eligibility criteria, the more frequent and longer were the delays in completing clinical studies [9]. Andersen also showed that volunteer retention rates are much lower among patients participating in more complex clinical trials. The authors cautioned that when volunteers terminate their participation early and are lost to follow-up, the validity of the study results may be compromised [10].

A 2008 Tufts CSDD study evaluated 10,038 unique Phase I–IV protocols designed by 75 pharmaceutical and biotechnology companies. The
protocols targeted a representative variety of therapeutic areas, and performance measures were adjusted to control for geographic area differences.
Tufts CSDD compared the performance of simple protocol designs to
more complex designs—those with a higher number of eligibility criteria,
unique procedures, conducted more frequently (see Figure 10.1). The
results indicated that the average overall clinical trial duration was 64%
longer for complex designs. Median cycle time from protocol readiness to
last patient/last visit increased by 73%. Enrollment rates for volunteers
who met the eligibility criteria for complex protocols were 21% lower
and retention rates were 19% lower than those for the simpler protocol
designs [11].

In addition to increasing the burden on resources involved with collecting, cleaning, managing, and storing data, bad protocol designs
adversely affect investigative site personnel. The 2008 Tufts CSDD study
found that the work effort required of study staff to administer procedures for complex protocols was substantially greater than that for simpler
protocol designs. Tufts CSDD computed a metric, referred to as work
effort units (WEUs), which are based on Medicare's well-known relative
value unit (RVU) approach to calculating reimbursement payments to

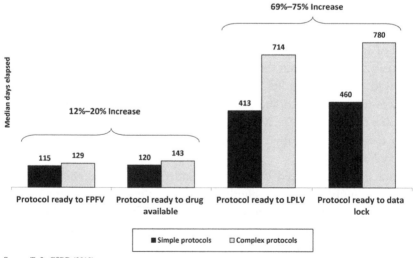

Source: Tufts CSDD (2012)

Figure 10.1 Comparing cycle times of simple and complex protocols.

physicians; RVUs are based on the estimated value of physicians' time and expertise in administering medical procedures. Procedures not assigned a Medicare RVU were assigned a WEU established by a panel of physicians at the Tufts University School of Medicine. The Tufts CSDD study found that, on average, the work effort to administer complex protocols, based on WEUs, was significantly higher than that required for simple protocols [11].

A subsequent 2011 Tufts CSDD study found that more complex protocols are associated with a significantly higher number of protocol amendments [12]. Protocol amendments are highly disruptive, causing significant unplanned expense and delays for research sponsors and unexpected burden for investigative sites. In this study, Tufts CSDD evaluated more than 3400 protocols provided by 15 middle and major pharmaceutical and biotechnology companies and found that each protocol was amended an average of 2.4 times, triggering nearly seven changes to the protocol design, at a realized direct cost of over $1 million per protocol and four months of incremental time to implement (see Figure 10.2). Tufts CSDD also found that more than 40% of protocols were amended prior to the first subject/first visit, and one-third of amendments were avoidable (see Figure 10.3). Importantly, complex protocols were amended nearly twice as often as were simple protocol designs.

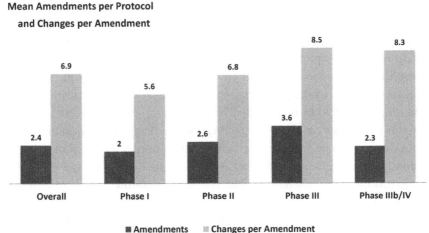

Mean Amendments per Protocol and Changes per Amendment

■ Amendments   ▨ Changes per Amendment

Source: **TCSDD 2010 analysis of 3,596 amendments and 19,345 changes**

Figure 10.2 Amendments and changes per protocol.

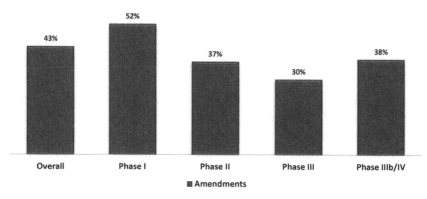

Percentage of Amendments Occurring before
First Patient First Dose

■ Amendments

Source: TCSDD 2010 analysis of 3,596 amendments and 19,345 changes

Figure 10.3 Protocol amendment timing.

4. THE SOLUTION: OPTIMIZING STUDY DESIGNS

A growing number of research sponsors and contract research organizations (CROs) have taken steps to optimize their protocol designs with the goal of reducing complexity and cost, improving feasibility, and gathering more meaningful clinical data. Many of these approaches are discussed at length in subsequent chapters in this book. Here we summarize a few key developments.

Many organizations are now referring to published benchmark data on protocol design characteristics in peer-reviewed journals. Some organization are also exploring the use of commercially available softwares and consulting services to evaluate their study design practices. Some sponsor organizations are looking for ways to improve study design feasibility by soliciting feedback from principal investigators, study coordinators, and patients to identify areas—prior to final protocol approval—in which protocol designs can be simplified, made easier to implement, and more convenient for participants. Feedback mechanisms include in-person meetings, focus groups, teleconferences, and the use of online social and digital media communities.

Sponsor companies and CROs are also revamping internal legacy protocol authoring practices. To that end, a new reference was made available for protocol authors called SPIRIT, an initiative designed to ensure that the purposes of protocol procedures are transparent and tied to core objectives and end points. SPIRIT checklists and guidelines were developed with input from 115 global multidisciplinary contributors from medical writing, journal editors, regulatory agencies, ethics committees, clinical research, and health care professionals.

SPIRIT 2013 called for simple, minimalist designs that are tied directly to core end points and objectives as defined by the CSR. Formatting conventions for various protocol elements (e.g., table of contents, glossary of terms, abbreviations) are also provided.

In a 2013 study, Tufts CSDD found that many major pharmaceutical companies have established formal governance committees charged with challenging clinical teams to improve protocol feasibility [13]. The creation of these committees signals a growing commitment among major pharmaceutical companies to adopt a more systematic and long-term approach to optimizing study design. Committees are positioned within their respective organizations as objective governance and assessment mechanisms, offering guidance and input into the existing protocol review process without requiring organizations to alter legacy study design practices and procedures.

The committees raise awareness within the clinical team of the impact that design decisions have on study budgets and on study execution feasibility. Committees typically provide input into the study design just prior to final protocol approval, and they routinely offer insight into how protocol designs can be streamlined and better "fit to purpose." Ultimately, internal facilitation committees may drive long-term change in study design practices.

Nearly all of the facilitation committees comprise cross-functional representatives who volunteer their time. Committee representatives come from a variety of functions, including clinical development, clinical operations, statistics, data management, medical writing, clinical pharmacology, regulation, safety, and pharmacovigilance, as well as finance and/or procurement. Although some committees have more expansive goals than others, all committees are charged with simplifying and streamlining protocols by reducing unnecessary procedures and the number of amendments. To meet these goals, committees assess the direct cost of performing noncore procedures. Some committees also look at core procedures that may be conducted more frequently than necessary.

Adaptive trial designs represent a potentially powerful approach to feasibility planning prior to protocol approval. Adaptive designs are all preplanned, typically through the use of trial simulations and scenario planning. The program team predetermines which clinical trial design elements will be modified and adjusted while the trial is under way based on the results of an analysis of interim data. Tufts CSDD has determined that approximately one of five (20%) late-stage clinical trials, on average, use simple adaptive design approaches. A much lower percentage—less than 5%—use more sophisticated adaptive approaches [14].

Study terminations due to futility are the most common simple adaptive design used, and they are becoming the most widely adopted approach. Sponsor companies have found that early terminations due to futility are relatively easy to implement and are likely to become standard practice in Phase II and Phase III studies, across all therapeutic areas. Sample size reestimation is also viewed by a growing number of companies as a relatively simple adaptive design to implement.

Adaptive trial designs hold considerable promise for optimizing study design. Depending on clinical trial scope, early study termination due to futility and sample size reestimation could save up to a hundred million U.S. dollars in direct and indirect costs annually for each sponsor company when the trial is actually terminated and on the sponsor's overall implementation of this adaptive approach across the development portfolio.

Perhaps the greatest impact from adaptive trial designs will come from improvements in late-stage clinical success rates. Even modest improvements in success rates for new molecular entities and new biologic entities represent billions of dollars in increased revenue potential for research sponsors.

In the short term, adaptive trial designs offer cross-functional teams direct insights into study design through scenario planning and trial simulation prior to finalizing the protocol. Rigorous up-front planning—similar to optimization practices for traditional study designs—is forcing organizations to challenge protocol feasibility prior to placing the protocol in the clinic.

5. THE NECESSITY TO OPTIMIZE PROTOCOL DESIGN

Between the 1980s and the mid-2000s, study design practices were largely influenced by scientific functions within pharmaceutical and biotechnology companies. Operating and logistical functions played a more passive role, focusing primarily on execution with only limited input into revising study designs to improve feasibility. At that time, companies reasoned that the short-term incremental cost of delays and inefficiencies would be more than offset by the commercial performance of the newly launched drug.

Since the mid-2000s, drug development costs and cycle times have continued to rise, whereas global market competition has intensified and economic conditions have worsened. Operating and logistical functions have been given greater leverage in improving protocol design feasibility. Moving forward, research sponsors will continue their efforts to optimize study design by working to achieve a better balance between good science and feasible, practical execution.

As the ultimate blueprint guiding new drug innovation, protocol design holds the key to fundamentally and sustainably transforming drug development performance, cost, and success. Optimized protocol design is essential to achieving higher levels of drug development performance and efficiency.

6. TAKE HOME MESSAGE

- Protocol designs have become increasingly more scientifically and logistically complex since the mid-1990s.
- Protocol design complexity is associated with poorer development performance and inefficiency (e.g., patient recruitment and retention rates are worse, study costs are higher, and average cycle times are longer with more complex protocol designs).
- A growing number of sponsor companies are implementing improvements in protocol design feasibility to positively influence development performance and efficiency.
- Study design optimization opportunities include identifying and reducing the number of noncore procedures, establishing internal mechanisms and external panels to review and challenge protocol feasibility, modifying protocol authoring practices, and adopting adaptive trial designs.

REFERENCES

[1] Getz K, Stergiopoulos S, Marlborough M, Whitehall J, Curran M, Kaitin K. Quantifying the magnitude and cost of collecting extraneous protocol data. Am J Ther 2013. Published ahead of print. April 9, 2013.
[2] Getz KA, Stergiopoulos S. Therapeutic area variability in the collection of data supporting protocol end points and objectives. Clin Invest 2014;4(2):125–30.
[3] Friedman L, Furberg C, DeMets D. Data collection and quality control in the fundamentals of clinical trials. Chapter 11. Springer Science and Business Media; 2010. pp. 199–214.

[4] Nahm ML, Pieper CF, Cunningham MM. Quantifying data quality for clinical trials using electronic data capture. PLoS One 2008;3(8):e3049. http://dx.doi.org/10.1371/journal.pone.0003049.

[5] Barrett J. What's behind clinical trial data. Appl Clin Trials 2009;18(1):22.

[6] Clark T. Data is king. Int Clin Trials. 2012;173:32–42.

[7] Ross S, Grant A, Counsell C, Gillespie W, Russell I, Prescott R. Barriers to participation in randomized controlled trials – a systematic review. J Clin Epidemiol December 1999;52(12):1143–56.

[8] Madsen S, Holm S, Riis P. Ethical aspects of clinical trials. Attitudes of public and outpatients. J Intern Med June 1999;245(6):571–9.

[9] Boericke K, Gwinn B. Planned to perfection. Int Clin Trials 2010;17(8):26–30.

[10] Andersen J, Fass R, van der Horst C. Factors associated with early study discontinuation in AACTG studies. Contemp Clin Trials 2007;28:583–92.

[11] Getz K, Wenger J, Campo R, Seguine E, Kaitin K. Assessing the impact of protocol design change on clinical trial performance. Am J Ther 2008;15:449–56.

[12] Getz K, Zuckerman R, Cropp A, Hindle A, Krauss R, Kaitin K. Measuring the incidence, causes, and repercussions of protocol amendments. Drug Inf J 2011;45:265–75.

[13] Getz KA, Kim J, Stergiopoulos S, Kaitin KI. New governance mechanisms to optimize protocol design. Ther Innov Regul Sci 2013;47(6):651–5.

[14] Kaitin KI, editor. The adoption and impact of adaptive trial design. Boston: Tufts Center for the Study of Drug Development; 2013. (Senior Leadership Brief).

CHAPTER 11

Data Mining for Better Protocols

Michelle Marlborough

Contents

1. THE NEED

Historically, protocol feasibility has been conducted via expert review of the protocol by key investigators, site staff, or even patient advocacy groups to determine things such as the scientific impact, the operational feasibility, whether the protocol is reasonable for the chosen patient population, and if there are adequate numbers of patients that meet the specified inclusion and exclusion criteria.

Although this method of feasibility is often very effective, it is typically conducted on a near final protocol, which means there is limited time to analyze and adopt feedback, and as such, detailed protocol feasibility is often considered a luxury that is conducted only on the largest and most important trials in a sponsor's portfolio.

Whereas input from sites and patients will always be an important process to include in the development of a protocol, it should not be considered the only option for protocol feasibility. Understanding how data on

Re-Engineering Clinical Trials
http://dx.doi.org/10.1016/B978-0-12-420246-7.00011-6

previous study performance and on the complexity and design of the study can be used to assess a study's feasibility and likelihood of success can enable sponsors to look at aspects of the protocol feasibility on an ongoing basis throughout the protocol authoring process.

Throughout the remainder of this chapter we discuss the design data and metrics that can be looked at to aid in protocol development.

2. THE SOLUTION

2.1 Access to Data

The most common sources of data used to conduct protocol feasibility are external, such as insurance data or electronic medical/health record data, which can help determine whether there are sufficient number of patients that meet the trial's eligibility criteria and where the highest concentrations of patients are. What many sponsors overlook is the huge amount of data they have internally available to them. Every organization that conducts clinical trials has data that can provide insight into the likelihood of success, including (but not limited to)

- enrollment rates for trials with similar inclusion/exclusion criteria
- dropout rates in studies utilizing specific clinical procedures
- most common reasons for amending a protocol in a specific therapeutic area
- how common a particular clinical procedure is in a specific therapeutic area

The challenge in leveraging this mountain of information is that all of the critical items needed to guide protocol design are buried deep in a series of unsearchable, disconnected word processing documents, spreadsheets, and operational systems.

A number of tools need to be in place to allow authors to drive smarter protocol design using both data from within their own organization and industry benchmark data; however, the biggest requirement is the need to be able to identify studies with a similar set of design characteristics. This can be achieved by the adoption of a structured approach to capturing the core protocol design information.

2.2 Structured Protocol Design

2.2.1 What Is Structured Protocol Design?

Structured protocol design simply means taking information that is typically written in a document and specifying it in a way that allows the metadata about a study to be captured. The most basic example of this is capturing a structured set of data about the type of trial being conducted: simply taking a protocol's title, which almost always contains many important pieces of metadata about the trial, and, instead of having a paragraph in a document that reads "A Phase 3, Multicenter, Double-Blind, Randomized, Placebo-Controlled, Parallel-Group Study to Evaluate the Safety and Efficacy of Drug X in Patients with Disease Y," capturing this as a set of properties as is shown in Table 11.1.

You then have a searchable set of data about the trial that was conducted.

2.2.2 Advanced Structured Design

Although having some basic information about the study can aid with data mining to truly be able to start using data to assess the impact of design on feasibility, it becomes important to be able to more closely match the design of the study with previous designs, and so the structured capture of the core clinical concepts of a trial design (eligibility criteria, objectives, end points, schedule of activities) and the relationships between them become more important.

Mapping procedures conducted at a specific time point to the end point the data supports and subsequently to the objective of the study supported creates a line of sight that, as we discuss later in the chapter, can be used in conjunction with internal data and industry benchmarks to ensure an optimally designed protocol.

Figures 11.1 and 11.2 provide a simple example of how components of a trial design that are typically spread across protocol sections can be

Table 11.1 Example of structured trial metadata

Phase	3
End-point classification	Safety and efficacy
Masking	Double blind
Indication	Disease Y
Allocation	Randomized
Intervention	Drug X
Intervention model	Parallel group

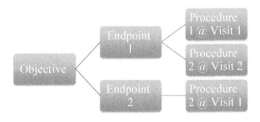

Figure 11.1 Generic visual representation of concept relationship.

Objectives	End points	Timepoints	Procedure
To evaluate the safety and efficacy of drug x in the treatment of patients with severe to moderate psoriasis	The proportion of subjects that achieve >75% in PASI between baseline and week 12	Baseline	PASI
		Week 1	PASI
		Week 2	PASI
		Week 3	PASI
		Week 4	PASI
		Week 5	PASI
		Week 6	PASI
		Week 7	PASI
		Week 8	PASI
		Week 9	PASI
		Week 10	PASI
		Week 11	PASI
		Week 12	PASI
	Incidence of adverse events	Baseline	AE Assessment
		Week 1	AE Assessment
		Week 2	AE Assessment
		Week 3	AE Assessment
		Week 4	AE Assessment
		Week 5	AE Assessment
		Week 6	AE Assessment
		Week 7	AE Assessment
		Week 8	AE Assessment
		Week 9	AE Assessment
		Week 10	AE Assessment
		Week 11	AE Assessment
		Week 12	AEAssessment

Figure 11.2 Expanded line of sight example.

visualized (and subsequently structured) to identify the relationships between them.

2.2.3 Options for Collecting Structured Design Information

There are many options for collection of the most basic structured design information, from as simple as setting up existing systems, such as a clinical trial management system or document management system, to collect the information to keeping a simple database of protocol IDs and their basic properties to allow suitable protocols for comparison to be identified during the development of new protocols.

The collection of more advanced structured design data is not as straightforward; organizations have two primary options: adoption of a structured protocol design tool or implementation of a database in which to capture such information. The benefits of having such a repository, though, are huge, not just for assessment of the design itself, but also for the benefits that can be gained from having easily machine-readable, and therefore usable, pieces of protocol information.

Structured design information can be used automatically across the many systems that need to understand the protocol design and also for activities such as submission to disclosure registries.

2.3 Adding Operational Data

Design data on previous studies can be vitally important in determining if a protocol design is likely to be feasible; however, in combination with historical operational and performance data, they become even more potent.

The following operational data and metrics would ideally be available for analysis alongside the design data:

- Number of protocol amendments
- Reason for amendments
- Enrollment rate
- Dropout rate
- Number of protocol deviations by type
- Number of low/zero-recruiting sites

2.4 Importance of Master Data

There are two key master data components that need to be taken into consideration when hoping to use data mining in protocol design. First, it is critical that there is a master data record for the protocol/study and the sites used across trials. Protocol design information, operational data, and site performance data will probably be collected from various systems, and identifying the same study and site is critical. The other key area of importance is the ability to identify clinical procedures across protocols and to be able to associate key information, such as cost, difficulty to complete, and burden to both patient and site. One option for procedure master data is to ensure that procedures are connected to a common code such as the American Medical Association Current Procedural Terminology code.

2.5 Using Data for Protocol Optimization

There are many ways in which the data discussed so far can help in designing a better protocol, from simply ensuring that the design is not unusual to advanced algorithms to predict the design's impact on enrollment rates. This section discusses some of the simplest uses of the data.

2.5.1 Avoiding Abnormal Designs

A simple assessment of the frequency of the procedure relative to previous studies or standard of care data can quickly identify areas that may

Procedure Benchmarks - By phase 2 / PAIN

Procedures (7) ▼	Average US Cost ($)▼	Complexity ▼	Study Frequency▼	% of Studies▼	Benchmark Average Frequency▼	Benchmark Frequency Range▼	Specificity ▼
Adverse Events Assessment	27	0.2	12	100	9	3-25	GSP
Clinical Chemistry	73	0.3	18	8	2	2-2	GSP
Demographic information	50	0.2	2	NA	NA	NA	
Informed Consent Process	75	0.2	4	100	1	1-2	GSP
Inpatient Vitals	56	0.4	20	16	7	1-20	GSP
Review Concomitant Meds	25	0.2	2	95	10	1-26	GSP
Single Drug Level	25	0.2	20	29	8	2-15	GSP

GSP - Indication Group/Phase
TSP - Therapeutic Area/Phase
▉▉▉ Out of Benchmark Range
▒▒▒ Above Average

Figure 11.3 Example of procedure frequency review.

have an impact on site or patient willingness to participate, especially if it is a particularly complex or invasive procedure (Figure 11.3).

The same procedure frequency data can be used to determine if a procedure is particularly unusual in a specific phase and indication, which will mean increased training or more difficulty in finding high–performance sites.

Additionally, simply comparing the operational outcome of the trial in terms of site performance, enrollment rates, etc., for trials with similar characteristics can quickly provide a good indication as to the likely success of the study.

2.5.2 Streamlining Protocols

The Tufts study on quantifying the magnitude and cost of extraneous protocol data [1] showed that in a typical trial approximately 25% of the procedures are not associated with a key primary or secondary objective, safety, or regulatory requirement. Each unnecessary procedure conducted increases the complexity of the study, making it harder to execute at site and less appealing to a patient to participate. Using the structured data to analyze the cost and complexity of each objective and end point can ensure that protocols are better designed and that effort is appropriately aligned with the most important goals of the study (Figures 11.4 and 11.5).

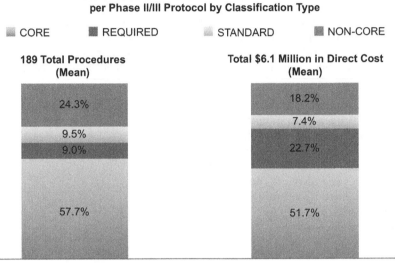

Figure 11.4 Distribution of procedure by purpose.

Study Design Metrics - Summary

	Category	Procedure Cost (per Subject) ($)	% Cost of Study	Complexity	% Complexity of Study
▶ To evaluate the effect of multiple daily consumptions of grapefruit	Primary objective	1,326	38.2 %	6.1	34.3 %
▶ To evaluate to safety of a single 0.6 mg dose of Fixitol	Secondary objective	297	8.6 %	2.2	12.3 %
▶ Regulatory	NA	75	2.2 %	0.2	1.1 %
▶ Screening	NA	50	1.4 %	0.2	1.1 %
▶ Unassociated	NA	1,724	49.7 %	9.1	51.1 %
Total		**$3,472**		**17.8**	

Figure 11.5 Alignment of cost and complexity by objective.

3. SWOT

Strengths	Weaknesses
• Ability to use data to assess feasibility during protocol design process ensures that every protocol can have feasibility completed	• Large management effort required to change protocol authoring process • Requires authors to work with tools other than Microsoft Word

Opportunity	Threats
• Data-driven feasibility at time of protocol design will reduce the number of amendments required • Reduction in unnecessary procedures and therefore complexity will reduce cost of trial, reduce cycle times, and increase likelihood of enrollment	• None

4. APPLICABLE REGULATIONS

None.

5. TAKE HOME MESSAGE

To conclude, building a database of historical design and operational data will enable:

- Protocol design feasibility to be built into the authoring process by surfacing industry benchmarks and historic performance data;
- An understanding of the purpose of each and every procedure in the protocol, which can lead to a reduction in complexity and can have a direct impact on study execution metrics.

REFERENCE

[1] Getz KA, Stergiopoulos S, Marlborough M, Whitehill J, Curran M, Kaitin KI. Quantifying the magnitude and cost of collecting extraneous protocol data. Am J Ther April 9, 2013.

CHAPTER 12

It's All in the Literature

Tatiana Gasperazzo, Johannes Lampe

Contents

1. THE NEED

A careful literature study, that is, an in-depth engagement with the knowledge available in the scientific community, has always represented the foundation for any and every scientific activity. Decisions are made and research protocols are designed based on the already available literature, the state-of-the-art knowledge covering all that has been done in a specific field in the past. For more than 350 years, communicating research findings by means of journals and other publications has been the center of scientific research, making it possible for other researchers to build upon previous work by others, to put one's own work under scrutiny and refine it, and to finally make one's own contribution to the general knowledge, offering new ideas and questioning established ones [1]. The main functions of scientific journals have been enumerated by Henry Oldenburg, the first Secretary of the UK Royal Society and creator of its *Philosophical Transactions*, and comprise registering research findings, their timing, and the responsible person(s); reviewing and confirming research findings before they are published;

Re-Engineering Clinical Trials
http://dx.doi.org/10.1016/B978-0-12-420246-7.00012-8

propagating the new knowledge; and maintaining a record of the findings for the long term [1].

For the Organisation for Economic Co-operation and Development (OECD) [2], research data can be defined as "factual records (numerical scores, textual records, images and sounds) used as primary sources for scientific research, and that are commonly accepted in the scientific community as necessary to validate research findings."

1.1 The Available Information Sources

Since the advent of the Internet, many important changes have taken place in the way investigational data are published. Among others, these new forms include open access archives, Internet publications, conference proceedings, and the rapid expansion of Google Scholar, Thomson Reuters's SCIE and SSCI, and Elsevier's Scopus [3].

In a study of the Scopus database by Wani and Gul [4], of a total of 25,482 publications, most were journals and journal articles (93.51%), followed by conference proceedings (2.96%), trade journals (2.74%), and book series (0.77%). Other sources of data, followed by examples, are external experts (academic clinical consultants), in-house experts (project teams), specialized consultancy companies (Pharsight), strategic company consultants (McKinsey & Co., The Boston Consulting Group), databases (Thomson Reuters, MEDLINE, ClinicalTrials.gov, Cochrane Central Register of Controlled Trials, EMBASE, PubMed), specialized commercial reports (Datamonitor), and others (press releases, congress contributions such as posters and presentations, conference proceedings, university repositories, etc.).

In investigational efforts, specialized data sources are typically consulted and can vary greatly, as shown earlier. It is precisely this variation in the shape of data sources that is responsible for their complexity, as simple comparisons among datasets provided by each distinct source can often not be done simply. Such analyses face the drawback of not addressing all aspects of the data, which are thus only partially covered. The reasons for this are mainly three: data complexity, data volume, and data heterogeneity. These aspects are described in greater depth in the following section.

1.2 The Challenges in Handling Scientific Data

It is not possible to discuss the available literature without mentioning "big data." According to Mike 2.0 [5], big data can be primarily defined by its size, but "big" refers to big complexity rather than to large volume. Still, complex datasets naturally tend to grow rapidly, so that big data can quickly become truly massive. In comparison to analytics, big data similarly aims to gain knowledge from the available data, using it advantageously for profit. However, big data is defined by some key characteristics, namely volume, velocity, and variety [6]. These principles, first mentioned by Doug Laney in 2001 [7] and normally used in the universe of enterprises, can be equally applied to science and medicine. A comparison between the fields can be made, as shown in Table 12.1.

Table 12.1 The principles of entrepreneurial big data [8] applied to the scientific/biomedical field [1,5,6]

	Enterprises	Science/Biomedicine
Volume	As of 2012, about 2.5 exabytes of data are created each day, a number that is doubling about every 40 months. There are more data crossing the Internet every second than there were in the whole Internet at the end of the twentieth century.	At an annual increase of about 5% and a doubling time of 13–15 years, by 2030 the number of works will amount to 2 million new ones each year.
Velocity	For many applications, the speed of data creation is even more important than its volume. Obtaining information in real time (or nearly so) enables a company to react much faster than its competitors—an invaluable competitive edge.	Traditional peer-reviewed journal publishing greatly delays the availability of research results, which may take months to become accessible, and then upon payment. This format does not keep up with the current speed of research and produced results. Alternative publishing options, such as open access, represent a way of accelerating the distribution of scientific results, not only to researchers, but also to the industry.
Variety	Among others, big data takes the form of messages, updates, and images posted to social networks; readings from sensors; and GPS signals from cell phones. Many of the most important sources of big data are relatively new.	Scientific data can have many formats, for instance, journal articles, press releases, Congress contributions (posters, presentations), conference proceedings.

Using big data leads to better predictions, and these, to data-driven and thus better decisions. This allows managers to decide on the basis of evidence rather than intuition [6], which is useful—or indeed essential—for the planning and successful execution of clinical trials or scientific research.

1.2.1 Data Complexity

In the past decades, the components of biomedical studies have grown in number and variety of aspects (e.g., significance of specific study outcomes, relevance of certain patient characteristics). Considering all of these factors in a single analysis has become necessary, as medical research and clinical practice are now expected to be guided by the sum of all relevant and sound evidence [9]. This data complexity implies that increasingly more problems must be considered simultaneously—and therefore represents a hurdle for successful analyses of the clinical data that can be hardly overcome.

1.2.2 Growing Data Volume

Active researchers from the academic community or research-intensive companies have a very large number of journals at their disposal, at any time and from any place. However, at the fast development pace of both research and the online environment, these professionals require more: permanent online access to the nearly 2 million new articles published each year, in addition to all those produced in the past, as well as the possibility of using novel tools and services for analyzing, organizing, and handling the newly acquired knowledge load [1].

Price [8] was the first author to publish quantitative data about the growth of scientific literature, covering the period from 1650 to 1950. For this evaluation, the first data analyzed were the numbers of scientific journals. This analysis yielded a growth rate of approximately 5.6% per year, doubling every 13 years. For 1950, the number of journals recorded was around 60,000; for the year 2000, the forecast was of about 1 million publications [3,8]. This way, Price predicted an annual growth of 4.7% and a doubling time of 15 years for the present time.

Indeed, the relative annual growth of publications over the past 30 years has amounted to an average of about 4%. Already at an annual increase of 5% in scientific publications, by 2030 the number of works will amount to 2 million new ones each year [10]. PubMed alone contains more than 23 million citations from the biomedical literature [11]. In addition, a multitude of other information types exists, as described earlier.

1.2.3 Data Heterogeneity

Heterogeneity of the data relates to the variation in the content of data sources. In clinical literature, for instance, these differences may be disease features (e.g., stage or severity), patient features (e.g., age or ethnicity), intensity or timing of interventions, and study design features, such as duration and outcome measures, which comprise the most challenging of the nonuniformities [12]. Overcoming this heterogeneity is a staggering challenge if no standardizing techniques are applied to find the common basis of all datasets, making them comparable and finally enabling conclusions to be derived.

1.3 The Classical Way of Handling Data and Its Limits

Investigation of the literature usually leans either on "hand searching" or on search engines. As the first method, though maybe the most precise, is also the most time-consuming, a number of strategies have already been published suggesting possible combinations of terms to be included in or excluded from the search, which should at last yield the most accurate list of results, containing the literature most relevant to the search intention (e.g., [13–15]). Finding the optimal search terms is thus the key for these procedures.

In 2005, an analysis was carried out to define an optimal search strategy on the MEDLINE database "for retrieving sound clinical studies on prevention or treatment of health disorders" [15]. The authors tested combinations of search terms, compared with best-single- and best-multiple-term searches, concentrating either on sensitivity or on specificity. Despite hence validating new empirical search strategies, which retrieved up to 99% of scientifically sound therapy articles, the authors affirm that no single search strategy will perform perfectly, for several reasons that include indexing inconsistencies in terms and methods. They recommended that the most specific search be used when looking for a few sound articles on a topic and the most sensitive one when carrying out a more extensive search for trials.

These examples show that the classical search ways present great barriers to obtaining accurate, sensitive, and specific result combinations. This may result in suboptimal achievement of goals that depend on good data and that are viewed as essential for a successful investigation outcome and consequent gain in competitive edge: research, clinical development (phases I/II/III/IV), marketing, indication-specific knowledge, indication-comprehensive scientific overview, scientific detail, proprietary data, and publicly available data. In this sense, a much stronger advantage will logically be obtained if the investigational aspects, among those mentioned, can be addressed simultaneously in the research phase, because as much information as possible concerning a topic can be thus regarded. Nevertheless, most of the above-mentioned consultancy sources do not cover all these aspects—mostly, they rely on only one or a few of them [16].

On a related note, Kola and Landis [17] assessed the average success rate for all therapeutic areas in a 10-year period (1991–2000) for 10 big pharmaceutical companies in the United States and Europe. The assessment revealed that this rate lied by approximately 11%—in other words, of nine compounds, only one made it through to development and got approved by the respective regulatory authorities. The main causes for this daunting attrition rate in the clinic in the year 2000 were lack of efficacy (accounting for approximately 30% of failures) and problems with safety (toxicology and clinical safety, adding up to about a further 30%). Other authors have found that a considerable proportion of the causes for attrition in drug development was due to reasons other than economic and scientific ones (Figure 12.1) [17,18]. Would a more thorough assessment of the available biochemical literature have improved this rate, if only it had been possible to gather all the relevant information and not miss out on the most important data?

As shown by the examples earlier, the classical search approach of scientific and biomedical literature, generally insufficient, has by now reached its

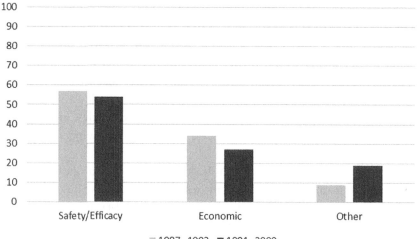

Figure 12.1 Reasons for attrition in drug development from 1987 to 2000. *Adapted from [16,18].*

limits. Even though more innovative strategies exist to handle the amount of data, these analyses face the drawback of not addressing all aspects of the information, which is hence only partially covered. The reasons for this are mainly three: data complexity, data volume, and data heterogeneity. Together, these aspects make it hardly possible for a single expert to cover the whole abundance of data.

2. THE SOLUTION

Data have been considered more and more important as an output of research, so that increasing interest exists in how to support researchers in their more effective management of data and guaranteeing their availability to others for use in their own research or other purposes [2]. Solutions have already been proposed for each of the points listed: complexity, data volume, and data heterogeneity. These solutions mainly consist of systematic analyses, meta-analysis, computational and sensing technologies, and the multidimensional method. The advantages and disadvantages of each method are presented in the SWOT analysis in the following section.

2.1 Automated Analyses

To override the complexity of the data, systematic automated analyses have been developed. Publishers have moved toward the use of the online environment and "semantic web" technologies to improve the presentation of journal articles—a strategy also known as "semantic publishing." Among others, this is done by enriching the text with interactive figures and "semantic lenses," which commute tables into graphs or animate diagrams; by providing links to term or concept definitions and additional information about them, as well as on relevant people or institutions; by providing direct links to all the listed references and to the full datasets underlying the article; and finally, by including machine-readable metadata [1].

S: The literature research procedure in this method is greatly simplified, owing to the use of automatic screening based on a selection of skillfully chosen search terms.

W: Search algorithms do not work as precisely as highly adapted searching "by hand," possibly resulting in incomplete assessments.

O: This method may contribute to the decision-making process of pharmaceutical companies, at little cost or effort, for problems of low complexity.

T: Decisions based on incomplete assessments may lead to failure in the research and development (R&D) process or market placement of a compound.

2.2 Meta-Analysis

Meta-analysis is one of the techniques adopted to handle the pressure for timely, informed decisions in the fields of public health and clinical practice, in view of the explosion of available information [18]. It is frequently adopted by pharmaceutical companies and the academic world.

S: Meta-analysis can support or lead to rejection of a proposed hypothesis by gathering and scrutinizing data sources as varied as patents and research articles. It further allows mining and analyzing large datasets in the various scientific and social areas, delivering new knowledge [19].

W: Meta-analyses do not cover all the necessary perspectives of the available literature.

O: By delivering new knowledge, this method has the potential to improve the R&D process for problems of low complexity.

T: Decisions based on incomplete assessments, relying on a proposed hypothesis, may lead to failure in the R&D process or market placement of a compound.

2.3 Computational and Remote-Sensing Technologies

For handling very large volumes of data, help has come in the shape of computational and remote-sensing technologies. The gathering and increasingly sophisticated analysis of data from various sources has driven the business of public and commercial sectors alike: the infrastructure making ready-to-use data available is now recognized as the foundation for successful research [1]. Text-mining tools are available to analyze and process the information contained in various journal articles or other sources so as to extract, manipulate, and generate new relevant information [19].

S: Systematic data entry brings collected data to a common basis, thus overriding its intrinsic heterogeneity [19].

W: The method is not yet used on a large scale, especially owing to the complexity of shaping publications to be available for text mining, as well as to high entry costs for those lacking the necessary technical skills. Moreover, data mining cannot work if information is not offered uniformly or explicitly.

O: Standardization and process optimization (SOP-controlled data entry and analysis) are feasible possibilities in this method, which can be employed productively by pharmaceutical companies and academia. Text mining presents great potential for increasing the efficiency, effectiveness, and quality of research, uncovering thus far unknown connections between underlying data and developing new knowledge, ultimately contributing, among others, to the enhancement of drug discovery [19].

T: Decisions based on incomplete assessments may lead to failure in the R&D process or market placement of a compound.

2.4 Multidimensional Method

Despite all the mentioned advantages and progress brought about by the newest developed techniques (e.g., meta-analyses and text mining), none of them succeeds in fully addressing the whole data complexity, as discussed earlier. In view of this difficulty, one of the most suitable approaches to addressing the key challenges (i.e., complexity, volume, and heterogeneity) met by pharmaceutical, medical technology, and life science companies in the R&D process is the multidimensional method. The core of this method is differentiation: using a compound's key scientific features needed in the market—safety and efficacy—as a foundation to discover its successful "niche" in the market. Differentiation is responsible for more than 50% of the commercial success of new drugs in the market [16].

S: The technique successfully covers all essential aspects by combining highly standardized search and identification of relevant literature with quality-controlled extraction of information from the datasets, its entry into a relational database, and a multidimensional analysis and in-depth interpretation of the results. This set of procedures allows the inclusion of large data volumes, as well as standardization of data of heterogeneous nature, making it possible to handle and overcome information complexity. The product of this process is a report highly customized to provide the necessary knowledge on the basis of all available information in a comprehensible way [16].

W: Owing to the broad coverage of the method, additional efforts are necessary in comparison to other methods.

O: A multidimensional analysis enables companies to make evidence-based decisions, minimizing the risk of failing compounds and devices; to obtain the broadest possible product label; to assess the product pipeline and product portfolio; and to optimize study designs. The systematic and objective approach not only covers proposed hypotheses, but also allows one to address questions that would otherwise not have been brought up.

T: None identified.

3. APPLICABLE REGULATIONS

Regulations are not applicable to the literature screening methods described here.

4. TAKE HOME MESSAGE

Owing to the complexity of data, their quantity, and their heterogeneity, the traditional form of scientific literature analysis has long reached its limits and demands innovative approaches. The solutions are given and consist of standardization, process optimization, and systematic data analysis, leading to the ultimate goal: product differentiation and consequent market success. These approaches exceed the limits of typical expert knowledge, not intending to replace it, but rather to relieve highly specialized and highly paid experts from routine tasks. This way, they provide experts with the necessary freedom to solve more essential content-related challenges. Moreover, these solutions offer cost-effective results and fact-based arguments, providing data reports that are unbiased, objective, and quantitative.

REFERENCES

[1] Finch DJ. Accessibility, sustainability, excellence: how to expand access to research publications. Report of the Working Group on Expanding Access to Published Research Findings; 2012.
[2] OECD. Principles and guidelines for access to research data from public funding. OECD; 2007.
[3] Larsen PO, von Ins M. The rate of growth in scientific publication and the decline in coverage provided by science citation index. Scientometrics 2010;84:575–603.
[4] Wani Mu-A, Gul S. Growth and development of scholarly literature: an analysis of SCOPUS. Libr Philos Pract (e-journal) 2008;217.
[5] Mike 2.0. Big data definition; 2014. [accessed 22.01.14]. http://mike2.openmethodolo gy.org/wiki/Big_Data_Definition.
[6] McAfee A, Brynjolfsson E. Big data: the management revolution. Harvard Business Review; 2012.
[7] Laney D. 3D data management: controlling data volume, velocity, and variety. Application Delivery Strategies – META Group; 2001.
[8] Price DJS. Science since Babylon. New Haven: Yale University Press; 1961.
[9] Sutton AJ, Higgins JPT. Recent developments in meta-analysis. Stat Med 2008; 27:625–50.

[10] Neuroskeptic. Science: growing too fast? discover magazine blog; 2012. [accessed 25.01.14]. http://blogs.discovermagazine.com/neuroskeptic/2012/09/30/science-gro wing-too-fast/#.Ut_Ty_swdlY.

[11] PubMed, http://www.ncbi.nlm.nih.gov/pubmed; 2014. [accessed 25.01.14].

[12] National Health and Medical Research Council (NHMRC). How to review the evidence: systematic identification and review of scientific literature [Handbook series on preparing clinical practice guidelines]; 1999.

[13] Dickersin K, Scherer R, Lefebvre C. Identifying relevant studies for systematic reviews. BMJ 1994;309:1286–91.

[14] Robinson KA, Dickersin K. Development of a highly sensitive search strategy for the retrieval of reports of controlled trials using PubMed. Int J Epidemiol 2002;31:150–3.

[15] Haynes RB, McKibbon KA, Wilczynski NL, Walter SD, Were SR, for the Hedges Team. Optimal search strategies for retrieving scientifically strong studies of treatment from Medline: analytical survey. BMJ 2005;330:1179.

[16] Lampe and Company. The L-matrix method; 2014. [accessed 04.04.14] http://www.lampeandcompany.com.

[17] Kola I, Landis J. Can the pharmaceutical industry reduce attrition rates? Nat Rev Drug Disc 2004;3:711–5.

[18] DiMasi JA. Risks in new drug development: approval success rates for investigational drugs. Clin Pharmacol Ther 2001;69:297–307.

[19] McDonald D, Kelly U. The value and benefits of text mining. JISC 2012.

CHAPTER 13

What Makes a Good Protocol Better?

Peter Schüler, Clara Heering

Contents

> *If you want to improve study protocol quality, you first need to deactivate the copy-and-paste function in Word for those writing them.*
> **INC Research's COO Alistair Macdonald, private communication, 2014**

1. THE NEED

Study protocols are the backbone of individual clinical trials. However, K. Getz (see Chapter 10) gives clear evidence from Tufts' data that numerous study protocols are not fit for purpose, with 22% of all collected data-points only adding more noise than clarity to the compounds' profiles, e.g., they do not contribute to the primary or key secondary endpoints. The key reason may, in fact, be that protocols are still typically not developed based on a well-defined process, but by a staff working under time pressure and often using older protocols as a "template" for a fast and simple copy-and-paste exercise.

The initiative of "risk-based monitoring" from Food and Drug Agency (FDA) and European Medicine Agency (EMA) also spot over complex protocols as a main reason for low quality trials.

The EMA Reflection paper on risk-based quality management in clinical trials, November 2013, states: "This paper intends to open up the

Re-Engineering Clinical Trials
http://dx.doi.org/10.1016/B978-0-12-420246-7.00013-X

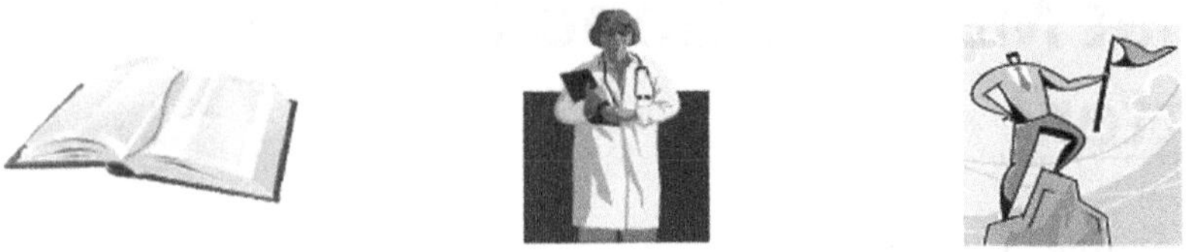

High Quality Protocol	+	Good Site Selection	=	High Chance of Successful Trial

Figure 13.1 A high-quality protocol, combined with adequate study sites, is the prerequisite of a successful study. *Modified from Metrics Champion Consortium (2011).*

discussion on approaches to clinical trials to new thinking, in order to facilitate the development of proportionate clinical-trial processes. Areas that are most often raised as causing particular concern are the design and complexity of the study protocols and data to be collected..."

FDA (Oversight of Clinical Investigations—A Risk-Based Approach to Monitoring, August 2013) says: "During the past two decades, the number and complexity of clinical trials have grown dramatically. These changes create new challenges to clinical trial oversight, particularly increased variability in clinical investigator experience, site infrastructure, treatment choices, and standards of health care, as well as challenges related to geographic dispersion. [...] The most important tool for ensuring human subject protection and high-quality data is a well-designed and articulated protocol. A poorly designed or ambiguous protocol may introduce systemic errors that can render a clinical investigation unreliable despite rigorous monitoring. Additionally, the complexity of the trial design and the type and amount of data collected may influence data quality." This concept is illustrated in Figure 13.1.

2. THE SOLUTION

Study protocols need to fulfill a variety of objectives—and only some of these are nowadays incorporated in a typical protocol (also see reference [1]).

Nowadays typically addressed:
- In line with ICH-GCP (E6; R1) Section 6 (Clinical Trial Protocol and Protocol Amendments).

Nowadays typically not fully addressed:
- Identify potential study risks (scientific and operational) and proactively mitigate these through improved study design.

- Give reasons for any requested activity or restriction, so site staff not only has to "follow orders" but also understands the rationale.
- Involve potential trial subjects and investigators in the design so studies are better fit for those that need to comply with them.
- Enhance consistency across multiple protocols, e.g., agree on one way of causality assessment for Serious Adverse Events (related and not related) instead of using lots of categories with different wording in every study, which only causes confusion.
- Limit the study complexity as much as possible by reducing the number of secondary endpoints, subject selection criteria, assessments, and visits.

This enhanced approach is most needed for indications with a long-lasting treatment period, tough subject-selection criteria, and a wide range of required assessments—or in short, complicated studies.

The answers to the questions below should support the review of how helpful the protocol is in avoiding potential errors which could be made by site staff.

1. For each inclusion/exclusion criterion:
   a. Is the rationale for each criterion clear?
   b. Is the process for verifying each criterion clear?
   c. Is the process for documenting the verification of each criterion clear?
   d. What are acceptable ranges for each criterion, are these in line with clinical practice?
2. For the investigational product:
   a. Is the instruction for dispensing and accountability clear?
   b. Is drug accountability supporting immediate feedback to the investigator/patient in case of errors in dosing?
   c. Are the code break rules clear?
   d. Is there a risk in errors of dispensing because of an overly complex dosing schedule?
   e. Are the instructions to maintain oversight clarified?
   f. Are there ways to simplify the process to avoid errors?
3. For each procedure (event) in the protocol:
   a. What is the difference between the procedure and standard practice across the geographies in which the study will be conducted?
      – For each geography, describe the difference and highlight how this may induce error; verify if changes can be made to minimize the risk of error.

   b. Is the timeline for review of diagnostic/safety results clarified? (e.g., central lab data review).
- Is this realistic, is there an acceptable range of days?
- Are the centralized services clearly describing accountability for reporting of alert values?
- Are there ways to simplify the process?

   c. Are diagnostic services for the study potentially provided by satellite structures?
- If so, what oversight is expected of the principal investigator?
- What can be done to limit complexity?

   d. Patient questionnaires:
- Is there an option to have these in electronic format?
- Are these validated?

   e. Is the sequence of events in the protocol causing concern?
- Is the burden in time acceptable for the patient population?
- Are the proposed tools and volume of questionnaires acceptable for the patient population?

The Metrics Champion Consortium (MCC, www.metricschampion. org, 2011) created a checklist that shall support the proper analysis of study protocols for design quality. The checklist also includes items about involvement of sites in the design. For more details, see Figure 13.2.

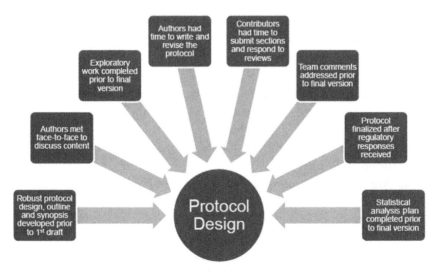

Figure 13.2 Not only the internal content defines a protocol quality, but also factors such as time and team-cohesiveness during the design process. *Modified from Metrics Champion Consortium (2011).*

Even rather simple key indicators, such as the word count of inclusion and exclusion criteria or concomitant medication sections, give an easy view on a protocol's complexity.

Last, but not least, methods also described in this textbook such as failure mode and effect analysis (FMEA), and lean and shop floor management are very adequate to better manage the process of protocol writing and avoid unnecessary review cycles and fruitless time pressure on the writing team with the attempt to still keep the target dates.

Even at the level of operational details, many protocols are not fully thought through. The safety sections of 20 randomly selected phase II and III protocols from 20 different sponsor companies in five core therapeutic areas (oncology, CNS, cardiovascular, metabolic diseases, and GI) that were finalized in 2006 and 2007 were reviewed for optimized criteria for description of safety data collection and assessment (EU DIA, Barcelona, 2008). None of the protocols described all core criteria: (1) the duration of adverse events (AE) and serious adverse events (SAE) collection, (2) what constitutes an adverse event of special interest, (3) what events should be assumed as "always serious," and (4) how to assess the term "clinically relevant" for lab abnormalities. Only nine of 20 defined "adverse events of special interest" and what is meant by "clinically relevant safety events," and eight clarified how to address progression of the underlying disease. How to assess relatedness was managed very inconsistently, even though "Council for International Organizations of Medical Sciences (CIOMS) VI working group [2] recommends that the investigator be asked to use a simple binary decision for drug causality (related or not related)." Protocols requested the investigators to decide between on average four categories (ranging from two to seven), with three protocols not providing any specification.

3. TABLE/CHECKLIST

3.1 Frequent Operational Imprecisions in Study Protocols

- Endpoints
  Can primary endpoints be captured as planned? Pay attention to scales (validated in all planned regions/languages?), surrogate endpoints, biomarkers (accepted by authorities?), mixed endpoints (defined how to evaluate as primary?), outcome studies (patient drop-outs considered? Is a separate Informed Consent Form (ICF) wording needed to allow long-term follow-up?), and practicality (invasive assessments tolerated by pts and Independent Ethics Committee (IEC)/Institutional Review Board (IRB)?).

- Visits and assessments

Are any "standard of care" assessments allowed during prescreening prior to ICF signature?

When is rescreening allowed? Which procedures (including re-signing the informed consent form) need to be repeated?

Are the procedures per visit doable for the given patient population (e.g., outpatients, elderly, and children) and the site staff or would these cause stress and exhaustion?

- Stopping rules

Are stopping rules described for (1) individual subjects, (2) parts of the trial, and (3) the entire trial?

When does one withdraw a subject due to "noncompliance"?

What types of noncompliance are acceptable (e.g., brief episodes of drug interruption for up to two weeks)?

When does one withdraw a subject based on a protocol deviation?

- Subject selection criteria

Challenge vague terms such as history of, current, clusters, repeated, etc.

For laboratory criteria, does the protocol use the same units which are used by the laboratory (usually SI units, but in certain situations or countries conventional units can also be used)?

For any hard threshold (e.g., >10.0), challenge the client if they are sure about that hard cutoff. As an alternative, consider a term like "any result between 8.0 and 12.0 needs to be confirmed by the medical monitor case by case prior to enrollment."

- Study drug/Experimental treatment

Do clear instructions exist for dose-titration (if applicable), including options for both up- and down-titration?

What does one do concerning episodes of drug interruption and withdrawal?

Is there a risk of withdrawal or rebound phenomena?

Is drug packaging adequate for the population (e.g., no childproof caps in an elderly population)?

Are appropriate actions described if the subject misses one dose (also described in the subject information) and in case of overdose?

Did relevant nondrug "treatment(s)" get excluded (e.g., cognitive training in dementia studies)?

- Concomitant drug

Are reasons given for excluding certain drugs or therapies (e.g., "interaction with CYP3A4," or "affects efficacy endpoint")?

It needs to be clear what drug is excluded for patient safety reasons. Patients violating such an exclusion most probably need to stop experimental therapy immediately for safety reasons.

Are washout periods stated?

Are these easy to follow, e.g., do not differ from drug to drug? Try to limit complexity to only three periods: short-, mid-, and long-term washouts. The washout time frames should be in relation to either the screening or the baseline visit.

- Assessments

    What is the allowed variability of visits or assessments (e.g., ± 3 days)? Is that reasonable?

    Is there any definition for what assessments may be missed without triggering a protocol deviation; which ones are crucial (for efficacy and safety)?

    Does there exist descriptions of each assessment in adequate detail so there is no ambiguity about what is expected from the site (e.g., when measuring blood pressure: once, in sitting or standing position)?

- Lab

    Can a local lab data be used for a confirmation test or other urgent safety parameters; how will local lab data be captured and documented?

    Do the procedures for blood sampling need to be described (peripheral versus central access)?

    Should subjects come fasted or for a set time?

    In case any parameters can be assessed by several lab methods, a statement concerning which method is acceptable should be provided (e.g., lipid levels measured or calculated).

    In pediatric studies and in some progressive indications, the volume of sampled blood needs to be kept as small as possible.

- Safety

    When should adverse events and SAEs be collected (start and stop time points, e.g., start the collection with signing the ICF or with the first dose)?

    Should "adverse events of special interest (AESI)" be defined?

    How does one report the worsening of underlying disease or elective surgery?

    Will withdrawals for reason of suffered AEs be captured?

    Will descriptions of procedures for rechallenge and follow-up and for any further assessments for withdrawals given?

    Is the follow-up period long enough to capture any withdrawal or rebound phenomena?

---

4. SWOT

Strengths: Better written protocols will enhance compliance with the requirements and improve enrollment rates and data quality.

Weaknesses: Not all potentially interesting questions will get answered in a single study. That may make additional studies necessary. It will take more time to create such a protocol and also will frustrate some mainly academically interested contributors since their questions may not get answered.

Opportunities: It's possible to make studies cheaper and more "fit for purpose," thus, also increasing the probability of a positive result.

Threats: In case competent authorities request additional supportive data after first review, the clinical database may not hold such additional data in a streamlined and slimmed-down design that collects fewer (initially not needed) data-points.

5. APPLICABLE REGULATIONS

ICH-GCP (E6; R1) Section 6.

EMA Reflection paper on risk-based quality management in clinical trials, November 2013.

FDA Oversight of Clinical Investigations—A Risk-Based Approach to Monitoring, August 2013.

6. TAKE HOME MESSAGE

Most existing study protocols fulfill the ICH-GCP requirements, but are not fit for the purpose. They tend to be over complex, not providing any reasoning for the requirements to the site staff, thus leaving them "in the dark." Imprecise and overloaded protocols are, however, a main risk for slow enrollment and data variability and, therefore, for a failed study. The attempt to streamline the development process should start with better planning and implementation of a defined protocol development process that deserves that name. That would also give more room for less site monitoring efforts, which will contribute to major cost savings.

REFERENCES

[1] Schüler P. Writing better protocols. GCPJ 2004;11(4):22–3.
[2] Geneva. Management of safety information from clinical trials (CIOMS VI); 2005. Section IVc.

CHAPTER 14

The Clinical Trial Site

Brendan M. Buckley

Contents

1. THE NEED

The success or failure of a clinical trial ultimately depends on how closely investigators and their staff follow the protocol. Therefore, it is a fundamental challenge in all trials to identify, contract, train, and support good trial sites. These must be capable of recruiting to target, retaining study subjects, and conducting the trial to a high standard of compliance.

Traditionally, investigator sites are identified for invitation to participate in trials based on databases that reflect the accumulated experience of the sponsor or Clinical Research Organisation (CRO). These are generated from sites previously used and from local knowledge of hospitals or clinics known to be interested in research. Recruitment Web sites are often used as entry points for new sites into these databases. Additionally, local franchises of the sponsor company may involve local key opinion leaders as high-profile investigators for marketing purposes in case the product gets on the market. A number of service companies exist that focus on identifying investigators by accumulating data from publicly accessible databases such as PubMed and clinicaltrials.org and specialty lists of senior clinical staff on hospital and university Web sites. Published sources, such as those of the WHO and the U.S. Centers for Disease Control and Prevention, may sometimes allow the identification of "hot spots" of disease prevalence. Patient organizations are an important source of intelligence through their Web sites and otherwise, especially for rare diseases and orphan drug development. There has been considerable interest in the

Re-Engineering Clinical Trials
http://dx.doi.org/10.1016/B978-0-12-420246-7.00014-1
145

use of social media as a means of investigator and site recruitment. However, its actual use has up to now been low, with less than 3000 "hits" on searching the term "clinical investigator" in LinkedIn at the time of writing (2014). Furthermore, trials that employ social media for patient recruitment are in a small minority [1], although this may improve as smarter and more attractive models are evolved.

Having identified potential trial sites, it is then necessary to determine their capability of executing a particular protocol through a detailed feasibility questionnaire either on paper or through Web-based systems. This is an expensive labor-intensive exercise and it typically results in sites overestimating their capabilities for recruiting subjects. The flaws in this system are illustrated clearly by the number of sites that fail to recruit any or more than a few subjects once the study commences.

What is clear is that the present model for site selection is not working very well. Consensus in the industry is that about 10–20% of trial sites enroll the majority of subjects and 10–20% of sites do not enroll a single patient (see Trizna, C., Chapter 9 this volume). The cost of initiating a site is estimated at about $10,000 to $30,000, whether or not it subsequently recruits any subjects. Although sites that recruit nobody may be shut down, those that recruit very few subjects generally need to be maintained, at an estimated cost of around $1500 per month. As well as the waste of time and money entailed in poorly recruiting sites, about 70% of trial sites do not recruit on time. Drs. Getz and Kaitlin (Chapter 1, this volume) have documented the delays typically found in study recruitment.

The pool of potential investigators appears to be shrinking in the United States, where the number of new investigators declined by 10% between 2002 and 2007, although this has been more than countered by the increasing supply of active new investigators outside the United States. This has been reflected in a major geographic shift, with the proportion of U.S.-based principal investigators declining from 96% of the total global pool of FDA-regulated investigators in 1990 to 54% in 2007 [2].

2. ENABLING STAFF AT CLINICAL TRIAL SITES TO PERFORM WELL

It is probably reasonable to expect that no investigator or trial site staff member wants to perform inadequately in a trial. Whereas motivations for acting as an investigator may vary, it is to be expected that respect for subjects in any trial is to the fore and that their safety is paramount. Nevertheless, the actual standard of investigator performance achieved in most trials is disappointing. Figures published for 2013 by the Office of Scientific Investigations of U.S. FDA's Center for Drug Evaluation and Research (CDER) show that, of 349 clinical investigator inspections, 3% had official action indicated and 43% had required voluntary action [3]. The kinds of inspection findings for which official action needs to be taken are shown in Figure 14.1 and the distribution of findings for which either voluntary (46%) or official action (3%) had to be taken is shown in Figure 14.2. The FDA's annual statistics show that these patterns did not change greatly over the decade from 2003 to 2013. Noteworthy among these are that protocol violations comprise the most common findings, and consistently it is found that deficient recording of informed consent from subjects comprises around 10% of adverse findings. There is no reason to assume that sites that have not been randomly inspected by regulators are performing any better than those that have been.

A fundamental issue in attempting to ensure high standards of performance at trial sites lies in the fact that many trials, especially from Phase IIb onward, are conducted mainly by investigators whose primary job is to deliver a clinical service to patients. With the exception of specialized commercial sites, trials are generally a voluntary addition to the core job of most investigators. For this majority of sites, conducting clinical trials is a peripheral task that is subsidiary to clinical service delivery, with its pressures and regular crises; these always take priority over trial-related activity. Against

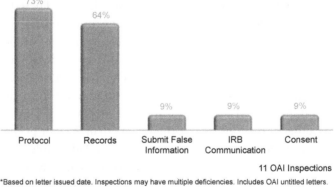

11 OAI Inspections

*Based on letter issued date. Inspections may have multiple deficiencies. Includes OAI untitled letters. (OSI database as of January 31, 2014).
Note that this does not denote number of inspections completed, but rather number of inspections report evaluated and closed in FY2013.

Figure 14.1 Frequency of clinical investigator-related deficiencies based on post-inspection correspondence issued: official action indicated (OAI) final classification* (full year 2013). *Figure courtesy of U.S. FDA CDER.* http://www.fda.gov/downloads/About FDA/CentersOffices/OfficeofMedicalProductsandTobacco/CDER/UCM256376.pdf.

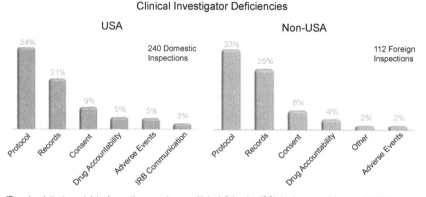

Clinical Investigator Deficiencies

*Based on letter issued date. Inspections may have multiple deficiencies (OSI database as of January 31,2014). Note: this does not denote number of inspections completed, but rather number of inspection reports evaluated and closed in FY2013.

Figure 14.2 Frequency of clinical investigator-related deficiencies based on postinspection correspondence issued* (full year 2013). *Figure courtesy of U.S. FDA CDER.* http://www.fda.gov/downloads/AboutFDA/CentersOffices/OfficeofMedicalProductsandTobacco/CDER/UCM256376.pdf.

this background, maintaining close compliance with every aspect of a protocol throughout the duration of the trial is difficult given realities such as the ever-increasing intricacy of trials, the growth in number and complexity of procedures to be performed, and trial site staff turnover.

Investigator meetings have been the usual way of trying to train investigators and site staff to perform specific trials for decades. These have never been shown to be effective and there are many reasons to believe that they are largely a waste of money, and a considerable amount of money at that. The problems with investigator meetings are obvious and in outlining them, here I am drawing on my personal experience of several decades as an investigator. First, there is the problem of taking time off from clinical service to attend, particularly if significant travel is entailed. Many trials with which I have been involved have gathered less than 20% of primary investigators together and the meetings have been attended mainly by site coordinators as well as by subinvestigators whose involvement may be short-lived. Meetings are often held months before many sites will see their first screenee, often before Institutional Review Board approval. By the time the first subject appears, it is likely that little of what has been communicated at the meeting will be remembered. Meetings usually attempt to pack large quantities of information into a short time: the term "death by PowerPoint" has been used many times about the format. Typical meeting components,

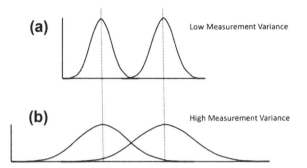

Figure 14.3 Effect of measurement variance on a comparison of two treatments. In (a), the variances in both treatments are low and there is a clear difference between them. In (b), the variances are large, for instance, because of differences in how well and precisely individual trial sites make the measurements, so the treatments do not appear to be significantly different even though the means are the same in both circumstances.

for instance, detailed instructions about handling blood samples for the central laboratory, are almost impossible to remember even immediately afterward. There is probably some merit in being able to network with trial sites at such meetings but even that may be frustrated if they are held in an attractive location that lures some of the participants away to see the sights. Of course, there is often turnover of site staff in the course of a trial, especially if it goes on for more than a year. Those new staff who come on board during the trial cannot benefit from investigator meeting attendance. In summary, a realistic view of investigator meetings is that they provide a signature list as "evidence of training" but are otherwise wasteful and ineffective.

Lack of effective site training is a major contributor to problems in trials and there are many ways in which this may contribute significantly to failure of a drug's development. A basic reason relates to the power calculations, which are the fundamental mathematical expression of a trial's design. This calculation assigns a predicted or assumed variance to the measurements that are being compared between active and comparator groups. If the trial sites together do not make these measurements exactly as the protocol specifies, the variance is likely to be greater than that assumed in the design and the trial may fail to show a significant difference between the trial treatment and the comparator (Figure 14.3).

Clinical sites may often conduct a number of different trials in parallel, with different sponsors and CROs. Thus, it is not surprising that confusion may arise. Anyone who has visited or worked at a trial site will be familiar with the large quantity of paper stored in binders from various studies, from which the extraction of a specific piece of information in a hurry is challenging.

Three major problems arise from poor or forgotten training of site staff that can cause serious damage to a trial. These comprise (1) enrollment of subjects that breach inclusion/exclusion criteria, (2) incorrect management of adverse events, and (3) misinterpretation of efficacy signals that lead to inappropriate action. A common feature of all three is that they occur during "live" interaction with the subject and, once that is over, the errors cannot be corrected later by a CRA. Although published data on enrollment errors is scanty, rates in multicenter intensive care medicine trials, for instance, have been reported ranging from 9.4% (159/1690) [4] to 16.5% (77/464) [5]. There is often the phenomenon of turning a blind eye to inclusion or exclusion criteria in the name of compassion, so that a patient with an unmet need may have access to a study. For example, patients with fewer than 3500 white blood cells per microliter may be specifically excluded from a cancer trial but an investigator may choose in breach of this to include a needy patient with a count of 3200, justifying this on the basis of "clinical judgment."

Incorrect management of adverse events, which does not strictly follow the risk management process detailed in the protocol, may be harmful to subjects and very damaging to the treatment being trialed. The following scenario illustrates the problem. A study subject in a Phase IIb oncology trial of a targeted therapy phones her study nurse on Friday afternoon to report the recent onset of diarrhea. Being away from her trial office, the nurse gives the best advice that she can think of, which is to temporarily stop taking the study medication, drink plenty of fluids, and phone back on Monday morning. The protocol, however, is specific that the subject should suspend taking the study medication, commence loperamide, maintain hydration with a specified water and electrolyte solution, and come in person as an outpatient within 24 h to the site for further evaluation. The nurse returns to work on Monday to discover that the patient has been admitted for intravenous fluid replacement because of collapse secondary to severe dehydration. Thus, an adverse event has been allowed to become a serious adverse event, shifting the balance of risk and benefit against the drug.

Misinterpretation by sites of the potentially positive effects of a treatment may result in serious consequences for a trial. An example relates to a trial in which an effective treatment for a cancer caused a marked rise in its diagnostic biomarker in the subjects' blood after the first cycle of treatment, resulting from tumor lysis. However, despite specific instructions in the pro-tocol to the contrary, some sites interpreted this as indicating accelerated progression of the tumor and withdrew the subjects from the trial. Because sufficient cases of this occurred, all of which involved the active treatment arm, the trial was void.

Basic to the three categories of error just described is that all of them can potentially compromise patient safety. It is a clear indictment of present systems of training that this can be permitted to persist. Monitoring of trials, occurring as it does long after trial visits have occurred, cannot fix any of these three problems, which are irrevocably set once a subject completes the trial visit or phone interaction at which they have occurred. They can be prevented only by ensuring that investigators and their staff are properly and continually trained.

3. THE SOLUTION

It is a matter for debate whether there should be an industry-wide effort to develop a comprehensive database of investigators and trial sites that would be accessible to all sponsors and CROs, participating as a consor-tium in its construction and maintenance. This would seem to be in the overall interests of accelerating drug development and therefore to the benefit of patients. The concept recognizes that most trial sites work with a variety of sponsors and CROs already. However, competitive pressure forms a formidable barrier to this kind of sharing of resources and com-panies are usually reluctant to pool a resource that they have built up with much effort and cost. Competition for trial sites and subjects is evident particularly in therapeutic areas in which a number of trials of similar therapies compete for a confined pool of patient participants. Examples of this are frequent in oncology, particularly for similar targeted therapies directed at highly specific tumor molecular subtypes and also for efficacy studies on biosimilars.

It could be said that existing approaches to investigator trial site selec-tion are based on the application of business processes rather than of science. They largely entail the aggregation of information from disparate systems that are accessed more opportunistically than systematically. The process of engineering a better way of selecting sites should entail "(t)he creative application of scientific principles to design or develop structures, … processes, … utilizing them singly or in combination; or to construct or operate the same with full cognizance of their design; or to forecast their behavior under specific operating conditions…" [6]. Thus is defined "engineering."

An engineering approach to site selection would seek to utilize the enormous quantity of data that exists about study sites and patients in various repositories. Among the most important of these are electronic medical records. As more institutions move to electronic medical records, there should be a great opportunity to mine these to discover valuable data about demographics of disease distribution, where diseases are treated, who treats them, how they are treated, and what are the outcomes. These should help point to where the best sites should be found for clinical trials. However, there are significant practical barriers to this approach. Many different electronic record systems exist, their heterogeneity making the reliable aggregation of data for a single analysis difficult. Second, access to medical records is regarded as highly sensitive and is tightly controlled. In the United States the "HIPPA Act" [7] and in the European Union the General Data Protection Regulation [8] strictly limit access to records. Nevertheless, there are efforts to use this resource in a manner that is fully compliant with individual privacy rights and the law. A third issue is that adoption of electronic record systems has been slow. A study in 2013 found that only 44% of U.S. hospitals surveyed report having and using what they define as at least a basic electronic health records system. And although 42% met all of the federal stage 1 "meaningful use" criteria, only 5% met the broader set of stage 2 criteria [9]. Use elsewhere in the world, with some national exceptions, is likely to be no better than in the United States. A caution here is that the minority uptake of electronic records systems and their uneven distribution throughout the world makes their use as a major means of trial sites selection liable to cause bias in trials by drawing recruitment from a population subset that may not be truly representative of the whole.

Pharma companies, CROs, and electronic data capture (EDC) providers all control very large trials databases. Activity information about trial sites is often buried in these, such as their therapeutic area competences, human resource numbers, and recruitment metrics. In addition, there is valuable information about performance quality, for example, query rates, Serious Adverse Event (SAE) reporting compliance, laboratory sample requirement compliance, and even perhaps protocol deviation rates. Using these sources and employing a "big data" approach, it should be possible to test a series of hypotheses on the correlation of activity with performance as well as with demographics. This approach is already in development and is likely to become the norm in the near term. It goes some way to moving the business process to an engineered approach because, by its nature, it enables continuous feedback, testing of the underlying assumptions, refinement of the algorithms that drive it, and the incorporation of new data sources and knowledge as these become available.

Accepting that traditionally conducted investigator meetings are inadequate in training investigator site staff to ensure patient safety and data integrity, then alternative means must be substituted.

The Internet provides a powerful means to train and support trial staff. This can be self-paced, targeted at different roles on site, and available throughout the trial to accommodate new staff starting midtrial. However, many training providers simply present slide shows and "talking head" videos on the Internet and these are not the answer. No attempt to provide Web-based training that can be run, minimized and silenced, in the background while the "trainees" check their e-mails, can be regarded as more than a futile gesture. At a minimum, training should be intelligent, highly interactive, concentrated on problem areas, and focused on getting trainees to solve trial-relevant scenarios. To allow certification of users, it should be evaluated and tracked. Although many sponsors are still content to allow Web-based training systems as well as investigator meetings to be optional and to rely on staff training signoff at site initiation visits, it is difficult to reconcile this with the spirit of Good Clinical Practice (GCP) and the Declaration of Helsinki. If potential trial subjects were fully informed of how poorly some of their investigators are trained to execute the protocol, they might well be discouraged.

Even with the best pretrial training, the reality is that many trial sites see only a few trial subjects per month and often do so while conducting other studies in parallel. In that environment, even when staff have been demonstrably well trained before commencing a trial, it is not easy to maintain competence throughout a long trial in the best motivated sites. There has been annual double digit growth in the complexity of protocols and in the numbers of procedures to be performed at visits. Many protocols require site staff to become experts in managing several diverse portals for EDC and interactive web-based randomisation system (IWRS) from various vendors, for central laboratories, and other centralized assessments. Multiple user names and passwords come with the job. Study-specific devices must be mastered. Site staff may need to administer rating scales and perform functional tests (such as 6-min walks) that are not part of their usual clinical practice in the therapeutic specialty. They must take the right blood samples in the correct tubes and ship them at the proper temperature. Perhaps the greatest challenge is in quickly distinguishing the procedures in one trial from those of another. Once the equipment and procedures for a trial are learned and applied, the next patient through the door may be in another trial altogether. Therefore a system of support and ready reference that can be accessed quickly is needed, so that a study nurse or investigator can quickly find out for any specific visit what must be done, all that must be done, how it should be done, and where it should be recorded. The traditional binders full of paper do not provide this. A number of providers have addressed this in combination with training, of which the widely used Firecrest Clinical® is the most comprehensive. Overall, it is fundamental to the concept of training, in any sphere, that it should be effective, evaluated, and continuing.

Surprisingly, given the importance of study site staff competence, there has been little formal evaluation of training methods published, probably reflecting complacency with the status quo despite all evidence. A fairly simple correlation between the number of sites' interactions with an online training and support tool and the occurrence of protocol deviations points to a definite effect of the tool on quality. Figure 14.4 shows in one trial how sites' interactions with a study-specific training and visit-by-visit guide

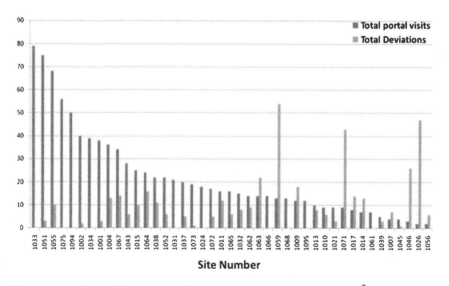

Figure 14.4 Effect of frequency of interactions by sites with Firecrest® study-specific training and support portal (in red) on the rate of protocol deviations in each site (green). *Data courtesy of Firecrest Clinical Ltd (an ICON plc company).* (For interpretation of the references to color in this figure legend, the reader is referred to the online version of this book.)

influence their protocol deviation rate, demonstrating that about 80% of deviations are committed by the sites having the lowest quintile of usage.

4. TAKE HOME MESSAGE

The reengineering of the process of training and supporting trial sites has got to leave behind systems that are demonstrably ineffective and wasteful in favor of a systematic and comprehensive process based on the application of modern instructional design and communications technology. It is time to rethink fundamentally the process for instructing site staff, for maintaining and growing their competence trial-long, and for supporting them visit by visit to avoid error. We owe it to trial subjects for their better protection and to the proper use of investment that we enable new treatments to be given an error-free and fair trial.

- An enormous quantity of data exists about study sites and patients in various repositories. Among the most important of these are electronic medical records.
- Pharma companies, CROs, and EDC providers all control very large trials databases.
- Using these sources and employing a big data approach, it should be possible to test a series of hypotheses on the correlation of activity with performance as well as with demographics.
- These should help point to where the best sites should be found for clinical trials.

5. SWOT

1. Strength: Sites are primarily introduced to deliver good quality work. Big data plus more interactive training shall enable one to pick the best possible sites and train them for the specific study.
2. Weaknesses: Not all useful data are available because of data protection limitations. Not all scientifically competent sites are interested in also applying the appropriate technologies to increase their trial competence. In the United States, the HIPPA Act [7] and in the European Union the General Data Protection Regulation [8] strictly limit access to records. Adoption of electronic record systems has been slow.
3. Opportunity: Economic pressure on the sites will enforce more professionalism in trial conduct.
4. Threats: All data available are historic, and thus may no longer reflect the current site status.

6. APPLICABLE REGULATIONS

- Health Insurance Accountability and Portability Act 1996, Public Law 104–191, 104th Congress of the United States of America.
- European Commission. Proposal for a regulation of the European parliament and of the council on the protection of individuals with regard to the processing of personal data and on the free movement of such data (General Data Protection Regulation), COM(2012) 11 final, 2012.

REFERENCES

[1] Getz K. Drug sponsors tread cautiously using social media to aid clinical research. Tufts Cent Study Drug Dev Impact Rep March/April 2014;16(2).

[2] Getz K. Current investigator landscape poses growing challenges for sponsors. Tufts Cent Study Drug Dev Impact Rep January/February 2009;11(1).

[3] http://www.fda.gov/downloads/AboutFDA/CentersOffices/OfficeofMedicalProduct sandTobacco/CDER/UCM256376.pdf.

[4] Macias WL, Vallet B, Bernard GR, Vincent JL, Laterre PF, Nelson DR, et al. Sources of variability on the estimate of treatment effect in the PROWESS trial: implications for the design and conduct of future studies in severe sepsis. Crit Care Med 2004;32:2385–91.

[5] Sprung CL, Finch RG, Thijs LG, Glauser MP. International sepsis trial (INTERSEPT): role and impact of a clinical evaluation committee. Crit Care Med 1996;24:1441–7.

[6] Engineers' Council for Professional Development. Canons of ethics for engineer. New York: Engineers' Council for Professional Development; 1947.

[7] Health Insurance Accountability and Portability Act 1996. Public law 104–191. 104th Congress of the United States of America.

[8] European Commission. Proposal for a regulation of the European parliament and of the council on the protection of individuals with regard to the processing of personal data and on the free movement of such data (General Data Protection Regulation). COM; 2012. 11 final. 2012.

[9] DesRoches CM, Charles D, Furukawa MF, Joshi MS, Kralovec P, Mostashari F, et al. Adoption of electronic health records grows rapidly, but fewer than half of U.S. hospitals had at least a basic system in 2012. Health Aff August 2013;32(8):1478–85.

Alternative Study Designs

CHAPTER 15

Do We Need New Endpoints in Clinical Trials: Surrogate and Biomarkers

Erich Mohr

Contents

1. THE NEED

Current challenges with low productivity and the attendant greater costs of drug development pose increasing economic risks for the world's pharmaceutical and biotechnology companies. New drug applications, both new molecular entities and new biological entities, approved on an annual basis by the U.S. Food and Drug Administration (FDA) were at their lowest point in the time period from 2005 to 2010 relative to the last 25 years [1]. Development costs, on the other hand, have risen steeply, with estimates at over 1 billion US dollars for the development of a new medication from discovery to market [2]. The combination of these two trends requires a major redesign of the traditional approach to drug development, away from large mega trials, typically with a major focus on patient-reported outcomes (PROs), to more objective, biologically based outcomes. This will assist both with the definition of precise target populations and with circumscribed, highly specific, biologically derived endpoints of clinical trials. Continuation of drug development utilizing traditional approaches will drive expense levels of new medications to unsustainable heights. Current health care models will, therefore, no longer be sustainable. Pharmaceutical

Re-Engineering Clinical Trials
http://dx.doi.org/10.1016/B978-0-12-420246-7.00015-3
159

industry price to earnings ratios, as well as share prices, have remained largely unchanged during most of the first decade of the twenty-first century [3]. Indeed, health care costs across the world are continuing to rise, [4] making novel approaches mandatory, which take full advantage of the unprecedented explosion in the human knowledge base, particularly in the life sciences and, broadly speaking, in the area of informatics and biomedical engineering, coupled with the increasing interaction of these fields.

2. THE SOLUTION

Recent advances in the biomedical sciences have shifted the longer term focus in drug development away from clinically based outcome measures, including PROs with all their attendant issues in terms of validity, reliability, and changing parameters based on the stage of disease, to a more biologically based approach. The emergence of surrogate markers, measures which typically represent a biological metric of a specific underlying pathological condition, and a potential change of this metric as a result of a medical intercession has greatly enriched the tool kit of drug developers. Particularly in the area of central nervous system (CNS) therapeutic development, there is a continuing heavy reliance on PROs, obtained by testing or interview-based outcome measures. Many, if not most of these metrics, are subject to considerable variability, based on the education and experience of the test administrator and the circumstances of test administration, including their timing and the environment of administration.

Study failures with large-scale studies in Alzheimer's disease (AD), with compounds with well-established mechanisms, proven design parameters, and adequate power, were deemed to be related to lack of deterioration of placebo patients relative to actively treated subjects [5]. The effects of inter-rater reliability are of prime importance in this context. A recent review paper on this subject asserted that a study's power in differentiating actively treated subjects from those on placebo is principally related to three factors: sample size, mean difference between actively and placebo-treated subjects, and the amount of testing variability [6]. This was supported by the assertion that a reduction of reliability from a perfect $R = 1$ to 0.5 will double the required sample size, or less dramatically, but equally impressively, an improvement in reliability from 0.7 to 0.9 will decrease sample size requirements by more than one-fifth [7].

In addition, factors like rater bias, reflective of enrollment pressures, may yield reports of greater pathology at study entry than would have been assessed at a different stage in the study [6]. Expectancy bias may also play a major role. Expert neurologist raters demonstrated markedly greater accuracy in ratings of Alzheimer patients over time when tapes were labeled accurately in terms of temporal sequence, as opposed to mislabeled tapes, where the order of baseline and endpoint was intentionally reversed [8]. In addition, the assertion reviewed by Kobak [6] that ratings by different raters over time rather than the same rater yielded significantly greater separation between actively and placebo treated patients and ultimately resulted in less of a placebo response, supports the notion that careful evaluation of PROs, in particular, in pivotal trials is required.

These observations, including the issue of the influence of tester variability as well as increasing costs for repeat training of testers across large numbers of sites, have spawned an entirely new approach to the administration of clinically based outcome measures, such as video conference–based ratings and the like. Centralized expert rating and monitoring services are now being used to address, at least in part, the challenges of sensitivity and variability with PROs attempting, in particular, to increase their sensitivity in the development of new therapeutic CNS agents [6,9].

While representing an improvement over traditional approaches, many of the challenges of the PROs in terms of diagnosis, patient selection, prognosis, and finally, outcome measures remain. Integration of biomarkers and, ultimately, surrogate markers into the therapeutic drug life cycle have the potential to significantly reduce the cost of drug development, increase efficiency, and have an impact on the cost of attrition of candidates during the development process [4]. Population enrichment through enhancement of diagnostic accuracy and potentially definition of more precise target (sub) populations will be greatly facilitated by new biomarkers. In addition, their use may guide dose selection in the case of the more traditional oral agents, as well as determination of concentration, in the case of emerging, advanced, localized delivery approaches such as convection enhanced delivery [10], which, by way of a pressurized infusion system, allows for a precisely targeted distribution of a defined volume of infusate in a specific CNS target [10]. Furthermore, risk benefit ratios may be enhanced by introducing more objective measures which might also facilitate review and exchange of ultimate assessments between the various regions of the world [11]. This makes an increasingly strong case for the use of biomarkers and surrogate markers, particularly in the early stages of drug development (Figure 15.1) [3].

The terms biomarker and surrogate marker are often used interchangeably in the literature. However, a biomarker marker is typically a physical

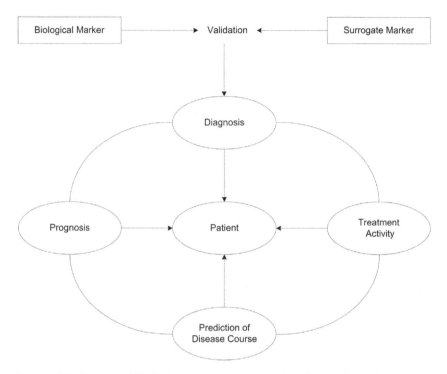

Figure 15.1 The use of biological and surrogate markers in the drug development process.

metric of an underlying pathological state, including a condition's modification by a therapeutic intercession. Whereas, a surrogate marker is a biomarker which has advanced to the point of a more defined validation [12]. In more general terms, a defined set of biomarkers which function as validated substitutes or are complementary to PROs can be classified as surrogate markers, the term literally meaning "to substitute for" [13], especially when they function as a substitute for a clinically relevant endpoint in predicting the outcome of a therapeutic intercession [14].

Key to the successful introduction into the clinical trials landscape are both the sensitivity and specificity of a biomarker or surrogate marker. Sensitivity describes the ability of identifying patients with a disease based on a positive test result. Whereas, specificity reflects the ability to correctly identify people free of a disease by the absence of this biomarker.

Pittsburgh Compound B (PIB positron emission tomography (PET) scan) is an example of a potentially useful biomarker, which in the face of good sensitivity shows relatively poor specificity [15,16], therefore, limiting its potential diagnostic utility. Another example, in the area of AD, is Aβ42 [15]. Levels of this biomarker are significantly reduced in the cerebrospinal fluid (CSF) of patients with the clinical diagnosis of AD [17,18], and low CSF Aβ42 levels show a relationship with high levels of amyloid in neocortex and hippocampus [15,19]. In the area of Parkinson's disease, the traditional, clinically based, diagnostic triad of tremor, rigidity, and bradykinesia, adding postural instability in the later stages, may be supplemented by a whole array of emerging biomarkers. These include α–synuclein, the principal component of Lewy bodies, manifested, for example, by increased expression of α–synuclein in skin fibroblasts in affected patients [20]. Other potential markers of disease progression reflected by nonspecific measures are oxidate stress and [14] neuroimaging measures, such as radiotracer neuroimaging of the nigrostriatal system with 18F-fluorodopa PET [14].

In traumatic brain injury (TBI), protein profiling has been a major focus of biomarker research [21]. One of the most studied markers in this context is S100B, which shows some correlation with the extent of injury, as well as neurologic outcome [22]. A whole array of other biomarkers with varying prognostic utility have been put forward, particularly for prognostic purposes [21]. In addition, it has been proposed that certain genetic predisposition, such as inheritance of the APOE-e4 allele, is associated with poor functional outcome in TBI, making this a potentially useful prognostic biomarker [23].

Finally, in terms of actually established endpoints, surrogate markers are perhaps most established in metabolic medicine, where development programs of lipid-altering drugs have long had their basis in the observation that elevated low-density lipoprotein (LDL) levels have a highly consistent relationship with the emergence of cardiovascular disease [24]. Therefore, there is a more than decade of regulatory history of approval of compounds based on the inhibition of absorption of cholesterol, representing a major example of the successful use of surrogate endpoints in the development of new compounds [24].

Biomarkers are currently classified as "exploratory," "probable valid," or "known valid" [25]. It is the latter two categories of probable valid and known valid which are of most interest in the current context. Probable valid is defined as "a biomarker that is measured in an analytic test system with well-established performance characteristics for which there is a scientific framework or body of evidence that appears to elucidate the physiologic, toxicologic, pharmacologic, or clinical significance of test results" [25]. A known valid biomarker, on the other hand, is defined as "a biomarker that is measured in an analytic test system with well-established performance characteristics and for which there is widespread agreement in the medical or scientific community about the physiologic, toxicologic, pharmacologic, or clinical significance" [25].

Established biomarkers or, ultimately, surrogate markers typically serve several separate and distinct purposes.

Diagnosis: One or several biomarkers or surrogate markers may have a confirmatory role in the diagnostic process, particularly in disease entities which are heterogeneous and typically rely on clinical parameters. An example is AD, where among other parameters alterations in CSF markers may aid diagnosis [15,26,27]. Identification of carriers of the ApoEe4 allele establishes their increased risk of developing late-onset AD [28].

Parkinson's disease, where an array of genetic, blood, CSF, and neuroimaging markers may serve as an adjunct diagnostic differentiator to the current clinical metrics [14], is another example where these biomarkers play an increasingly important role in diagnostic identification of patients who may profit from ever more sophisticated but highly invasive therapeutic intercessions [29]. This certainly holds true across the whole spectrum of neurological diseases and includes even smaller disease entities, such as inflammatory and auto immune disorders, particularly when involving the CNS [30].

An example of the relationship between pathophysiology and biomarkers is shown in Figure 15.2.

Prognosis: These are biomarkers, and once validated, surrogate markers, typically of the prodromal stage of a disease which inform on the likelihood of development of a specific disease state [31] and its progress, in a stage-dependent manner [28].

Prediction: Biomarkers or surrogate markers in this category classify patients by the likelihood of a response to a particular therapeutic intercession, although not necessarily predictive of a meaningful therapeutic effect [32] or predict long-term outcome. Examples include the previously discussed S100B biomarker in serum levels of those affected by TBI [21] or other markers in AD [33]. This category plays an increasingly important role as the drug development process moves away from the "one size fits all" approach to a more individualized approach [4]. The requirement to streamline clinical trials and the ability to classify patients on the basis of their potential benefit to a novel therapy not only accelerates the development process, but will lead to the desired outcome of failing ineffective therapies early and increase the likelihood of success in the latter stages of

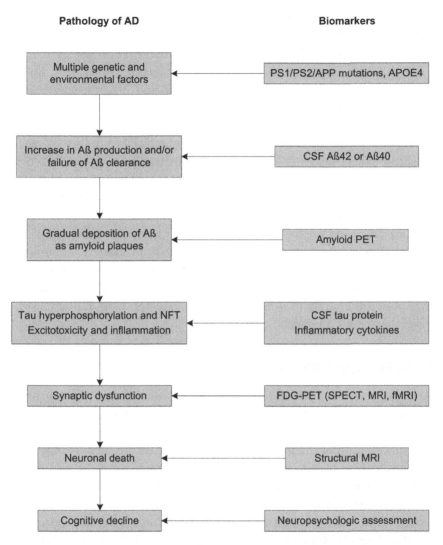

Pathology of AD

Biomarkers

Multiple genetic and environmental factors ← PS1/PS2/APP mutations, APOE4

Increase in Aß production and/or failure of Aß clearance ← CSF Aß42 or Aß40

Gradual deposition of Aß as amyloid plaques ← Amyloid PET

Tau hyperphosphorylation and NFT Excitotoxicity and inflammation ← CSF tau protein Inflammatory cytokines

Synaptic dysfunction ← FDG-PET (SPECT, MRI, fMRI)

Neuronal death ← Structural MRI

Cognitive decline ← Neuropsychologic assessment

Figure 15.2 Correspondence between biomarkers and neuropathology processes [15]. PET, positron emission tomography; CSF, cerebrospinal fluid; AD, Alzheimer's disease. *Reprinted by permission.*

the clinical trial process, thereby avoiding the potentially most hazardous and costly type of development failure. Therefore, it is increasingly likely that biomarkers and, therefore, surrogate markers will become an integral part of clinical trials [34,35].

Activity: Biomarkers and surrogate markers play a key role in this category, as they are used to provide a more accurate and objective assessment of outcome than the PROs now typically used in late-stage clinical trials, particularly in the CNS arena and, perhaps equally important, to ensure target engagement [3]. In fact, use of CSF biomarkers in patient selection in a trial simulation that identified appropriate subjects across 19 trials showed a reduction in sample size and trial costs by 67% and 60%, respectively, relative to a clinical trial with patients with minimal cognitive impairment, unselected on the basis of a biomarker [28].

While these uses of biomarkers and surrogate markers are by no means exhaustive, their emergence is beginning to materially affect both the drug development landscape as well as the approach of regulatory agencies in establishing criteria as to what is needed to show clinically meaningful changes as a result of a specific therapy.

This new landscape has resulted in a number regulatory publications that seek to establish guidelines both for the medical and scientific community and industry on how to best employ this new tool kit in terms of nosology in general, diagnosis in particular, and in the most general terms, and perhaps most importantly, in assessing changes in patient status resulting from a novel therapeutic approach.

3. APPLICABLE REGULATIONS

Recently, both the FDA and the European Medicines Agency have issued guidance documents of how to deal with biomarkers related to drug or biotechnology product development, ranging from general guidance of regulatory qualification of the proposed biomarkers, if used to support regulatory decision making [11], to specific uses of biomarkers as part of enrichment designs of disease-specific clinical trials, such as AD [36]. Indeed, the FDA's Center for Drug Evaluation and Research (CDER) has undertaken a number of formal processes to provide guidance in terms of analytic validation of specific Drug Development Tools (DDTs) [37]. The FDAs Critical Path Initiative identified the fact that scientific advances in the biomedical sciences have not enriched the drug development process as fully as might be desirable. Accordingly, several guidance documents for industry were issued by the FDA [11,37]. Qualification and review of new DDTs, including biomarkers, represents a significant activity of CDER and has led to assignments of specific offices within CDER to lead the required applicable process [37]. These qualification processes do not only cover the proposed biomarkers themselves, but may also entail review and qualification of the devices required to perform the measuring procedure. However, importantly, qualification of the

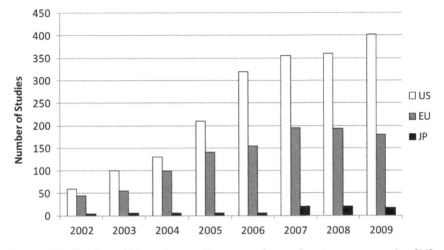

Figure 15.3 Number of biomarker studies grouped according to sponsor region [38]. *Reprinted by permission.*

proposed biomarkers and the devices used to assess these biomarkers are typically two independent processes and will need to be treated as such [37].

The Japanese context is more complicated. While Japan ranks second after the United States in terms of pharmaceutical market size of an individual country, its share of clinical studies involving biomarkers and surrogate markers is exceedingly small and far behind the more prevalent use of these tools in the United States and the European Union based on sponsored studies. Therefore, the Japanese regulatory landscape is less developed in that regard while, of course, being part of and adhering to the International Conference on Harmonization (Figure 15.3) [11].

4. TAKE HOME MESSAGE

- Drug development suffers from low productivity and is too expensive.
- PROs have limits in terms of validity and reliability.
- Biomarkers and their validated counterpart, surrogate markers, can enrich populations, make outcomes more certain, predict disease course, and reflect the impact of proposed treatments, which makes the development process more productive and efficient.
- The regulatory process lags behind the pace of scientific discovery, but qualification guidelines and active regulatory involvement have sought to encourage the discovery and development of biomarkers and surrogate makers and their integration into the development process.

- Market size does not necessarily reflect integration of biomarkers and surrogate markers into the development process, with large regional differences in their use and, therefore, ultimately, application in disease management, with the United States and the European Union leading the world.

5. SWOT

Strengths: Biomarkers and their validated form of surrogate markers can serve to enrich study populations, provide prognostic metrics in the prodromal stages of disease (thereby enabling pre-symptomatic treatment approaches), predict disease course (with attendant optimization of intervention), and provide outcome measures for the assessment of a specific therapeutic intercession.

Weaknesses: As a young and highly dynamic field, there is variable buy-in for the use of these markers in the scientific community, and the frequent absence of comprehensive validation makes their utility in terms of replacing PROs limited.

Opportunities: Rapid development, validation, and widespread use of biomarkers and surrogate markers can render major advantages to pharmaceutical and biotechnology developers in terms of enhancement of productivity, speed, and, ultimately, cost of development.

Threats: In spite of significant regulatory advances, particularly in the United States and the European Union, replacement of PROs by biomarkers and surrogate markers, or even their supplementary use, is not universally accepted and may well not be a "safe course" from a regulatory perspective for the development of a specific drug or biologic.

6. CONCLUSION

The use of biomarkers and, ultimately, surrogate markers in clinical trials is fueled by an ever increasing knowledge base in the areas of molecular biology, imaging, biochemistry, informatics as well as biomedical engineering and the ever greater overlap of these fields. The use of these new tools is mandatory, both from a cost-control perspective as well as a productivity and efficiency viewpoint, to ensure that the development of new medicines stays competitive and that the implementation of new medical and scientific knowledge is not hampered first and foremost by cost considerations and limitations of the reliability of assessment instruments. The ensuing improvements in productivity will ensure that the development process is healthy and is limited principally by the boundaries of medical knowledge.

REFERENCES

[1] Khanna I. Drug discovery in pharmaceutical industry: productivity challenges and trends. Drug Discovery Today 2012;17(19–20):1088–102.

[2] Munos B. Lessons from 60 years of pharmaceutical innovation. Nat Rev Drug Discovery 2009;8(12):959–68.

[3] Paul SM, Mytelka DS, Dunwiddie CT, Persinger CC, Munos BH, Lindborg SR, et al. How to improve R&D productivity: the pharmaceutical industry's grand challenge. Nat Rev Drug Discovery 2010;9(3):203–14.

[4] Organisation of Economic Co-operation and Development. Policy issues for the development and use of biomarkers in health. Paris: OECD; 2011.

[5] Gold M. Study design factors and patient demographics and their effect on the decline of placebo-treated subjects in randomized clinical trials in Alzheimer's disease. J Clin Psychiatry 2007;68(3):430–8.

[6] Kobak KA. Inaccuracy in clinical trials: effects and methods to control inaccuracy. Curr Alzheimer Res 2010;7(7):637–41.

[7] Perkins DO, Wyatt RJ, Bartko JJ. Penny-wise and pound-foolish: the impact of measurement error on sample size requirements in clinical trials. Biol Psychiatry 2000;47(8):762–6.

[8] Quinn J, Moore M, Benson DF, Clark CM, Doody R, Jagust W, et al. A videotaped CIBIC for dementia patients: validity and reliability in a simulated clinical trial. Neurology 2002;58(3):433–7.

[9] Kobak KA, Kane JM, Thase ME, Nierenberg AA. Why do clinical trials fail? the problem of measurement error in clinical trials: time to test new paradigms? J Clin Psychopharmacol 2007;27(1):1–5.

[10] Bobo RH, Laske DW, Akbasak A, Morrison PF, Dedrick RL, Oldfield EH. Convection-enhanced delivery of macromolecules in the brain. Proc Natl Acad Sci USA 1994;91(6):2076–80.

[11] United States Food and Drug Administration, Center for Drug Evaluation and Research. Guidance for Industry. E16 biomarkers related to drug or biotechnology product development: context, structure, and format of qualification submissions. Geneva: ICH; 2011.

[12] Katz R. Biomarkers and surrogate markers: an FDA perspective. NeuroRx 2004;1(2):189–95.

[13] Biomarkers Definitions Working G. Biomarkers and surrogate endpoints: preferred definitions and conceptual framework. Clin Pharmacol Ther 2001;69(3):89–95.

[14] Morgan JC, Mehta SH, Sethi KD. Biomarkers in Parkinson's disease. Curr Neurol Neurosci Rep 2010;10(6):423–30.

[15] Wu L, Rosa-Neto P, Gauthier S. Use of biomarkers in clinical trials of Alzheimer disease: from concept to application. Mol Diagn Ther 2011;15(6):313–25.

[16] Jack Jr CR, Lowe VJ, Weigand SD, Wiste HJ, Senjem ML, Knopman D, et al. Serial PIB and MRI in normal, mild cognitive impairment and Alzheimer's disease: implications for sequence of pathological events in Alzheimer's disease. Brain 2009;132(Pt 5):1355–65.

[17] Vemuri P, Wiste HJ, Weigand SD, Shaw LM, Trojanowski JQ, Weiner MW, et al. MRI and CSF biomarkers in normal, MCI, and AD subjects: diagnostic discrimination and cognitive correlations. Neurology 2009;73(4):287–93.

[18] Schoonenboom NS, van der Flier WM, Blankenstein MA, Bouwman FH, Van Kamp GJ, Barkhof F, et al. CSF and MRI markers independently contribute to the diagnosis of Alzheimer's disease. Neurobiol Aging 2008;29(5):669–75.

[19] Strozyk D, Blennow K, White LR, Launer LJ. CSF Aβ 42 levels correlate with amyloid-neuropathology in a population-based autopsy study. Neurology 2003;60(4):652–6.

[20] Hoepken HH, Gispert S, Azizov M, Klinkenberg M, Ricciardi F, Kurz A, et al. Parkinson patient fibroblasts show increased alpha-synuclein expression. Exp Neurol 2008;212(2):307–13.

[21] Dash PK, Zhao J, Hergenroeder G, Moore AN. Biomarkers for the diagnosis, prognosis, and evaluation of treatment efficacy for traumatic brain injury. Neurotherapeutics 2010;7(1):100–14.

[22] Unden J, Astrand R, Waterloo K, Ingebrigtsen T, Bellner J, Reinstrup P, et al. Clinical significance of serum S100B levels in neurointensive care. Neurocrit Care 2007;6(2):94–9.

[23] Manley GT, Diaz-Arrastia R, Brophy M, Engel D, Goodman C, Gwinn K, et al. Common data elements for traumatic brain injury: recommendations from the biospecimens and biomarkers working group. Arch Phys Med Rehabil 2010;91(11):1667–72.

[24] Psaty BM, Lumley T. Surrogate end points and FDA approval: a tale of 2 lipid-altering drugs. JAMA 2008;299(12):1474–6.

[25] Goodsaid F, Frueh F. Biomarker qualification pilot process at the US food and drug administration. AAPS J 2007;9(1):E105–8.

[26] Hu WT, Chen-Plotkin A, Arnold SE, Grossman M, Clark CM, Shaw LM, et al. Biomarker discovery for Alzheimer's disease, frontotemporal lobar degeneration, and Parkinson's disease. Acta Neuropathol 2010;120(3):385–99.

[27] Choi YS, Choe LH, Lee KH. Recent cerebrospinal fluid biomarker studies of Alzheimer's disease. Expert Rev Proteomics 2010;7(6):919–29.

[28] Vellas B, Hampel H, Rouge-Bugat ME, Grundman M, Andrieu S, Abu-Shakra S, et al. Alzheimer's disease therapeutic trials: EU/US task force report on recruitment, retention, and methodology. J Nutr Health Aging 2012;16(4):339–45.

[29] Palfi S, Gurruchaga JM, Ralph GS, Lepetit H, Lavisse S, Buttery PC, et al. Long-term safety and tolerability of ProSavin, a lentiviral vector-based gene therapy for Parkinson's disease: a dose escalation, open-label, phase 1/2 trial. Lancet January 2014;10. Early Online Publication.

[30] Dale RC, Brilot F. Biomarkers of inflammatory and auto-immune central nervous system disorders. Curr Opin Pediatr 2010;22(6):718–25.

[31] van Rossum IA, Vos S, Handels R, Visser PJ. Biomarkers as predictors for conversion from mild cognitive impairment to Alzheimer-type dementia: implications for trial design. J Alzheimer's Dis 2010;20(3):881–91.

[32] Cudkowicz ME, Katz J, Moore DH, O'Neill G, Glass JD, Mitsumoto H, et al. Toward more efficient clinical trials for amyotrophic lateral sclerosis. Amyotroph Lateral Scler 2010;11(3):259–65.

[33] Hampel H, Prvulovic D. Are biomarkers harmful to recruitment and retention in Alzheimer's disease clinical trials? an international perspective. J Nutr Health Aging 2012;16(4):346–8.

[34] Thal LJ, Kantarci K, Reiman EM, Klunk WE, Weiner MW, Zetterberg H, et al. The role of biomarkers in clinical trials for Alzheimer disease. Alzheimer Dis Assoc Disord 2006;20(1):6–15.

[35] Dickerson BC, Sperling RA. Neuroimaging biomarkers for clinical trials of disease-modifying therapies in Alzheimer's disease. NeuroRx 2005;2(2):348–60.

[36] European Medicines Agency, Committee for Medical Products for Human Use. Qualification opinion of Alzheimer's disease novel methodologies/biomarkers for PET amyloid imaging (positive/negative) as a biomarker for enrichment, for use in regulatory clinical trials in predementia Alzheimer's disease. London: EMEA; 2012. EMA/CHMP/SAWP/892998/2011.

[37] United States Food and Drug Administration, Center for Drug Evaluation and Research. Guidance for industry. Qualification process for drug development tools; 2010. Silver Spring, MD [Draft Guidance].

[38] Hayashi K, Masuda S, Kimura H. Analyzing global trends of biomarker use in drug interventional clinical studies. Drug Discov Ther 2012;6(2):102–7.

CHAPTER 16

On the Measurement of the Disease Status in Clinical Trials: Lessons from Multiple Sclerosis

Martin Daumer, Christian Lederer

Contents

1. THE NEED

There are two fundamentally different approaches in the assessment of the disease status of a patient: the pathophysiological approach and the phenomenological approach.

When measuring the disease status in multiple sclerosis (MS) clinical trials, the pathophysiological approach is represented by MRI techniques, whereas the phenomenological (clinical) approach currently consists of a variety of scores from clinical tests (e.g., expanded disability status scale (EDSS), multiple sclerosis functional composite (MSFC)), symptom counts (relapses), and patient-reported outcomes.

In MS, these approaches lead to inconsistent results ("clinicoradiological paradox").

The notion of clinicoradiological paradox makes the implicit assumption that both the pathophysiological and the clinical approaches are valid and meaningful. The solution of the paradox is that currently used clinical

Re-Engineering Clinical Trials
http://dx.doi.org/10.1016/B978-0-12-420246-7.00016-5

171

outcomes are not valid and that MRI outcomes are clinically not meaningful.

The currently accepted (European Medical Agency (EMA), Food and Drug Administration (FDA)) outcome in phase III trials is the so-called "sustained progression" in EDSS, although the designer of this scale recommended not to use it in clinical trials; Kurtzke was right [1]. Similar concerns hold for the MSFC that was promoted as a scale with less deficiencies compared to the EDSS [2].

Symptom counts (relapses) are an accepted outcome in phase III trials, although there exists evidence that the occurrence of relapses might counterintuitively even predict a benign disease course [3].

MRI was introduced in the field around 1990.

1.1 Mystification of Surrogates

Meanwhile, authorities have been repeatedly confronted with the claim to accept MRI as a "surrogate." The concept of surrogate markers was introduced to obtain evidence concerning the efficacy of a treatment earlier or less costly, not to relax the demands of evidence. Prentice [6] originally defines a surrogate endpoint as a "response variable for which a test of the null hypothesis of no relationship to the treatment groups under comparison is also a valid test of the corresponding null hypothesis based on the true endpoint." In the same paper, Prentice states (without proof) three formal criteria for surrogacy in the context of a survival model that then have be extended to more general models (still without proof, now mutated to a new set of four criteria that still are called "Prentice criteria"). Begg and Leung [7] give examples where the application of these criteria leads to inconsistencies with the demand formulated in the original Prentice criterion. This type of inconsistency can frequently be found in the published results of an entire research program aiming to establish the surrogacy of MRI parameters in MS: typically, the surrogacy is "concluded" from data that show a marginal effect on the original outcome together with a huge effect on the MRI outcome [8].

2. THE SOLUTION

From a pragmatist point of view, an outcome in MS should
1. have an obvious link to a typical patient's well-being in daily life
2. be quantifiable with current technology with sufficient signal-to-noise ratio to allow for manageable sample sizes.
   Walking ability in daily life clearly fulfills (1).

Concerning (2), in the past a reliable quantification of daily life, walking ability, was not possible, either by questionnaires [9] or by clinical short-term tests [10].

Recent advances in using microelectronic devices allow to continuously monitor human motion in daily life for an extended period (≥10 days). With sensor location close to the center of mass, algorithms have been developed to compute certain aspects of walking ability, in particular steps and walking speed for each step.

These algorithms have been repeatedly validated, both for MS patients in clinical environment [11] and healthy individuals in daily life [12,13] (Figures 16.1 and 16.2).

3. SWOT

3.1 Strength

Mobile accelometry is currently a robust, rather cheap, and easy-to-apply technology. It may get introduced as primary endpoint in all diseases that affect mobility.

3.2 Weaknesses

The influence of seasonal variation and environmental factors has not yet been studied in detail. For pathological gait, the signal-to-noise ratio in

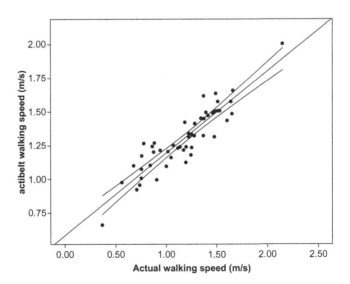

Figure 16.1 Association between gold standard walking speed and walking speed from actibelt® in patients with mild and moderate MS [11].

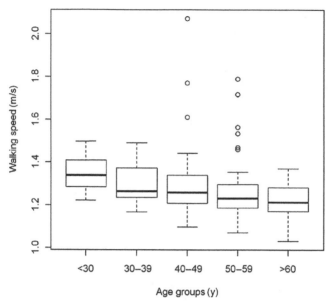

Figure 16.2 Relationship between walking speed and age in healthy individuals [12].

step detection and speed estimation is currently too low to be recommended in clinical trials. For trials studying the effect of exercise therapy, the methodology has not yet been established to disentangle intervention and effect.

3.3 Opportunity

It is up to the industry to establish and fully validate this surrogate endpoint in coming phase II studies, thus making it fully acceptable for pivotal trials.

3.4 Threats

Failure as surrogate endpoint during the validation or nonacceptance by authorities for other reasons.

4. TAKE HOME MESSAGE

The following topics should receive special attention in the further development of mobile accelerometry:

- Standardization (in particular, sensor position)
- No preprocessing of the raw signal

- Ecologically valid gold standards (treadmill data may not suffice)
- Fully automatic extraction of parameters (e.g., gait speed, falls)
- Free annotated databases (in particular, falls)

5. APPLICABLE REGULATIONS

- Patient-reported outcomes guidance for industry, EMA scientific advice
- Either norms related to consumer electronics or EN60601.

REFERENCES

[1] Ebers GC, et al. Disability as an outcome in MS clinical trials. Neurology 2008;71(9):624–31.

[2] Rudick RA, Cutter G, Reingold S. The multiple sclerosis functional composite: a new clinical outcome measure for multiple sclerosis trials. Mult Scler 2002;8(5):359–65.

[3] Scalfari A, et al. The natural history of multiple sclerosis, a geographically based study 10: relapses and long-term disability. Brain 2010;133(7):1914–29.

[4] Unger L. Ueber multiple inselförmige Sklerose des Centralnervensystems im Kindesalter. Wien: Toeplitz & Deuticke; 1887.

[5] DeLuca GC, Ebers GC, Esiri MM. Axonal loss in multiple sclerosis: a pathological survey of the corticospinal and sensory tracts. Brain 2004;127(5):1009–18.

[6] Prentice RL. Surrogate endpoints in clinical trials: definition and operational criteria. Stat Med 1989;8(4):431–40.

[7] Begg CB, Leung DHY. On the use of surrogate end points in randomized trials. J R Stat Soc Ser A Stat Soc 2000;163(1):15–28.

[8] Sormani MP, et al. Combined MRI lesions and relapses as a surrogate for disability in multiple sclerosis. Neurology 2011;77(18):1684–90.

[9] Helmerhorst HJ, et al. A systematic review of reliability and objective criterion-related validity of physical activity questionnaires. Int J Behav Nutr Phys Act 2012;9(1):103–57.

[10] Albrecht H, et al. Day-to-day variability of maximum walking distance in MS patients can mislead to relevant changes in the expanded disability status scale (EDSS): average walking speed is a more constant parameter. Mult Scler 2001;7(2):105–9.

[11] Motl RW, et al. Accuracy of the actibelt® accelerometer for measuring walking speed in a controlled environment among persons with multiple sclerosis. Gait Posture 2012;35(2):192–6.

[12] Schimpl M, et al. Association between walking speed and age in healthy, free-living individuals using Mobile Accelerometry—a cross-sectional study. PLoS One 2011;6(8):e23299.

[13] Schimpl M, Lederer C, Daumer M. Development and validation of a new method to measure walking speed in free-living environments using the actibelt® platform. Plos One 2011;6(8):e23080.

CHAPTER 17

Generating Evidence from Historical Data Using Robust Prognostic Matching: Experience from Multiple Sclerosis

Martin Daumer, Christian Lederer

Contents

1. THE NEED

Multiple sclerosis (MS) is a chronic inflammatory disease of the central nervous system. The etiology is not well understood. The disease course is frequently "relapsing remitting" and then tends to transform in a "secondary progressive" phase. To assess the status of the disease, various outcome parameters are used: on the one hand, parameters from magnetic resonance imaging (MRI), in particular the number and volumes of visible lesions in the brain and the spinal cord which are, however, not accepted as outcome measures in phase III clinical trials. On the other hand, one uses the frequency of relapses and the so-called Expanded Disability Status Scale (EDSS), a score linked to disability that is in a wide range characterized by the gradual loss of walking ability.

There is no cure for MS. Several approved drugs modify certain aspects of the disease course favorably, although often coupled with unwanted side effects. In clinical studies exploring new candidates for more effective drug

Re-Engineering Clinical Trials
http://dx.doi.org/10.1016/B978-0-12-420246-7.00017-7

treatments, it is therefore problematic for ethical reasons to test against placebo. A test against one of the standard disease-modifying treatments would invariably lead to smaller effect sizes, hence, to larger sample sizes and costs. The dilemma applies to many other disease entities with approved therapies yet in the market.

2. THE SOLUTION

When the Sylvia Lawry Centre for MS Research (SLCMSR) was founded in 2001, one of its goals was to solve the placebo problem, i.e., how to create novel designs for MS clinical trials that use "virtual" placebo patients instead of real ones. This does not mean to simulate the pathophysiology of the disease course of a patient. A virtual placebo group is rather a mathematical–statistical method that allows to generate a similarly strong evidence for the efficacy of a drug like in a prospectively randomized controlled trial, but based on the comparison of a group of treated patients with a suitable "virtual" control group taken from a database instead of a "real" placebo group.

In the meantime, we have built the Ian McDonald database, which comprises information on more than 100,000 patient years from approximately 26,000 patients that were recruited in natural history studies, observational studies, and controlled clinical trials [1].

2.1 Virtual Placebo Groups and Robust Prognostic Matching

The first step in the attempt to compare real patient groups with virtual ones is to take into account the differences in the baseline characteristics. This can be done by matching a subgroup of the database or by means of a regression model. In general, matching procedures seem to be superior, not only for reasons of practicality but more for methodological reasons, to reduce the largely uncontrollable effect of errors in the assumptions about the statistical model [2].

Exact matching of the baseline variables is typically impossible. Therefore, it is necessary to define the "similarity" of two patients (p,q) with baseline variables $X=(X_1,...,X_m)$ and $Y=(Y_1,...,Y_m)$ by a distance measure $d(p,q)$. The selection process of a matching control group is thereby transformed into a combinatorial optimization problem: find, for a given group of patients $(p_1...p_n)$ a subgroup of placebo patients $(q_1...q_n)$ from the database, with the property sum $\sum |d(p_i,q_i)| = Minimum$.

A common distance measure is the so-called propensity score [3]. It was introduced to reduce the effect of treatment selection bias in observational studies. This effect can lead to the at-first-sight paradoxical result that the patient group with the worst disease course is receiving the treatment type and dosage that is considered to have the strongest effect (see [4] with some examples from oncology). The propensity score $b(X)$ is here defined as the conditional probability for a patient to receive a treatment given the patient's baseline covariates X and the metric d defined by $d(p,q) = |b(X)-b(Y)|$.

Rosenbaum and Rubin have shown [5] that the propensity score is a "balancing score" in the sense that conditional distribution of the covariates X, given $b(X)$, is the same for treated and untreated patients. However, this does not imply that the sample distributions between matched groups are similar: The baseline variables themselves are ignored in the matching procedure. In a study with a 1:1 randomization scheme, the propensity score would be ½, i.e., the distance d would be constantly 0 and the matching would be arbitrary. If one wants to match patients of a one-armed study against placebo patients from a database, the definition of the propensity score is not meaningful.

The method of *robust prognostic matching* was developed at the SLCMSR using a different robust metric that is also working for matching a single patient against multiple controls. The method was originally developed as a basis for an online analytical processing (OLAP) tool to predict the individual course of the disease for a given patient (Figure 17.1). The main reason not to use a regression model is the need to reduce the dependency on model assumptions. The predictions depend more on the model-dependent shape of the regression surface than on the underlying data, in particular around the less-populated edges of the dataset available for analysis, such that one may get bad predictions for patients with untypical covariates. Robust prognostic matching works as follows.

A regression model for the primary outcome is fitted. This model, however, is not directly used for the prediction, but is just used to distribute appropriate weights to the covariates used in the matching procedure.

The model coefficients $\beta = (\beta_1,\ldots,\beta_m)$ define a metric on the space of patients. The distance $d(p,q)$ between two patients (p,q) with covariates $X = (X_1,\ldots,X_m)$ and $Y = (Y_1,\ldots,Y_m)$ is defined by $d(p,q) = \sum |\beta_i| |X_i-Y_i|$. (Categorical variables are dummy coded or effect coded beforehand.) In the unrealistic case of a perfect model, one could use the metric $d'(p,q) = |\sum \beta_i(X_i - Y_i)|$; in the linear case, $d'(p,q)$ would be proportional to the difference of the expected outcomes. This metric would correspond to the method of matching with "prognostic scores," the mathematical properties of which have been studied in [6]. Matching with prognostic scores,

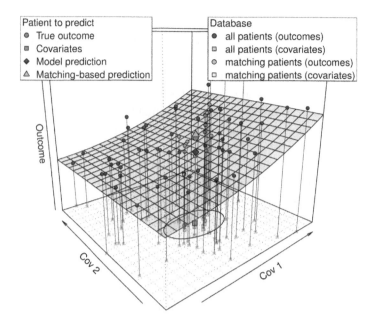

Figure 17.1 Schematic comparison between model-based and matching-based prediction: In model-based prediction, the outcome of a patient (characterized by covariates 1 and 2) is estimated by projecting the patient on the regression surface. Thus, the quality of the prediction depends strongly on the choice of the analytical functional form (e.g., selection of the link function in a glm), which is typically difficult to justify. The matching-based prediction takes the mean behavior of "similar" patients (located in the yellow ellipse). An analytical model is only used to estimate the relative predictive power of the covariates, determining the ratio of the main axes of the ellipse (ellipsoid in the multidimensional case).

however, would assume implicitly that the underlying model is good enough to justify the mutual cancellation of differences in different variables. The aim, however, was to be less dependent on model assumptions.

Using the metric d, one selects the n "nearest" patients. For simple numerical outcomes, one uses the mean of the outcomes of the matching patients for the prediction; more complex outcomes (such as Kaplan–Meier for survival times with censored data) make use of nonparametrical models.

In a recently conducted validation study, we could show that the long-term predictions of the OLAP tool for individual patients using robust prognostic matching are at least on par with the predictions of highly specialized MS neurologists [7]. For the pairwise matching of placebo patients, one also needs to solve the combinatorial problem to search controls that solve $\sum | d(p_i,q_i) |$ = *Minimum*. The method developed and implemented by the SLCMSR uses simulated annealing [8] for this purpose. Typically, in this method, one generates control groups that have a remarkably similar distribution of relevant covariates compared to the given group of patients (Figures 17.2 and 17.3).

2.2 Study Effects

Study effects describe the well-known fact that outcome measures can differ considerably between placebo groups, even in the absence of essential differences between the covariates of the patients. Reasons for this effect are differences in the quality of the studies (blinding), differences in definitions, and differences in unmeasured "hidden variables" (e.g., lifestyle, physical activity, nocebo effects) that affect the course of the disease. A virtual placebo group that would be considered as a basis for a marketing approval of a new drug would need to compensate for these study effects. Pocock suggests a methodology [8] that introduces an additional component of variability to take into account the study effects. This methodology assumes that (1) the variability of the study effect can be estimated reasonably well from historical trials, (2) the variability is smaller than the expected treatment effect, and (3) changes over time are negligible.

Although the Ian McDonald database seems to be perfect for exploring study effects, contractual obligations with data donors only allowed for partial performance of the necessary analysis.

Study effects in MRI data were described in [9]. A multivariate analysis showed, in essence, that for all commonly used MRI parameters, study effects have a much stronger influence than the known demographic and clinical predictor variables.

A recently conducted study [10] examined effects for relapse rates. It turned out that relapse rates observed in clinical trials decreased considerably over the last 20 years, being only partly explained by the change in the prestudy relapse rate, a known predictor variable. A possible explanation for this finding could be the changes in diagnostic criteria in 2001 and 2005 [11]. There were not enough data to decide if this trend continues or if a new plateau has been reached. Only seven studies were made available for analysis performed after 2001, and only four studies were made available for analysis after 2005; differences between these studies were considerably smaller than some treatment effects in studies with patients with relapsing-remitting MS (RRMS).

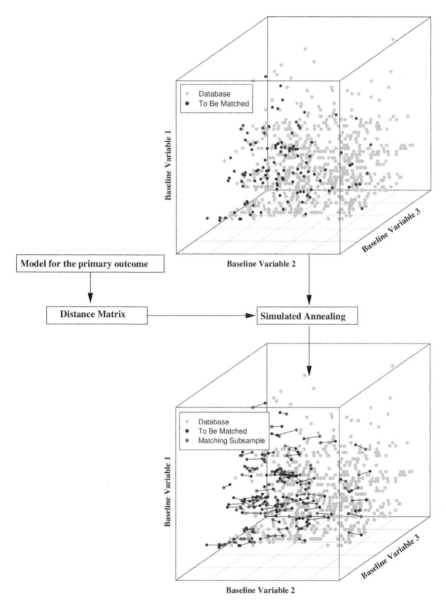

Figure 17.2 The matching algorithm can be used to select historical controls from a database that reflect the probable behavior of placebo patients.

If the small variability between studies can be confirmed with a sufficiently large number of trials, it seems feasible to replace real placebo groups of RRMS patients with virtual ones that are recruited only from studies that have been performed after the changes in diagnostic criteria had been

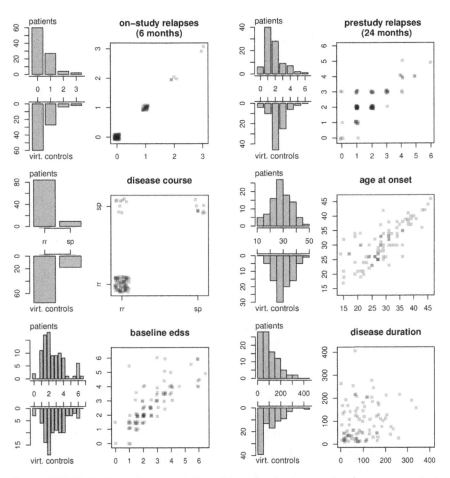

Figure 17.3 Typical matching result (matching of a short-term placebo group against the Ian McDonald database). Since relapses have strong predictive power, the corresponding points lie on the diagonal. The smaller the predictive power of a covariate, the higher the allowed tolerance (e.g., disease duration).

implemented. Study effects related to the outcome "sustained progression in EDSS" have not yet been analyzed thoroughly.

3. SWOT

We summarize using a SWOT (Strength, Weakness, Opportunity and Threat) model:

Strength: The biostatistical and bioinformatic methodology of robust prognostic matching to generate virtual placebo groups has been developed and has been tested successfully [7,12,13].

Weakness: On the basis of scientific results that have been obtained and published during the last years, we conclude that there will be no phase III trials in RRMS with EDSS progression as primary endpoint without a—treated or untreated—"real" control group in the foreseeable future. Sustained progression as a measure for unremitting deteriorations on the EDSS scale—the gold standard in clinical trials—is frequently actually not sustained, but rather a temporary fluctuation or a not-yet-completed recovery from a previous relapse [14,15]. For MRI parameters, it appears unlikely, at least in the near future, to use virtual placebo groups in phase III studies because study effects are too large.

Opportunity: In the context of relapse rates, virtual control groups have been used and are currently used in scientific/clinical research [16] to assist in difficult/borderline decisions for regulatory bodies (Bfarm report 2010 [17]), to increase the sample size using virtual controls, and for evidence-based decision support for the individual course of the disease [7,12].

If the results concerning the new plateau and the low intertrial variability of replase rates observed in the last years/decades can be confirmed, in our view it is possible to design one-armed trials with the reduction of relapse rate as primary outcome and virtual placebos as control. We are in dialogue with the regulatory bodies about this issue and related topics.

Threats: In the light of, at best, the very modest additional predictive value of standard MRI parameters for the disease course [18] and due to the unclear value of modern MRI parameters ("clinical radiological paradox"), it is most likely that MRI parameters will not be accepted as outcome in phase III trials by the authorities [19].

4. TAKE-AWAY MESSAGE

The concept of a virtual placebo group was introduced to circumvent the increasing ethical and practical problems related to recruiting placebo patients for clinical trials in MS. We capture this concept with mathematical–statistical procedures to generate evidence for the efficacy of a drug by comparing a treated group of patients with placebo patients from a database. To compensate for differences in the baseline characteristics between these patient groups, we developed the method of robust prognostic matching. The concept of a virtual control group reaches a fundamental limitation if study effects are of the same order of magnitude as the expected treatment effect.

Looking toward future improvement of clinical research, developments like the European Network of Centres for Pharmacovigilance and Pharmcoepidemiology of the European Medical Agency, and the Critical Path Institute [20,21] in the context of the Food and Drug Administration's "critical path initiative" [20], seem to be particularly interesting initiatives for assessing and exploiting the value of modern concepts for improved study design and large biomedical data warehouses/registries. The ongoing process of revising the current guidelines for MS trials seems to be a particularly suitable opportunity to create guidelines that include recent scientific findings.

REFERENCES

[1] Noseworthy J, Kappos L, Daumer M. Competing interests in multiple sclerosis research. Lancet 2003;361:350–1.

[2] Ho DE, Imai K, King G, Stuart EA. Matching as nonparametric preprocessing for reducing model dependence in parametric causal inference. Polit Anal 2007;15: 199–236.

[3] Rubin DB. Matching to remove bias in observational studies. Biometrics 1973;29: 159–83.

[4] Giordano SH, Kuo YF, Duan Z, Hortobagyi GN, Freeman J, Goodwin JS. Limits of observational data in determining outcomes from cancer therapy. Cancer 2008;112:2456–66.

[5] Rosenbaum PR, Rubin DB. The central role of the propensity score in observational studies for causal effects. Biometrika 1983;70:41–55.

[6] Hansen BB. The prognostic analogue of the propensity score. Biometrica 2008;95: 481–8.

[7] Galea I, Lederer C, Neuhaus A, Muraro P, Scalfari A, Koch-Henriksen N, et al. A web-based tool for personalized prediction of long-term disease course in patients with multiple sclerosis. Eur J Neurol 2013;20(7):1107–9.

[8] Pocock SJ. The combination of randomized and historical controls in clinical trials. J Chron Dis 1976;29:175–88.

[9] Schach S, Scholz M, Wolinsky JS, Kappos L. Pooled historical MRI data as a basis for research in multiple sclerosis – a statistical evaluation. Mult Scler 2007;13:509–16.

[10] Stellmann J, Neuhaus A, Herich L, Schippling S, Roeckel M, Daumer M, et al. Placebo cohorts in phase-3 MS treatment trials – predictors for on-trial disease activity 1990–2010. Plos-One 2012;7(11):e50347.

[11] Polman CH, Reingold SC, Edan G, Filippi M, Hartung HP, Kappos L, et al. Diagnostic criteria for multiple sclerosis: 2005 revisions to the "McDonald Criteria." Ann Neurol 2005;58:840–6.

[12] Daumer M, Neuhaus A, Lederer C, Scholz M, Wolinsky JD, Heiderhoff M. Prognosis of the individual course of disease - steps in developing a decision support tool for multiple sclerosis. BMC Med Inform Decis Mak 2007;7:11.

[13] Lederer C, Tang D, Otten S, Pohlmann H, Strobl R, Pinheiro J, et al. Identifying historical controls for MS follow-up studies in a large database – methodological considerations. Presentation ECTRIMS 2007, Prag 2007;11. 14.10.2007.

[14] Ebers GC, Heigenhauser L, Daumer M, Lederer C, Noseworthy JH. Disability as an outcome in MS clinical trials. Neurology 2008;71:624–31.

[15] Ebers GC. Commentary: outcome measures were flawed. BMJ 2010;340:c2693.

[16] Then Bergh F, Kümpfel T, Schumann E, Held U, Schwan M, Blazevic M, et al. Monthly
      i.v. methylprednisolone in relapsing-remitting MS – reduction of enhancing lesions,
      T2 lesion volume and plasma prolactin concentrations. BMC Neurol 2006;6:19.

[17] Bfarm-Bericht (2010), Bewertung der Expertengruppe Off-Label im Bereich Neu-
      rologie/Psychiatrie nach § 35b Abs. 3 SGB V zur Anwendung von Intravenösem
      Immunglobulin G (IVIG) im Anwendungsgebiet Multiple Sklerose. http://www.bfarm
      .de/cae/servlet/contentblob/1061976/publicationFile/(15.08.2012).

[18] Daumer M, Neuhaus A, Morrissey S, Hintzen R, Ebers GC. MRI as an outcome in
      multiple sclerosis clinical trials. Neurology 2009;72:705–11.

[19] http://www.ema.europa.eu/ema/index.jsp?curl=pages/news_and_events/events
      /2013/06/event_detail_000724.jsp&mid=WC0b01ac058004d5c3.

[20] http://www.c-path.org/index.cfm (15.08.2012).

[21] http://www.ema.europa.eu/ema/index.jsp?curl=pages/news_and_events/events
      /2013/06/event_detail_000724.jsp&mid=WC0b01ac058004d5c3.

CHAPTER 18

Studies with Fewer Patients Involved—The Adaptive Trial

Simon Day

Contents

1. THE NEED

Clinical trials, as traditionally implemented, involve long periods of time where no one knows what the results might be. Although such an approach (the classic double-blind trial) has the advantage of eliminating certain types of bias, it also means that if anything could be—or ought to be—usefully modified so the trial could better answer its intended question, the sponsor will be unaware of this and so not in a position to make such a change. Only after the trial has finished will any deficiencies become known, sometimes resulting in a trial being of little or no value. A simple example: if it became apparent that the dose being tested was wrong, it would seem sensible to be able to change the dose when this became apparent, rather than discovering it after the trial had finished. Another example might be to allow or disallow a concomitant medication partway through a study. Particularly in the context of disallowing a co-medication, it is worth considering what action we might take, early on in a trial, if an untoward adverse interaction were observed between the treatment under investigation and a sometimes-used co-medication. Clearly the trial cannot continue as it is, with future patients exposed to a risky and harmful

Re-Engineering Clinical Trials
http://dx.doi.org/10.1016/B978-0-12-420246-7.00018-9

combination of (individually unharmful) therapies. The trial could be stopped on safety grounds and a new trial initiated with exclusion criteria disallowing co-use of the other medication. This would clearly result in delays and increased costs to complete a new trial. It would also "waste" the information from patients in the first trial who were not taking the co-medication and would be exactly the sorts of patients recruited to a new trial. A compromise might be to start a new trial but include these eligible patients from the first trial in some sort of meta-analysis with the second trial. A neater and more efficient solution would be to continue the initial trial, but with appropriately restricted inclusion criteria. These are the beginnings of the ideas of adaptive design: some feature(s) of the design can adapt as the trial ensues. Having appropriate methodology (mostly statistical tools) and the operational ability to make changes midway through a trial may help sponsors to avoid many lost opportunities.

2. THE SOLUTION

2.1 The Scope for Change

The above scenarios raise the question of "what might we change?" In fact, numerous changes have been made to ongoing clinical trials for many years. Some have been good, others bad. Some have been wise, others foolish. Some may have seemed like a good idea at the time, but in retrospect have proven to be unfortunate mistakes. Some of these might fit into the term "adaptive design" (even though they had been used well before the term was even thought of); others may not be a good fit for that definition. The list below suggests some changes that do happen (from minor and commonplace, to more substantial, and on to extreme):

- Change of inclusion criteria
- Addition (or removal) of exploratory endpoints
- Change of method of measuring endpoints
- Change of timing of measuring endpoints
- Change of sample size (increase or decrease)
- Stopping at an interim analysis (after efficacy and safety have been established)
- Stopping at an interim analysis (from futility)
- Change of primary objective
- Change of primary endpoint
- Change of dose or dosing regimen
- Change of control or experimental treatment

Some of these look commonplace and are typically handled as protocol amendments. Some (the last few on the list) might seem extreme, and perhaps rather obscure.

What classifies as an "adaptive design," as opposed to a simple protocol amendment or something else? Consensus is lacking, but the Committee for Medicinal Products for Human Use (CHMP) Reflection Paper (CHMP/EWP/2459/02, October 2007) used this definition:

> *A study design is called "adaptive" if statistical methodology allows the modification of a design element (e.g. sample-size, randomisation ratio, number of treatment arms) at an interim analysis with full control of the type I error.*

This seems widely encompassing (any "modification of a design element") but restricts the definition only to cases where full control of Type I error can be assured. Control of Type I error is important, but the inclusion of this as a requirement within the definition may in fact be too restrictive.

U.S. Food and Drug Administration (FDA) guidance ("Guidance for Industry: Adaptive Design Clinical Trials for Drugs and Biologics") from February 2010 (although still in draft more than four years later) states the following:

> *For the purposes of this guidance, an adaptive design clinical study is defined as a study that includes a prospectively planned opportunity for modification of one or more specified aspects of the study design and hypotheses based on analysis of data (usually interim data) from subjects in the study.*

It then goes on to add:

> *Analyses of the accumulating study data are performed at prospectively planned timepoints within the study, can be performed in a fully blinded manner or in an unblinded manner, and can occur with or without formal statistical hypothesis testing.*

This definition does not require full control of type I error, although it certainly doesn't imply that such control is unimportant. It restricts itself to changes made "based on analysis of data … from subjects in the study," thus excluding changes made due to outside influences. An interesting example of changes based on outside influences might be a change to the primary endpoint (surely seen as a major change). If this were done in an ongoing double-blind study, because another study in the same indication had suggested that an endpoint other than the intended primary endpoint were more appropriate, then many would argue there is no risk in changing the endpoint for the ongoing study. This would be in stark contrast to a study that had completed (or was ongoing but unblinded) and where the primary endpoint failed to show any treatment effect. Subsequently changing the study's endpoint, and retrospectively declaring that as "primary," could introduce unacceptable bias.

The FDA definition also refers only to changes based on analyses "at prospectively planned timepoints." These are generally considered the ideal conditions under which adaptations should be made. In particular, adaptive designs are seen as offering potential solutions to pre–thought-out potential problems, not as reactive fixes to problems that were unexpected.

Another definition that has been proposed, and probably most widely quoted, is from the Pharmaceutical Research and Manufacturers of America: "*A clinical study design that uses accumulating data to decide how to modify aspects of the study as it continues, without undermining the validity and integrity of the trial*" [1,2]. This definition seems most broad: it makes no restrictions about control of type I error or preplanned versus post hoc adaptions; and it hints at data coming from within the study ("accumulating data") but does not exclude the influence of data external to the study.

2.2 How Does an Adaptive Design Work?

It seems a simple idea to watch and monitor the progress of a clinical trial and make changes to the design as it proceeds. In essence, this is the intent of the adaptively designed clinical trial, although the practicalities are far more complex. Indeed, it's almost as if we were turning our backs on well-learned lessons from the last 50 years or so, since Bradford Hill carried out his classic experiment testing the treatment of tuberculosis with streptomycin.

For several years, many trials have incorporated some form of "adaption," although that term may never have been used to describe them. Sequential trials (or more commonly, group sequential trials) incorporate one or more interim analyses where a decision is made to continue or stop a trial. Statistical "stopping rules" have been widely developed to account for the problem of interpreting P values when multiple significance tests on accumulating data have been carried out. Independent data-monitoring committees then typically make recommendations to the sponsor on whether the trial should continue. These data-monitoring committees— contrary to the usually accepted rules of a double-blind trial—are unblinded to the treatment allocation and see accumulating efficacy and safety results, although the sponsor does not. The decision to stop a trial early (if that is the recommendation) makes the trial adaptive in some sense: the intended course of the trial is changed along the way. Whether a group sequential study design should be called adaptive depends on your view as to whether complete termination of a study fits within the realm of modifying "aspects of the study *as it continues*." The emphasis has been added, but clearly a study stopped at an interim analysis is no longer continuing.

Introduced more recently has been the idea of "sample size reestimation." Here, partway through recruitment to a trial, an updated estimate is made of how many total patients will be needed to preserve some specified level of statistical power. Therefore, the total sample size may not be as was originally planned or expected; again, this is a form of adaption. This type of change is usually implemented without unblinding the trial and is usually quite uncontroversial—although many people don't consider an adaptive design because the study has not been unblinded. In other situations, such changes are made to unblinded data, and as with group sequential methods, independent unblinded data-monitoring committees are usually employed to look at the data and make recommendations, while the sponsor still remains blinded. The only modification is to the eventual total study size, but that is an aspect of the study design, and all three definitions of adaptive design noted earlier would encompass this.

Much closer to the ideas of adaptive design in the sense that we use the term today is the so-called "continual reassessment method" (CRM) [3]. This has been used since the early 1990s in phase I oncology studies where the purpose is to determine the maximum tolerable dose. It is inefficient to test many patients at each dose. Instead, after each patient has been treated based on toxicity response (unacceptable or not), the likely maximum tolerated dose is estimated and a decision made about which dose the next patient should be given.

Aside from these long-standing ways to adapt a trial as it goes, particularly with CRM designs, many adaptions tend to be superficially straightforward but methodologically (i.e. statistically) quite complex, as emphasized in the CHMP definition. Bias in statistical analysis—avoiding it, or adjusting for it—is a key methodological concern. Consider an example whereby midway through a trial we plan to make a change to the design. For the sake of illustration, assume it is to expand the inclusion criteria once we are satisfied that patients will not be at undue risk if we do so. In a landmark paper, Bauer and Köhn [4] set out how the analysis should be carried out.

Without showing all the details here, such analysis involves making a comparison between the treatment groups using patients recruited *before* the change, and calculating the P value for the treatment effect, which we call P_1. Then we do a similar analysis for the patients recruited *after* the change, and call that P value P_2. The correct P value for the comparison of the treatments for all patients must then be calculated from the combination of the two P values; we cannot simply ignore the fact that a change was made, and calculate a single P value for the entire dataset.

In fact, correct calculation of statistical significance seems to be one of the easier problems to solve. More difficult can be estimating how large the treatment effect is. Consider a parallel group trial that plans to recruit 500 patients. There are two potential new treatments ($Test_1$ and $Test_2$) and we wish to know which one best compares with placebo. The trial is designed in two stages (or cohorts). In stage one, we recruit 300 patients and randomize 100 to each of $Test_1$, $Test_2$, and placebo. We then determine which of $Test_1$ or $Test_2$ is best, and stop randomization to the "loser." We then recruit a further 200 patients, randomizing 100 each to the preferred Test compound and placebo. At the end of the trial, we have 200 patients treated with the preferred test compound, 200 treated with placebo, and a further 100 treated with the test compound that was dropped. A correct P value can be calculated as a combination of the two separate P values described above, but let us consider the estimation of the size of the treatment effect.

Assume $Test_1$ and $Test_2$ actually have identical effects in comparison to placebo (of course, we can never actually know this). Simply through random variability, after the first cohort of 300 patients has been evaluated (100 each on $Test_1$ and $Test_2$, as well as placebo), the response rates for these two treatments will be slightly different; perhaps 20 patients respond to $Test_1$ and 24 to $Test_2$. If we knew that both treatments were identical, we would use the full 200 patients to estimate the response rate(s) and conclude that 44 of 200 have responded, i.e., 22%. It should be obvious that even if the two treatments have identical effects, one of them will almost certainly appear to perform better or worse than the other (just by chance), and we will automatically select the one that appears to be best, therefore introducing bias into the final estimate of effect size. In this example, the apparently best test treatment showed a response of 22%. How big the bias might be in any particular trial is very challenging to determine. The extreme case of this scenario is the so-called "seamless phase II/III design," and is illustrated in Figure 18.1. Initially, successive cohorts of patients are treated with different doses. This part of the study might look like a typical phase II design and be referred to as the exploratory phase of the study. As the trial continues, ineffective or unsafe doses may be dropped and new doses taken up; during this exploratory phase, there may (or may not) be an active comparator. Eventually, when a satisfactory dose (or possibly more than one) has been determined, new patients are randomized to receive one of these active doses, a placebo, or possibly an active control treatment. This part of the study might

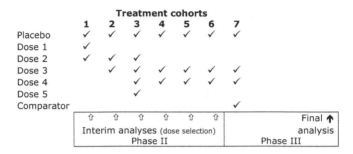

Figure 18.1 Schematic of a phase II/III adaptive trial design. Early in the study (during the phase II part), patients are randomized to receive either placebo or one of five possible active doses. After each cohort of patients completes its follow-up, an interim analysis is conducted to determine doses either to drop or add. After the sixth cohort (in this example) of patients has been tested, active doses three and four are selected and carried into the phase III part of the study. Here, patients in the seventh cohort are randomized to either placebo, one of the two active doses (three or four), or an active comparator.

look like a typical phase III design and be referred to as the confirmatory phase of the study. All of these changes would be part of a single clinical trial protocol, but one that can't specify at the outset which dose or doses will ultimately be compared with the active comparator, nor even how many patients will potentially be studied.

Such "seamless" designs need to be considered in one or another category, either operationally seamless or inferentially seamless. Operationally seamless means that the whole protocol is set out in advance, and successive patients can be recruited without any interruption as time goes by. It is assumed that drug supplies (possibly different doses, availability of active comparator, etc.) are all available as soon as required and as soon as decisions have been made about how the trial will continue. Inferentially seamless implies that the inference(s) or conclusions from the study will be based on the entire dataset; that is, on all patients who take part in the study. In effect, the phase II patients are used twice, once for dose determination and again for confirmation of effect. In contrast to this (using the example illustrated in Figure 18.1), we might use only the data from the part of the study akin to the "phase III part" for making final conclusions. Such an approach might avoid some of the bias in estimating the size of treatment effect described earlier in this section. A study can be operationally seamless with or without being inferentially seamless. If we do not try to make a trial inferentially seamless, then—although it is one ongoing trial—it bears much closer analogies to a phase II trial followed by a phase III trial and maintains the ideas of distinguishing between a learning phase and a confirming phase.

2.3 Objections to Adaptive Designs

The CHMP Reflection Paper makes the particular point that "the purpose of phase III is to confirm the findings from preclinical studies, tolerability studies, dose-finding and other phase II studies... To argue for design modifications in a phase III trial (or a late stage phase II trial supposed to be part of the confirmatory package) is then a contradiction to the confirmatory nature of such studies..." Indeed, the document is titled "Reflection Paper on Methodological Issues in *Confirmatory* Clinical Trials Planned with an Adaptive Design" (emphasis added). It is well-recognized that post hoc analyses of trial results can lead to substantial bias in their interpretation. Hence, there is very strong emphasis made, for example, in ICH E9 about prespecifying analyses and statistical analysis plans. Apparently, we now have a trial design that allows us to change design, endpoint, timing of assessment, choice of comparator, method of analysis (the list is seemingly endless), and yet still regard it as a confirmatory trial rather than an exploratory one. How can this be?

Perhaps the simple answer is that adaptive designs are not the panacea for treatments that do not work, or for poorly designed trials or development plans. Unfortunately, in the early days of using these sorts of trials, many proposals were methodologically poor and paid little attention to things like operational bias in ongoing studies or correct inference (either significance testing or estimation). Still, operational bias is often ignored, perhaps because it is difficult to quantify, and most of the research work on adaptive designs has been carried out by statisticians. As a consequence, issues of correct significance testing and estimation have taken prominence. But as outlined at the beginning of the chapter, there is an element of ignoring long-learned lessons from 50 years's experience conducting clinical trials. To help circumvent this, data-monitoring committees are being used more and more to inspect interim results and make recommendations for changes. Regulators (and sponsors) have substantial experience with operational aspects of data-monitoring committees—and regulatory guidance is extensive. However, it must be realized that data-monitoring committees are being asked to make bigger decisions in adaptive designs than in more traditional interim analyses: they may be recommending changes to inclusion criteria, endpoints, choice of comparator, or others. In a commercial setting, all of these points can have major implications on an eventual product label, and such decisions cannot be made independently of company business strategy. Yet, as soon as the sponsor is involved in making these decisions, the study may start to become unblinded. There is a potential paradox that the "more adaptable" a trial can be, the less acceptable it may be to the sponsor who cannot take part in the decision-making.

2.4 Potential Gains from Adaptive Designs

Objections and difficulties should not be dismissed lightly, but should be managed so that the potential gains from such designs can be realized. The obvious gain is that for a useful medicine, a trial that is initially not optimally designed to demonstrate its benefits can be changed along the way. This avoids the possibilities of (at best) having to redo trials, with the ensuing costs and delays in getting good medicines to patients. At worst, it avoids the possibility that a good medicine might be dismissed as ineffectual and discarded, when in fact it was the trial that was lacking, not the medicine.

A further time-saving opportunity is illustrated in Figure 18.2. Part (a) illustrates a typical (if simplified) example Gantt chart for a drug

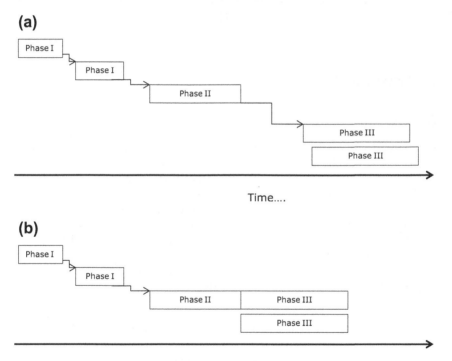

Figure 18.2 Typical Gantt chart showing a sequence of trials in the drug development plan. The transition between the different phase I trials, and from phase I to phase II, may still follow a traditional sequential path, with planning time or "white space" between them, as illustrated in both scenarios. Scenario (b) shows the white space eliminated between phase II and phase III—an opportunity provided via the use of a seamless phase II/III adaptive design—and the resulting time saved until completion of the phase III (and full development) program. Part (a) Traditional (sequential) drug development. Part (b) "Seamless" phase II/III design, eliminating "white space."

development program. It begins with phase I (perhaps several studies; other clinical pharmacology studies also might be carried out later during the development period). We then have phase II (here shown as just one study) and then phase III (shown as two studies, as is often the case). The important points to note are not the times when studies are ongoing, but the so-called "white space" between the end of each phase and the beginning of the next. Much time is used here on administrative issues such as regulatory and ethics approvals to carry out the next trial, as well as study "start-up" activities such as training investigators, preparing courier services, negotiating contracts, and many more. It is these "white spaces" that are great opportunities for elimination. Part (b) of Figure 18.2 shows the same trial durations, but phases II and III are put together, back-to-back, illustrating how (operationally) phase III can run seamlessly off the back of phase II.

3. SWOT ANALYSIS

Strengths	Weaknesses
• Knowledge of what is happening in a trial should be far more reliable than prior assumptions. • Trials that are potentially failing (as well as treatments that are potentially failing) can be identified much sooner than they can in a conventional fixed design.	• More time must be invested when designing a trial, to map out potential adaptions that might be needed. • Not all bias—particularly operational bias—can necessarily be eliminated from an adaptively run trial.
Opportunities	**Threats**
• Fewer trials should fail to answer the question they were designed to answer. • Effective therapies, tested in ineffective trials, should be a thing of the past if we can eliminate ineffective trials. • Software for simulating and implementing adaptive designs has been very quick to develop, allowing much easier design of adaptive trials.	• There have been many cases of poorly designed or poorly implemented adaptive trials. • Bad examples have made regulators cautious, leading to a conservative approach from many sponsors.

4. APPLICABLE REGULATIONS

The International Conference on Harmonisation of Technical Requirements for Registration of Pharmaceuticals for Human Use (ICH) E3 (Structure and Content of Clinical Study Reports), ICH E6 (Guideline for Good Clinical Practice), ICH E8 (General Considerations for Clinical Trials), ICH E9 (Statistical Principles for Clinical Trials), and ICH E10 (Choice of Control Group and Related Issues in Clinical Trials).

FDA "Guidance for Industry: Adaptive Design Clinical Trials for Drugs and Biologics" (draft, February 2010); FDA "Guidance for Clinical Trial Sponsors: Establishment and Operation of Clinical Trial Data Monitoring Committees" (March 2006).

CHMP Guideline on Data Monitoring Committees (EMEA/CHMP/EWP/5872/03 Corr, July 2005), CHMP Reflection Paper on Methodological Issues in Confirmatory Clinical Trials Planned with an Adaptive Design (CHMP/EWP/2459/02, October 2007).

5. TAKE HOME MESSAGE

Adaptively designed clinical trials allow the possibility to monitor the progress of an ongoing trial, in a blinded or unblinded manner, and make appropriate design changes as the trial progresses.

Such possible design changes should generally be prespecified and not simply reactive fixes to trials that are going wrong. Identifying and solving problems of bias are particularly paramount, and data-monitoring committees are being used more and more to help with this problem.

There are also benefits in efficiency to be gained.

REFERENCES

[1] Gallo P, Chuang-Stein C, Dragalin V, Gaydos B, Krams M, Pinheiro J. Adaptive design in clinical drug development – an executive summary of the PhRMA working group (with discussions). J Biopharm Stat 2006;16:275–83.
[2] Gallo P, Krams M. PhRMA working group on adaptive designs: introduction to the full white paper. Drug Inf J 2006;40:421–3.
[3] O'Quigley J, Pepe M, Fisher L. Continual reassessment method: a practical design for phase 1 clinical trials in cancer. Biometrics 1990;46:33–48.
[4] Bauer P, Köhne K. Evaluation of experiments with adaptive interim analyses. Biometrics 1994;50:1029–41.

CHAPTER 19

Connected Health in Clinical Trials: The Patient as Sub-Investigator

Brendan M. Buckley

Contents

1. CONNECTED HEALTH

The International Telecommunications Union has estimated that there were about 6800 million cellular subscriptions by people worldwide by the end of 2013, with an estimated 2700 million people using the internet [1]. This has enabled unprecedented opportunities for people both to share information about themselves and to have access to the enormous store of information and education on the internet. While social media have been the most rapidly and widely adopted form of this, there is a maturing opportunity for delivery of important aspects of healthcare through this instantaneous and bidirectional flow of information. Healthcare delivery has used a telehealth model for many years, whereby patients are placed in touch with remote caregivers by telecommunications. Such systems include remote dermatology clinics by videoconference, teleradiology, and telepathology, whereby images are transmitted for centralized, specialized interpretation. This has now evolved into a more innovative form in which mobile devices such as smartphones are used either as the originator or as intermediary to other mobile devices to transmit physiological information about the user to a

Re-Engineering Clinical Trials
http://dx.doi.org/10.1016/B978-0-12-420246-7.00019-0

central service. This "Connected Health," with its variant sometimes called "Mobile Health" or "mHealth," aims to optimize the efficient and relevant deployment of healthcare resources to the population and to empower people to better maintain their own health. Where disease is present, connected health allows patients to participate more actively in monitoring their status and enable them to better self-manage their own care in collaboration with their physicians and other medical caregivers.

The terms "connected health" and "mHealth" are broad, encompassing as they do two distinct forms. The first is a consumer-focused suite of devices and apps which are directed at enabling health and well-being, for instance, by tracking activity and exercise, providing assistance in healthy eating, and monitoring normal physiological functions such as heart rate, sleep patterns, and even emotions. In essence, these devices are worn for extended periods and have both wireless connectivity and "smart" internal processing ability. They are typically enabled by sensors such as accelerometers, microphones, light sensors, strain gauges, etc. Their use is often embedded in an ecology in which they are associated with the use of social media, sometimes with the inclusion of a form of game simulation and competition as reinforcements for their use. Typical examples are devices in the form of watches which continuously log measurements of time, speed, distance, heart rate, and gait cadence during athletic performance, allowing the wearer not just to monitor their own performance but also to transmit the data to social media sites which enter the data in virtual competitions. Such devices are now ubiquitous among serious recreational cyclists and runners. Simpler forms, such as wearable bracelets that communicate with smartphones, are also widely worn as a combination of fashion statement ("Look at me: I'm fit and healthy") and aid to healthy living.

A second form of connected health application is for use in assisting the management of illness and disease. Devices used in healthy and fitness-related applications may well be also used in disease monitoring, but particular requirements such as the measurement of ambulatory blood pressure (BP), blood glucose concentration, spirometry, oxymetry, etc., have generated a wide range of specific medical devices for these purposes. Many of these have been in use in "nonconnected" fashion for decades, the best example being blood glucose measurement which became "semiconnected" when it became possible to download the contents of instruments' memory to a personal computer. Connected mobile devices allow the collection of highly detailed patient data, if needed many times per day for blood glucose, compared with infrequent measurements made in the artificial setting of hospital clinics doctors' offices. The volume of data on a single person allows the determination of the normal range of that particular measurement for that individual and allows detection of deviations (possibly due to deterioration in the disease state) as well as comparison against population normative data for that patient.

It is likely that the impact of connected health will be greatest in relatively stable chronic disease. The overall prevalence of diabetes among a representative sample of Chinese adults has recently been estimated [2] as 11.6% with a prevalence of prediabetes of 50.1%, and this was extrapolated to suggest that about 114 million Chinese adults have diabetes and more than 490 million have prediabetes. The implications even for simply providing diabetes-trained physicians and nurses to deal with this problem are obvious. It is clear that conventional models of hospital clinic-based care, whereby all patients are seen at regular intervals, whether achieving good or bad diabetic control, are insupportable. However, a connected health model of care would allow triaging of patients, selecting for in-person medical review those whose diabetes is not at target.

About 30% of adults in the United States are hypertensive by conventional definition. As the most common reason to visit a doctor's office and a contributor to half of all cardiovascular disease-related deaths, it is estimated to cost in total more than $100 billion at present value [3]. Despite this and the clear evidence of benefit in prevention, less than half of individuals with hypertension have their BP under control [3]. BP monitoring at home has been feasible for many years with simple, reliable, and inexpensive devices, and these are now increasing being enabled with wireless connectivity to allow integration with smartphone apps, centralized monitoring, and databases. It is likely that the proper organization of this by healthcare systems would allow those with good BP control to be managed without needing clinic visits, while time and effort in clinic could be invested in those needing further intervention.

Where connected health systems are put in place, it is important to design them to be bidirectional, with information and education feedback to patients to allow them to recognize and modify the factors that adversely influence their condition. This could be achieved relatively simply in the examples given for diabetes and hypertension.

Connected health is still behind other sectors in the economy in which "online" has transformed personal communications, shopping, and banking. There are still relatively few examples of significant programs that are actually implemented at the time of writing. Among them is the long-established US Department of Veterans Affairs Home Telehealth Service, with the stated aim to make the home into the preferred place of care whenever possible. Veterans who have a health problem like diabetes, chronic heart failure, pulmonary disease, depression, or posttraumatic stress disorder are connected from the home to a VA hospital using land telecom lines to allow remote supervision by healthcare providers. In addition, the European Centre for Connected Health (ECCH) in the Public Health Agency of Northern Ireland has operated a telehealth system since March 2011 for people with cardiac and respiratory conditions, diabetes, and stroke. Further projects are active in Lombardia in Italy.

Studies are needed to validate whether connected health is delivering the benefits to patient care as well as has been anticipated, and such an evaluation is underway in the EU, to be completed in 2015. A potential problem with telemetric accelerometry measurement is data loss. For example, data loss occurred in home sleep studies in 4.7–20% of cases [4] and resulted in lower expected cost savings.

2. APPLICATION OF CONNECTED HEALTH IN CLINICAL RESEARCH

Some connected health approaches have already been quite well adopted in clinical research, although this has tended to be on a rather piecemeal basis with relatively small cohorts of subjects. These are employed in a sense as biomarkers of safety and/or efficacy of interventions. Actigraphy, the measurement and recording of movement, mainly employing accelerometry, has been used to study subjects' response to pharmacotherapies for sleep disturbance as well as clinical associations with sleep and [5,6] and is, undoubtedly, promising. However, conferences' poster presentations of studies have reported that consumer devices when trialed may not be adequately accurate compared with research-grade devices.

The technique might be used in a wide variety of fields beyond that of sleep monitoring in which it has been largely used up to now. Many diseases influence movement and patterns of activity. For example, there is growing interest in developing inexpensive and objective motor fluctuation evaluation methods for Parkinson's disease (PD). The effect of levodopa challenge on movement in patients with this condition has been described. Results showed that simple wrist-worn actigraphy lacked specificity, but suggested it may be suitable for dyskinesia assessment, although not for on-state and off-state evaluation [4]. Other neurological conditions may be conducive to monitoring by actigraphy. For example, depression is associated with psychomotor retardation and characteristic diurnal fluctuations in activity, so that it could be envisaged that trials of antidepressants might incorporate this modality. Similarly, Alzheimer disease may be associated with distinctive patterns of physical activity. The approach might be extended to trials of treatment in other neuromuscular diseases such as muscular dystrophy, motor neuron disease, and multiple sclerosis in some circumstances, particularly as it has the benefit of being tolerable for long periods of time and suits the need to observe patients with these diseases over timescales of years. The use of actigraphy in trials of treatments for the various kinds of arthritis may improve objectivity of assessment of joint mobility [7].

There are definite issues with the use of motion sensing in clinical trials in the settings suggested above. Most importantly, not enough data have been collected and published from patients with these conditions, nor are there adequate correlations with other measures of disease phenotypes. Analysis of such data that exist has not, to a sufficient extent, adopted the "big data analytics" approach which is required to make sense of the richness of the information content. Thus, we do not know enough yet to understand what may be a crucial subtle signal in the data and what may be just noise. Ideally, a mass effort might be made, mobilizing the resources of patient organizations, to gather and analyze crowd-sourced data using consumer-grade devices. This could form the basis for use in trials and in other clinical research. However, there are suggestions that consumer-grade actigraphy devices may not be precise or accurate enough for this purpose, and it is likely that differences between different device models may prevent generalization of any interpretive algorithms. The net result is that it is likely to be slow and painstaking to convince regulators to accept motion sensing data as valid surrogates of disease state and outcomes. Therefore, this aspect of engineering the clinical trial of the future will lag well behind the community adoption of motion-based wearable devices. It is urgent that the process of realizing their potential in developing better drugs faster begins immediately.

3. CONSUMER DEVICES IN CLINICAL TRIALS

A common issue in considering the use of consumer-connected health devices for clinical research is the heterogeneity of their firmware and software as well as the lack of standards governing them. Such devices, in general, have been designed and built for informal use, the results that they report are an end unto themselves, and not intended to support the supply of data for much more critical applications like the detection of the safety or efficacy of treatments for disease. This lack of standardization, reminiscent of the Betamax versus VHS debate three decades ago, further complicates their use. For somebody wishing to utilize them in a clinical trial, this results in the problem of rational selection of an appropriate model based on understanding of the relative precision and accuracy of competing brands. Furthermore, they will need to understand precisely what they report and the algorithms which they use to convert raw accelerometry data to their readout.

There is a lively ongoing debate about how such devices might be regulated if they are to morph from being consumer devices to supporting more serious healthcare purposes [8]. Currently, the FDA is responsible for ensuring that medical devices are safe and effective. However, a series of bills presented in the US Congress suggest growing sentiment for change in the status quo. Lobbying on the basis that a complex regulatory framework could inhibit future growth and innovation in a promising market has resulted in bills introduced in October 2013 and February 2014 that would exclude "clinical software" from FDA regulation [9]. However, drawing the line between the regulation of devices and mobile app software for supporting telehealth and those to scientifically support drug development is not straightforward. There is no obvious evidence of this issue being addressed urgently by the EU at present, where medical device regulation in general is being reviewed.

There are some instances of mobile devices being used in clinical trials for several years to gather data from patients [10]. Prominent among these are respiratory function devices to measure parameters like FEV_1 and FVC_1. A number of companies provide systems that trial subjects can use frequently in their own homes to make respiratory measurements, as well as collect e-diary and e-patient reported outcomes (ePRO) data. These are transmitted either by mobile telephony or through connection with home computers to a secure site for centralized analysis. It is of interest that, despite the success of home measurement in respiratory disease studies and the fact that they have been well established for a considerable time, the majority of drug trials in this area are still conducted conventionally at trial sites, presumably on the basis that sponsors wish to obtain laboratory quality, though intermittent, data at trial visits.

Home BP measurement became practical over two decades ago as inexpensive and simple to operate electronic devices became available. There are many clinical studies now listed on Clinicaltrials.gov using this, including quite a number of clinical trials of pharmacotherapy. However, this has not really been operated as a true telehealth-based trial and subjects still attend conventionally at regular study visits. Similarly, trials in diabetes often gather home blood glucose data, but these really only supplement other laboratory measurements made at trial center visits. Thus, while home-based respiratory function measurements in trials of asthma and COPD could be thought to represent an early form of connected health, home measurements of BP and blood glucose to date do not really fit the definition.

4. THE TRIAL SUBJECT AS SUB-INVESTIGATOR

People that participate in clinical trials as subjects often do so at significant inconvenience, particularly if the trial is of a preventive intervention or is in stable chronic disease. Simple logistical barriers exist which they have to overcome, such as taking time off work, traveling to the trial site, and dealing with the nontrivial matter of finding car parking when they get there. A trial may sometimes extend over several years, so it is not surprising that drop-out rates may be large, sometimes to the extent that the trial is compromised. Often, the subject is regarded as just that—somebody who is subject to the requirements and edicts of the protocol and of those who implement it. Lip service may be given to the idea that the subject is a true stakeholder, but this is frequently not really acted on. The general public applies the term "guinea pig" more often to describe trial subjects than we should be comfortable with.

It is clear that many protocols contain requirements for the collection of large amounts of information that never contribute to results or conclusions. There is a lot of anecdote about this, but a recent study evaluated of eight oncology trials with nine corresponding publications found that across all the publications a median of 96 data items (18%) were reported in each manuscript, ranging from 11% to 27% per trial. In 8 of the 18 categories, 4% or less of collected data items were used [11]. This is not alone wasteful of time and resources but is also an imposition on subjects for whom, were they to realize it was going to happen, would be unlikely to have consented. Trial data collected at sites also is subject to the well-documented errors of trial staff, necessitating the mass effort of monitoring and correction by clinical research associates (CRAs).

Many, if not most, patients with chronic stable disease are capable of generating and reporting their own data and, if the technology is appropriately designed, can do so with the same level of fidelity as can staff at a trial site. In this, the subject is acting as a true sub-investigator who is thereby much more deeply invested in the study and should be able to participate at much less inconvenience. I specify chronic stable disease as it is clear that studies of acute or unstable disease or those requiring complex clinical assessment or imaging still are required to be done at trial sites. By using appropriate connected health technologies that fully satisfy data standards such as 21CFR Part 11 and the guidelines on electronic source data [12,13], subjects may collect and report their own data, including clinical measurements and ePRO-type diaries, in a manner that ensures that a large part of the data collected in the trial does not require to be monitored because it is "source."

A typical example might be in a cardiovascular (CVS) outcomes trial with a new diabetes drug. Such trials are, in effect, mandatory unless sufficient data can be accumulated from elsewhere in the clinical development program to satisfy the requirement to show CVS safety. Such a trial has a fairly simple objective, namely to test the hypothesis that subjects randomized to the new drug have no more CVS adverse events than do subjects randomized to placebo against the background of best conventional standard of care. Conventionally, the designs of such trials are replicas of previous studies and require tens of thousands of subjects in a brute-force exercise. They usually entail subjects attending trial visits every few months, where blood for glucose, HbA_1c and lipid measurements are taken, as well as a variety of other "interesting" parameters (e.g., fasting insulin) that don't contribute to testing the trial's hypothesis. Trial visits will also collect data on BP and ECG, as well as items possibly like concomitant medications. Ultimately, however, all that matters is the determination at the end of the trial of whether there was an imbalance in CVS events between the two groups, and it is useful to know whether the drug achieved its objective of helping achievement of diabetic control.

In a connected health diabetes CVS outcomes trial, the subjects/sub-investigators would be recruited as normal by a trial site. On entry to the trial, they would measure their own blood glucose and BP several times a day and transmit the results via GSM or internet from the devices directly or via an intermediary smartphone-like device to a central monitoring database that could also transmit ePRO and relevant data from the "internet of things," such as wireless temperature sensors in the refrigerator, if relevant. Their data would be transformed by tracking algorithms to allow the clinical staff at their site to follow their progress, and central data monitoring staff from the sponsor or clinical research organization (CRO) could track their anonymized data. In addition, they would see their own data interpreted in a way that updated them on their own progress and gave them access to advice and continuing training. Those subjects with unsatisfactory diabetic control would be called to visit the trial site for assistance. There would be no regular trial visits: just those required for good patient care of the minority requiring it. Capillary blood would be sent on filter paper for essential measurements to a central laboratory, and ECGs could be done (to detect silent myocardial infarction) annually, not necessarily at the trial site if there was a more convenient location for the subject elsewhere. I estimate from some pilot data that only about 15% of subjects would need to be called to visit the trial sites after trial entry to fulfil the requirements for good patient care. As the other 85% are constantly being monitored by telemetry, their care should be no less, and the investigator's responsibilities under Good Clinical Practice (GCP) and the Declaration of Helsinki would be fulfilled.

The advantages of this approach are obvious. The density of the data on blood glucose would allow conclusions to be drawn regarding diurnal patterns of control and potentially allow each subject to be followed according to their own normative values rather than just by reference to the population distribution. The instantaneous data flow would allow adaptive approaches to the determination of sample size, potentially cutting down on subject numbers and time. The requirement for on-site source data monitoring would fall substantially as most data would be "source." Subject withdrawal is likely to be lessened due to improved convenience and better connection with the study. The net result is likely to be considerably less cost and greater speed of execution of the trial.

No new technology needs to be invented to allow execution of a connected health trial of diabetes. Everything already exists on the market as regulated medical devices already. There needs to be further developed a different kind of role in sponsors and CROs to allow centralized monitoring of large data streams on individual subjects. This role is already being developed to allow risk-based monitoring. Algorithms need to be developed to maximize information from the connected data sources, first probably by using "Big Analytics" to interrogate previously completed trials. Regulators will need to come to terms with this new model. All those involved in sponsoring, designing, and executing trials will need to recognize that the classic way of doing business in chronic disease trials is wasteful and needs radical change. This is probably the most difficult to achieve in our risk-averse industry. Unless change is embraced, the world will change without us.

Subjects who participate in trials are entitled to be acknowledged fully as stakeholders, who in their everyday lives as consumers often employ technology that is many years ahead of the cumbersome traditional way in which we have tested new treatments.

5. TAKE HOME MESSAGE

There continues to be a proliferation of smartphone applications and connected measuring devices that are directed to enabling consumers to monitor aspects of their physiology. At present, these largely revolve around exercise. However, the number of connected medical devices is also increasing.

- There is an increasing opportunity to gather rich data directly from trial subjects at home, displacing some of the traditional activities in trial sites.
- This may move trial subjects from their present, fairly passive role toward being, in a sense, sub-investigators.
- This is likely to increase the proportion of electronic source data gathered, with implications for monitoring and quality assurance.
- Consumer devices, for instance those based on accelerometers, lack common standards of data, sensitivity, accuracy, precision, or calibration. Their use at present to collect important or pivotal data on efficacy or safety in clinical trials would probably not satisfy usual regulatory standards.
- Regulation of the proliferating applications and devices which may cross over from consumer to medical devices will be challenging.

6. SWOT

1. Strength: Source data directly from patients will decrease and change traditional ways in which trials are monitored. Data will be richer, denser, and in considerably greater volume and will contribute to big data analytics systems.
2. Weaknesses: There are substantial challenges for standardization and regulation of devices and systems in clinical trials in a "connected world."
3. Opportunity: More subjects will be enabled to access trials and will be empowered to participate more actively as data gatherers.
4. Threats: Neglecting to address regulatory issues early and failure of regulators to organize for the challenges will delay and possibly confound this opportunity.

7. APPLICABLE REGULATORY GUIDANCE

US Department of Health and Human Services Food and Drug Administration. *Guidance for Industry: Electronic Source Data in Clinical Investigations.* September 2013.

EMA GCP Inspectors Working Group (GCP IWG). Reflection paper on expectations for electronic source data and data transcribed to electronic data collection tools in clinical trials EMA/INS/GCP/454,280/2010: 09 June 2010.

REFERENCES

[1] International Telecommunications Union. Measuring the Information Society 2013. Geneva: ITU; 2013.

[2] Xu Y, Wang L, He J, Bi Y, Li M, Wang T, et al. Prevalence and control of diabetes in Chinese adults. JAMA 2013;310:948–59.

[3] Centers for Disease Control and Prevention (CDC). Vital signs: prevalence, treatment, and control of hypertension—United States, 1999–2002 and 2005–2008. MMWR Morb Mortal Wkly Rep 2011;60:103–8.

[4] Perez Lloret S, Rossi M, Cardinali DP, Merello M. Actigraphic evaluation of motor fluctuations in patients with Parkinson's disease. Int J Neurosci 2010;120:137–43.

[5] McCleery J, Cohen DA, Sharpley AL. Pharmacotherapies for sleep disturbances in Alzheimer's disease. Cochrane Database Syst Rev 2014;21(3):CD009178.

[6] Paudel ML, Taylor BC, Diem SJ, Stone KL, Ancoli-Israel S, Redline S, et al. Association between depressive symptoms and sleep disturbances in community-dwelling older men. J Am Geriatr Soc 2008;56(7):1228–35.

[7] Manheim LM, Dunlop D, Song J, Semanik P, Lee J, Chang RW. Relationship between accelerometer-based measures of physical activity and the Yale Physical Activity Survey in adults with arthritis. Arthritis Care Res Hob 2011;63:1766–72.

[8] Cortez NG, Cohen JD, Kesselheim AS. FDA regulation of mobile health technologies. N Engl J Med 2014;371:372–8.

[9] The preventing regulatory overreach to enhance care technology act of 2014 (Protect Act). S. 2007. 113th Cong. 2nd Sess; 2014. http://beta.congress.gov/bill/113th-congress/senate-bill/2007.

[10] Partridge MR, Schuermann W, Beckman O, Persson T, Polanowski T. Effect on lung function and morning activities of budesonide/formoterol versus salmeterol/fluticasone in patients with COPD. Ther Adv Respir Dis 2009;3:1–11.

[11] O'Leary E, Seow H, Julian J, Levine M, Pond GR. Data collection in cancer clinical trials: too much of a good thing? Clin Trials 2013;10:624–32.

[12] U.S. Department of Health and Human Services Food and Drug Administration. Guidance for industry: electronic source data in clinical investigations. September 2013.

[13] EMA GCP Inspectors Working Group (GCP IWG). Reflection paper on expectations for electronic source data and data transcribed to electronic data collection tools in clinical trials EMA/INS/GCP/454280/2010: June 09, 2010.

CHAPTER 20

Studies Without Sites: The Virtual Trial

Miguel Orri

Contents

1. THE NEED

Participant recruitment is often a major barrier to the feasibility and timely completion of clinical trials. Trial participation is often limited by geographical constraints due to the number of eligible participants who live near trial sites, especially for uncommon medical conditions. In addition, a requirement for multiple visits to the clinical site and a limited number of time slots can create a funnel for trial enrollment and interfere with completion. This dilemma may be enhanced by fact that patients are not always fully engaged in clinical trials, and therefore patient data are not optimally obtained or processed. Although considerable attention is focused on monitoring of medical records and the transcription of those

Re-Engineering Clinical Trials
http://dx.doi.org/10.1016/B978-0-12-420246-7.00020-7

into case report forms, the information obtained from the primary source, the patient, could be improved through better patient engagement, particularly in the light of increasing complexity, which makes clinical studies burdensome for patients. Furthermore, the primary care physician (PCP), often the patients first and most trusted point of contact for healthcare, is mostly not informed about ongoing clinical trials or incentivized to refer patients to clinical trial centers as in most cases they are insufficiently informed about the treatment response of their patients, and in some healthcare systems are also financially disadvantaged by referring their patients to other physicians.

Given these challenges as well as increasing demands on site personnel lead to a decreased interest from investigators in trial participation and maintaining consistent quality across multiple sites can pose additional challenges for study teams. The operation of trial sites (i.e., site management, payments, and monitoring) accounts for most of the costs of conducting clinical trials [1]. The current clinical trial paradigm does not allow sustainable innovation, and a more efficient way of conducting clinical trials is needed to reduce their current cost, improve timelines, and optimize data quality.

In parallel with the contemporary challenges of clinical research, trends are emerging in healthcare that are largely driven by the proliferation of information on Internet. The centralization of specialized healthcare services is enabling the decentralization of basic healthcare, such as improved access and convenience offered by health clinics in retail locations [2]. In parallel with these challenges, the proliferation of health information on Internet is giving rise to the "e-patient," a patient who is engaged, empowered, and online. In 2012, 59% of U.S. adults searched for health information online [3]. The widespread use of mobile phones has decreased socioeconomic and age barriers to web access [4]. Groups of patients with common medical conditions and concerns are also organizing online to share data and initiate research activities [5].

Participatory patient-centered (PPC), web-based, clinical trials could increase patient access to clinical trials; streamline trial conduct; and facilitate rapid reporting of clinical signals and outcomes to regulators, healthcare providers, and patients. The key components of PPC web-based trials are listed in Figure 20.1. More rapid recruitment and the potential to reduce clinical site costs are strong incentives for pharmaceutical companies to conduct web-based trials, and greater availability and convenience will enable more patients to join PPC web-based trials.

- **Subject:**
  - Web-based recruitment
  - Web-based multi-media informed consent process
  - Web-based screening
- **Technology:**
  - Mobile communication device-based efficacy assessments (e.g. e-diary)
  - Interactive remote data capture via secure patient portal
  - Real-time data access for sites, monitors, and auditors
- **Investigator site:**
  - Coordinating function for virtual assessments: patient does not attend investigator site
  - Study drug delivery by overnight courier
  - Study physician/call center available 24/7 by e-mail and/or phone
  - Real-time safety data processing
  - Study data returned to subject

Figure 20.1 Key components of a PPC trial.

2. THE SOLUTION

2.1 The REMOTE Study

The Research on Electronic Monitoring of overactive bladder (OAB) Treatment Experience (REMOTE) study was the first virtual study conducted within the framework of an investigational new drug (IND) application under the supervision of the Food and Drug Administration (FDA) [6]. Although this study assessed a variety of novel concepts and new technologies for data capture and handling, one of the main aims of this study was to demonstrate that it can be conducted in a completely remote manner. However, the modular concept allows for a stepwise improvement of the clinical trial processes for a large number of clinical trials in all phases of clinical development.

In the REMOTE study, which was based in the United States only, potential participants were recruited using a variety of web-based sources, including targeted advertisements on online search engines and health websites; online communities with a potential interest in target disease; online patient advocacy groups, social media sites, and craigslist; as well as from healthcare organizations, community-based clinics, and commercial recruitment vendors.

Potential participants were initially screened for eligibility using web-based questionnaires and laboratory test results. Additional precautionary procedures were included to verify participant identification and screening. To minimize potential fraud, approval was obtained from eligible participants to perform a secure and confidential third-party online identity verification using personal information. The online identity verification process did not include financial or credit checks but used a public records-based service widely for online identity confirmation. To prevent hacking of trial websites, an e-mail confirmation process was required wherein a time-sensitive link was sent to the potential participant's e-mail address. Once e-mail confirmation and identity confirmation were completed, the participants completed the online informed consent process followed by screening questionnaires based on study eligibility criteria. Those who signed the informed consent document and met screening criteria were contacted by the investigator's study staff for a telephone discussion about the trial and review of the informed consent details. After these telephone calls, appropriate patients were countersigned into the study and scheduled for laboratory testing and physical examination. After the study investigator reviewed the test results, those who remained eligible were enrolled in the placebo run-in phase. At this point, participants were sent single-blind study medication by courier to their home. Participants also received a mobile feature phone with a custom application installed for entering e-diary data. Participants who remained interested and eligible were randomized via an interactive voice response/interactive web response system to double-blind treatment and followed up with mobile phone-based diaries and web-based questionnaires. Patients had access to a physician from the investigator team at all times.

2.2 Physician Engagement

In the REMOTE study, a national clinician network was used to do the physical examination and to provide a report to the investigator for his or her evaluation, similarly as this is often done with electrocardiograms in conventional studies. For many late-phase studies, such tasks including blood or urine sampling and simple safety follow-up examinations, which do not need study-specific training, could be performed by the patient's own PCP without making them investigators. This would keep the PCPs closely connected with their patients' treatment and up to date with the clinical trial progress while getting reimbursed for their services.

From a study site perspective, this new paradigm makes the conduct of clinical trials much more efficient. As protocols become more and more complex and requirements for training and documentation compliance become more burdensome, it can be difficult for site personnel to maintain their focus on a small number of participants on a part time basis while adhering to all protocol requirements. This new paradigm allows sites to become coordinating centers and dedicate staff to recruit large numbers of patients in a short timeframe, and a lot of the documentation can be entered by the participants themselves directly into the system. As clinical trial platforms become commercially available, study sites can use a single platform for the management of several studies as these get added in a modular manner, and at the same time most of the training and documentation could be handled by one system, which would enable sites to work more efficiently.

2.3 Recruitment

Potential subjects may be identified through many different sources that may be available on a local, regional, national, or study-wide level. Although most studies still rely on small investigator databases and several different advertising modalities, the virtual trial model offers itself up to web-based advertising, collaboration with large patient organizations, and regional or national health databases as they become more and more available.

To engage potential participants from the beginning, it is essential to make the recruitment process as patient friendly as possible. Long web-based questionnaires over multiple screens may not be the best way even if a helpdesk is at hand. At the early stage of recruitment, it is paramount to gain the interest of potential participants in a trial, which may be suitable for them, by providing the essential facts about the study and demonstrating that their concerns are being addressed, allowing them to identify with the study. It is self-evident that all the information provided does need ethics committee or institutional review board (IRB) approval before it is presented to potential trial participants.

Another way of making the process more patient friendly and efficient, by reducing duplication of work in determining the eligibility of a potential participant, may be to engage a recruitment vendor who can elicit patient eligibility using an approved study questionnaire over the phone and entering the data directly into the study database that can then be verified by the investigator. In this way, the burden is taken away from the participant.

2.4 Identity Verification

Although in conventional trials, the patient is often known to the investigator or at least the existence of a real person as well as the age group and sex can easily be identified, this poses a new challenge for virtual trials where additional steps are needed to ensure the integrity of the trial.

At least in the United States, there are vendors who use information from publicly available databases to verify a person's identity based on questions that can only be answered by the individual. This system is also used by banks and government agencies and allows for a high level of security. However, it requires a participant to enter personal information such as a national insurance number and address to be identified, and many participants might not be willing to enter such information over Internet specially at a stage when they do not even know whether they are eligible for the study. Furthermore, there might not be enough data publicly available for a person to be identified, or the participant might get answers wrong, which could automatically exclude the person from participation.

As it is important to ensure that the person who signs the informed consent is actually the person participating in the clinical trial, it is essential that this link can be established and documented. This may be accomplished through the use of a trusted healthcare provider such as the patient's PCP, a pharmacist, or a local laboratory who may be engaged in the clinical trial.

2.5 Informed Consent Process

To accommodate the virtual nature of a clinical trial, the informed consent process needs to be well thought through and may necessitate several steps depending on the type of research and potential risks for the participants. However, to enhance recruitment and retention and to provide better quality data for clinical trials, it is important to have a patient-centric informed consent process that leverages multimedia to thoroughly and consistently explain a study and to achieve a more knowledgeable and engaged patient. At the same time, this process needs to be well documented and compliant with International Conference on Harmonization good clinical practices and acceptable to regulatory agencies, IRBs, and ethics committees. Ideally, this is handled by a centralized process, enhancing the ease of retrieval of source data for inspections, audits, and monitoring.

In the case of the REMOTE study, each participant began the informed consent process by viewing and listening to an online automated slide presentation, in which the principal investigator described the essential elements of the trial, followed by a review of the full informed consent document online. Participants could print a hard copy of the informed consent document for easier viewing. Before signing the informed consent document, each participant was required to pass a multiple-choice test confirming the individual's understanding of the informed consent document. After the participant passed the informed consent document test and read and signed the informed consent document, each participant also received a phone call from study personnel who discussed the informed consent document with the participant, answered any questions about the informed consent document or the trial, reviewed subject-reported medications and medical history as appropriate, and addressed any concerns. If the individual fulfilled study eligibility requirements and remained interested in participating in the trial, the study investigator countersigned the informed consent document. Two hard copies of the electronically or hand-signed informed consent document were then mailed to the participant. One copy was for the participant's records and the second copy was to be given to the PCP or health professional, should they seek medical care during the study.

This process provides a real-time tracking option, a more consistent and standardized process across sites where both the information provided to subjects and the resultant understanding are well documented and allow for real-time remote monitoring and audit access. The flow of the informed consent process is illustrated in Figure 20.2. This process has also been acknowledged by the U.S. Department of Health and Human Services in a document on Considerations and Recommendations Concerning Internet Research and Human Subjects Research Regulations [7].

As the computer technology is developing at a fast pace and an increasing number of informed consent solution providers enter the market, more patient friendly tablet or even downloadable application-based solutions may be more prominent in the future not only for virtual trials but also as a better informed consent process for conventional studies. For global studies, country-specific requirements such as witness signatures or validity of electronic signatures need to be considered and incorporated as needed.

2.6 Dispensing Study Medication

The dispensation of study medication also needs careful planning in the virtual setting, and country-specific laws and regulations require consideration especially for investigational new drugs (INDs). In the United States, for example, federal regulations state that study medications under an IND application must be shipped to study investigators for administration only to participants

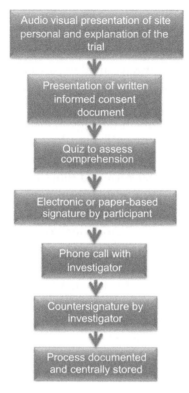

Figure 20.2 Electronic informed consent process.

who are under their direct supervision, an investigational product waiver of this requirement of 21 CFR 312.61 under 21 CFR 312.10 [8] may need to be requested by the sponsor of a clinical trial. Other countries may have requirements for drugs to be shipped from a depot or through a pharmacy. The chain of custody needs to be clearly documented, and some additional steps from the participant's side are needed to ensure the safe delivery and use of study medication. For example, once the study investigator has authorized the dispensation of trial medication possibly through an interactive response system, it may be sent to the participant's physical address using an overnight delivery service with a signature requirement. The participant then needs to confirm receipt of trial medication and the condition of the contents via the study computer portal. Receipt of this confirmation may trigger the start of a treatment phase. In each phase of the study, used and unused study medication bottles can be returned by each participant to the investigator site by courier using a preaddressed stamped envelope. Once received at the investigator site, study drug will be subject to the usual reconciliation and destruction process.

2.7 Web-Based Computer System

One of the key elements of the virtual trial setting is a computer portal designed for electronic data capture directly from the participant who may enter consent and study related data as well as for the data captured at the assessments throughout the study. This may include patient reported outcomes, and data from other linked up devices such as glucometers, blood pressure cuffs, or weighing scales, to name just a few. These data will be accessible to the investigator in the portal, and the investigator will review these to assess the eligibility or the progress of a subject. The review of screening data may also include medical history, physical examination, and laboratory reports from the PCP, which may be entered into the portal. The investigator can review all these data, and this review may also be documented in the portal. As these electronic clinical trial platforms are developing at a very fast pace, newer systems allow for patient recruitment, site management, clinical trial management and reporting all to be performed on the same platform allowing for even more efficiencies in the conduct of clinical trials.

It is important that the computer system is compliant with all applicable guidances and regulations, appropriately tested and validated, and retained in accordance with relevant record retention requirements.

2.8 Electronic Data Capture

The electronic remote data capture is another key elements of virtual trials that may be used in a large number of conventional clinical trials to improve data quality and accessibility. It requires some up-front investment of time and resource to define the system requirements, similar to a well-designed electronic case report form. The fundamental difference is that participants can enter data directly into the system with the option for logic checks at the time of data entry; this capability may substantially improve data quality and reduce the need for monitoring of source data at the trial site, leading to data queries, as the data have been entered directly into the system by the participant, reducing the risk of data transfer errors. Any remaining data queries can be addressed in real time as the data can be monitored as soon as they have been entered, enabling the investigator and sponsor to get faster access to safety signals on a patient and study level. The real-time access to the data by the investigator also allows the site personnel to follow up on missing data immediately and therefore potentially improve the data quality. It may also lead to substantial time saving at the end of the study as database lock may be achieved soon after last subject last visit rather than several weeks later as is often the case in conventional studies. The data flow for a virtual trial model is illustrated in Figure 20.3.

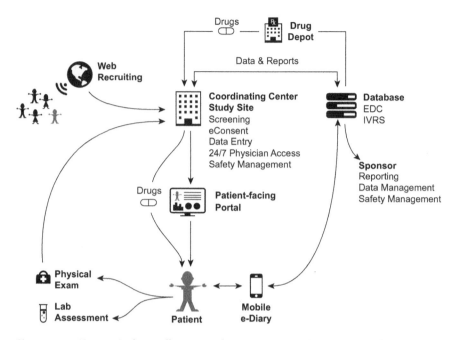

Figure 20.3 Electronic data collection and management. ECD, electronic data capture; IVRS, interactive voice response system.

2.9 Safety Monitoring

As in other trials conducted by community-based research sites rather than physician practices, the Clinical Trial Coordinating Center in a virtual study provides medical care for the subjects in the trial by referring subjects to their own PCP, a specialist, or emergency care as appropriate. This should be explained to the participants in the consent document.

As in conventional clinical trials, all adverse events are reportable from the time that the subject provides informed consent, either directly by the subject, the PCP, or any other treating healthcare professional.

The time of awareness of an adverse event by the sponsor is the time of receipt of the initial report at the call center or the computer portal.

All adverse events have to be followed up as appropriate by the investigator to obtain information adequate to determine the severity, causality, and outcome of the event and to assess whether it meets the criteria for classification as a serious adverse event. It is therefore necessary to have a process in place that ensures the investigator has access and documents his review of all reported adverse events within 24 h.

2.10 Patient Engagement

Although this concept enables the patient to participate without geographic limitations mainly from the comfort of their home and at the time of day that is convenient to them, it is not in itself a guarantee for patient engagement and compliance; therefore, it is essential that this subject is addressed separately. In the absence of a face-to-face interaction with the investigator, the computer interface used has to be simple, intuitive, trustworthy, and suitable for the study population. An Internet-based study website that requires the use of a web browser with several access steps may not be suitable for an elderly population, particularly in less developed countries, whereas a study in adolescents might offer itself up to a game-like application to engage participants in the flow of the study. To make the system as easy as possible for the participant to access, computer tablets may be the best solution as they can be preprogrammed to allow for access with the push of a single button while the connectivity to Internet or Cloud may be established in the background. Although currently it may be advisable to provide participants with a preprogrammed device, one can well imagine that with increasing penetration of smart phones, a downloadable clinical trial application might be a viable alternative for virtual clinical trials in the near future.

Apart from the technical aspects, an effort should be made to keep the participants informed of their progress to encourage them to perform all study-required tasks as needed. Again, the direct real-time access to the subject via a tablet of phone-based communication device allows the investigator team to remind the participants of upcoming assessments or request any missing data in a timely manner while reinforcing the message that their contribution is important and appreciated. The device can also be used to provide participants with information about the study or their disease, but provisions should be made to give the participant control of how much information they want to receive.

Each study population will respond to different ways of engagement, and this needs to be considered at an early stage of the trial design.

Finally, it is part of this model to provide individual study data back to participants at the end of the study in an electronic format, which would allow them to share the data with their healthcare provider and to add it to their personal health records.

2.11 Applicable Regulations

The first completely virtual clinical trial under an IND application has been successfully conducted while adhering to all ICH GCP principles and all applicable FDA regulations. In contrast to the sometimes assumed inertia from regulators toward innovation, this new study paradigm received a lot of interest and support both from the FDA as well as from European regulatory agencies, indicating their willingness to consider new approaches to safely and efficiently conduct clinical trials. However, virtual trials are still a new entity; therefore, it would be advisable to engage regulatory agencies early in the planning stages for a new study, as each study will be assessed on its own merit, and in other jurisdictions regulators may be more apprehensive to this innovative approach.

It is also important to assess telemedicine and prescribing laws for each country where the study is to be conducted. In the United States, for example, prescribing laws are not governed by federal law and therefore each individual state has its own and often very different legislation and interpretation of drug dispensation in the framework of a clinical trial. Telemedicine and prescribing laws in some legislations may not be supportive of virtual trials. There is also often a lack of clarity on the regulation of virtual clinical trials, and future changes are likely to occur. Further consideration should be given to the rules and regulations of the governing bodies for physicians in each participating country that in some instances do not allow doctors to diagnose or prescribe medicines to patients they have not personally seen and examined, without the risk of loosing their license to practice.

Finally, Institutional Review Boards and Ethics Committees may not be familiar with the virtual trial setting, and proactive and collaborative communication approaches may be the best way to address potential concerns and built confidence in this new model.

2.12 Generalizability

Completely virtual trials, at this point, may only be suitable for a limited number of late-phase clinical trials where the safety profile of a medicine has been established. At the same time, it is those large postapproval phase IIIb and IV trials where the biggest efficiencies can be achieved. There is also an increasing demand for real-world data, necessitating more of these large trials, often requiring 10,000 patients or more, which can be facilitated by the virtual trial setting with the opportunity of realizing substantial efficiencies. The regulatory authorities, such as FDA and some European agencies, have been supportive of this innovative approach and generally encourage the pursuit of innovative and more efficient ways of conducting clinical trials.

Although some of the above-mentioned considerations focused on clinical trials under an IND application, most principles equally apply for trials with approved drugs and many elements of this model might be even more attractive for noninterventional trials.

It needs to be emphasized that the virtual trial model by no means is an all-or-nothing decision. Many of the individual elements can be incorporated in a large number of clinical trials at all stages of development to improve data quality, patient engagement, and efficiency. Prime examples are the improved informed consent process and the remote data capture directly from the participant with the benefit of real-time data availability.

3. SWOT

1. Strengths

Virtual trials are designed for those most relevant: the patients. This has a positive impact on recruitment, retention and data quality. The concept enables trials with a reduced number of sites and remote monitoring which can lead to substantial cost savings.

2. Weaknesses

Not every trial is suitable to be conducted completely virtual. Overall complexity in planning at the sponsor end may initially be higher while the teams become familiar with the new electronic clinical trial platforms.

3. Opportunities

The growing population of "digital native" patients that are easily using modern communication tools and also seeking more independence in their lifestyle will prefer a "virtual" over a site-based study.

4. Threats

The lack of direct face-to-face contact with the investigator may not be the preferred option for elderly patients.

4. TAKE HOME MESSAGE

Virtual clinical trials are there to stay. Either in their entirety or as elements of a more conventional model, there is a potential for substantial benefits for patients, investigators, healthcare providers, and sponsors. Patient engagement is paramount for recruitment, retention, and data quality and needs to be thoroughly considered, both in studies with and without face-to-face interaction. The infrastructure and technology needed for virtual clinical studies is readily available, and the first virtual study has been successfully conducted. Regulatory authorities are supportive of this innovative approach as long as the fundamental patient rights, confidentiality, and safety are not compromised; however, the suitability of virtual trials needs to be assessed on a case-by-case basis. Even in a more conventional clinical trial setting, the available technology allows for substantial improvements in patient recruitment, consent, engagement, and retention; and data collection and handling as well as site selection and management can be substantially improved, potentially resulting in improved data quality, reduced timelines, and significant cost savings.

REFERENCES

[1] Eisenstein EL, Lemons 2nd PW, Tardiff BE, Schulman KA, Jolly MK, Califf RM. Reducing the costs of phase III cardiovascular clinical trials. Am Heart J 2005;149(3):482–8.

[2] Christensen CM, Grossman JH, Hwang J. The innovator's prescription: a disruptive solution for health care. New York: McGraw-Hill; 2009.

[3] Fox S, Duggan M. Health online 2013. Pew Research Center's Internet & American Life Project; January 15, 2013. Available at: http://pewinternet.org/Reports/2013/Health-online.aspx.

[4] Smith A. Mobile access 2010. Pew Research Center's Internet & American Life Project; July 7, 2010. Available at: http://pewinternet.org/Reports/2010/Mobile-Access-2010.aspx.

[5] Wicks P, Vaughan TE, Massagli MP, Heywood J. Accelerated clinical discovery using self-reported patient data collected online and a patient-matching algorithm. Nat Biotechnol 2011;29(5):411–4.

[6] Orri M, Craig HL, Bradly PJ, Anthony JC, Steven RC. Web-based trial to evaluate the efficacy and safety of tolterodine ER 4 mg in participants with overactive bladder: REMOTE trial. Contemp Clin Trials July 2014;38(2):190–7.

[7] Considerations and recommendations concerning internet research and human subjects research regulations, with revisions final document, approved at SACHRP meeting. March 12–13, 2013. Available at: http://www.hhs.gov/ohrp/sachrp/mtgings/2013%20March%20Mtg/internet_research.pdf.

[8] Investigational New Drug Application. Code of federal regulations Title 21, Volume 5, Chapter I, Part 312 (21CFR312). Food and Drug Administration. Available at: http://www.accessdata.fda.gov/scripts/cdrh/cfdocs/cfcfr/CFRSearch.cfm?CFRPart=312&showFR=1.

From Data to Decisions

CHAPTER 21

Re-Engineering Clinical Research with Data Standards

Wayne Kubick

Contents

1. THE NEED

Research and discovery are inherently creative processes. And creativity wants to know no bounds. The prospect of imposing standards on any aspect of research is thus likely to be greeted with some resistance no matter how compelling the potential benefits may seem to be.

And this was also the case with the initial efforts to introduce the use of data standards for clinical research studies beginning in the 1990s. It was not just a battle of the free-range versus fences, but grounded in fundamentally differing attitudes about the relative roles of different participants in the research process and how they should work together. Only a statistician can truly understand data. Some said, "You just can't trust the clinician to interpret complex data appropriately." Who knows what evils or pestilence would be unleashed if we unlock the Pandora's box of secrets by making

Re-Engineering Clinical Trials
http://dx.doi.org/10.1016/B978-0-12-420246-7.00021-9

research data, using universally standardized formats and terminologies, widely available and understandable to just about anyone?

Fortunately, in a data-transaction-driven world, attitudes do change. Imagine how difficult it would be to sequence genomics data if science hadn't agreed to represent DNA using the fundamental CATG alphabet. In the case of clinical research, data were commonly captured on CRFs or in batch transfers of lab data, such an alphabet, syntax, and a set of terminologies were provided though the Clinical Data Interchange Standards Consortium (CDISC) [1].

1.1 The Early Days

Data standards were hardly a hot topic among industry and regulatory executives back in 1997. Most pharmaceutical sponsors and contract research organizations (CROs) were using one of a very small number of available commercial clinical data management systems on a mainframe or mini-computer—or else building their own. Remote data entry was an unproven, unreliable, and costly alternative. Statisticians worked entirely with a text editor in SAS. Some companies viewed their systems as a competitive advantage and guarded their libraries, tools, and practices closely. And many clinical researchers, like most other scientists, had learned their craft with spreadsheets on a PC. When designing a study, you are focused on the how to prove a hypothesis through a protocol document—organizing your data was just something you did to report your results at the end, one study at a time. Of course, these were the salad days for pharmaceutical companies, who were enjoying their place in one of the most profitable industries of that time and could afford to take their time and worry about putting data together for, say, an integrated summary of safety once they were ready to prepare their regulatory submission.

Some early initial attempts at data standardization arose around regulatory submissions. As new drug applications (NDAs) became increasingly large and complex, FDA began to realize that it would be difficult to sustain a timely review process working with paper alone. Even if there was enough time, there wasn't enough room to store all the paper—or find that one specific page you needed for a specific question at just the right moment. This recognition led to the development of computer-assisted new drug applications (CANDAs) in the mid-1990s [2]—an attempt to put regulatory submissions on personal computers that could be delivered to FDA along with a truckload of paper. Because of the immense volume of information in an NDA, CANDA workstations often were the size of a Volkswagen, with two large CRT monitors, a hefty personal computer, multiple tapes, magnetic and optical disk drives, and a printer on one or more over-sized carts. Though most CANDAs were focused on searchable text and scanned images, a few did include database search and query tools as well. Usually the notion of standards was limited to file format—WordPerfect and tagged image file format (TIFF), maybe SAS, and eventually portable document format (PDF). The European DAMOS program tried to explore data structures, but didn't get very far since data was not required for European submissions, and DAMOS did not find traction in the United States where *data* was required. But the computers were difficult for reviewers to use, often crashed, and the lack of usable common standards meant the promise of CANDAs was not realized. Eventually, the FDA ran out of patience—and room—for the carts.

Meanwhile, CDISC was just getting established as a group of people who saw the need for data standards met together at a Drug Industry Association meeting in 1997 to discuss what they could do about this [3]. CDISC efforts initially focused on the development of a glossary of terms [4] commonly used in clinical research—a significant prerequisite for getting a conversation going. But an opportunity to do something more directly involved with data arose when FDA issued a new set of guidance documents in 1999 [5] to encourage submission of regulatory data in electronic format. These guidance documents specified the use of PDF file format for documents and SAS Version 5 Transport format for data and also described some tips for how to organize the information in a submission. Since sponsors were still of the mind to avoid standardization at that time, the arrival of an FDA guidance stating that they wanted electronic data submissions and saw the benefits of organizing data in a consistent manner, suddenly drew some industry attention. A small group of volunteers from CDISC saw the advantage of this guidance and how it could be leveraged to move forward on data standards, resulting in the creation of a metadata model for describing submission data [6]. Before long, CDISC had developed a complete set of detailed specifications for organizing submission data [7] Study Data Tabulation Model (SDTM), Standard for Exchange of Non-Clinical Data (SEND), Analysis Data Model (ADaM), and Define.xml) as well as a standard for exchanging Case Report Form (CRF) data between disparate clinical data management systems, the operational data model (ODM), and a laboratory data exchange standard. With the later addition of the Clinical Data Acquisition Standards Harmonization (CDASH) standard for case report form data and a Protocol Representation Model, CDISC was able to provide a complete set of standards (Figure 21.1) to represent and exchange

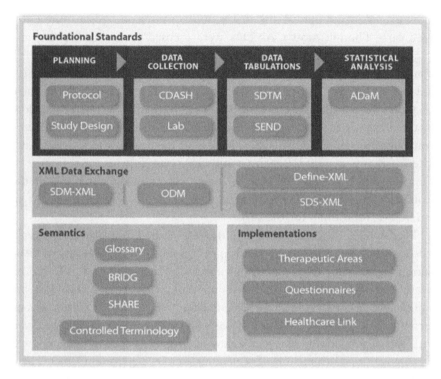

Figure 21.1 CDISC data standards. http://www.cdisc.org/standards-and-implementations – *used with permission.*

nonclinical and clinical data across the entire clinical trial process. Table 21.1 depicts an overview of the principal CDISC standards currently available.

2. THE SOLUTION

2.1 Realizing the Benefits of Data Standards

In July 2004, then FDA Commissioner Lester Crawford announced that FDA would accept CDISC SDTM datasets from sponsors in regulatory submissions [8]. Though the announcement did not specify that this would be a regulatory requirement, a notice of proposed rule change to require SDTM data was posted in the Federal Register a few years later [9]. While the initial announcement provided tangible evidence that sponsors would eventually need to provide data standards to FDA, there was no clear implementation timeline, so many reacted with a wait and see attitude. Those who chose to begin using SDTM sooner were faced with the realization that they'd most likely have to begin by converting existing legacy data into

Table 21.1 Overview of principle CDISC standards for clinical research

Research application area	CDISC standard	Description	Current version/ date	Other relevant standards
Foundational				
Study planning	Protocol representation model (PRM)	BRIDG-based model representing standard protocol content elements and relationships	V1 2010	None
Data collection/study conduct	CDASH	Clinical data acquisitions standards harmonization—describes basic data collection fields for CRF data with guidelines, best practices	V1.1 2010	None
Data collection/study conduct	CDASH SAE supplement	CDASH standard describing basic data collection fields for ICH E2B SAE data with implementation guidelines, best practices	V1 2013	ICH E2B HL7 ICSR
Data collection/study conduct	LAB	Standard model for the acquisition and interchange of clinical lab data between lab and sponsor/CRO recipients	V1.0.1 2003	HL7 v2 lab message LOINC
Submission/analysis	ADaM models	Analysis data model—describes fundamental principles and standards for creating analysis datasets and metadata ADaM time to event model ADaM adverse event model	V2.1 2009[a] V1 2013 V1 2013	None
Submission/analysis	ADaM IG	Implementation guide that describes standard data structures, conventions and variables used with the ADaM model	V1 2009	None

Continued

Table 21.1 Overview of principle CDISC standards for clinical research—cont'd

Research application area	CDISC standard	Description	Current version/date	Other relevant standards
Foundational (SDTM family)				
Submission/tabulation	SDTM	Study data tabulation model describes principles of representing clinical and nonclinical tabulation data	V1.4 2013 V1.3 2012[a]	None
Submission/tabulation	SDTMIG	SDTM implementation guide for human clinical trials (drug products and biologics)	V3.2 2013 V3.1.3 2012[a]	
Submission/tabulation	SEND	Standard for exchange of nonclinical data: SDTM IG to represent data from nonclinical studies	V3.0 2011[a]	
Submission/tabulation	SDTMIG-MD	SDTM implementation guide for medical devices—to represent data from clinical trials using medical devices	V1.0 2012	
Submission/tabulation	SDTMIG-AP	SDTM implementation guide for associated persons—to represent data about persons who are not study subjects (family, caregivers)	V1.0 2013	None
Foundational (XML data exchange)				
Study planning	Study design model (SDM-XML)	XML schema specification based on ODM for representing clinical study design, including structure, workflow, and timing	V1 2011	HL7 study design structured document (DSTU)

Data collection/study conduct	ODM	CDISC standard for the regulatory compliant acquisition, exchange and archive of clinical trials data and metadata	V1.3.2 2013	None
Submission metadata	Define-XML	XML schema specification to describe metadata for SDTM, SEND, and ADaM submission datasets	V2.0 2013[a]	None
Submission/dataset exchange	Study dataset-XML	XML schema specification for representing study datasets associated with Define-XML metadata	V1 Draft 2013	SAS V5 Transport
Semantics				
Semantics	Glossary	Glossary with definitions of acronyms and terms commonly used in clinical research	2011	None
Semantics	Controlled terminology	Controlled terminology to support CDISC standards such as SDTM, CDASH, and ADaM (in partnership with NCI EVS)	Quarterly; Pkg 16 2013	MedDRA, SNOMED CT
Semantics/model	BRIDG	Biomedical research integrated domain group—UML model of the semantics of protocol-driven clinical research	V3.2 2012	None
Semantics/metadata	CDISC SHARE	CDISC metadata repository—electronic source for all CDISC standard metadata and terminology	R1 2014	NCI CaDSR

Continued

Table 21.1 Overview of principle CDISC standards for clinical research —cont'd

Research application area	CDISC standard	Description	Current version/date	Other relevant standards
Implementations				
Study planning > submission/analysis	Therapeutic area standards	User guides describing how to apply CDISC foundational standards with controlled terminologies on clinical studies in specific disease areas	Ongoing since 2011	Various ontology and common data element libraries
Study planning > submission/tabulation	Questionnaires	SDTM implementation guide supplements with annotated CRFs and controlled terminology for representing data from questionnaires commonly used in clinical studies	2013	None
Study planning > conduct	Healthcare link	A suite of CDISC and IHE standards and "enablers" to improve the workflow of clinicians doing research leveraging electronic health records and research systems	Ongoing since 2004	None

[a]Specification in FDA guidance.
http://www.cdisc.org/standards-and-implementations – used with permission.

SDTM, which required significant data transformation and validation challenges. While SDTM might eventually become more familiar to regulatory reviewers than any individual sponsor's proprietary data habits and enable reviewers to use standardized review, visualization, and analysis tools to look more deeply into the data, the effort of conversion was initially viewed as an added cost and risk factor, which was compounded when SDTM had to be aligned with analysis datasets [10].

In 2006, a Gartner report predicted that while total adoption of data standards from the start would eventually save billions, the return on investment would decrease by 60% if only adopted at the submission stage [11]. But the SDTM standard [12] was designed for representing tabulation data for the commonly used domains that were typically included with most clinical studies that had been traditionally sent to FDA as long listings in PDF format—and not necessarily optimized for capturing data on CRFs. To fully capitalize on the benefits of applying standards from the start, sponsors would need structured protocol-level information [13] and standardized CRF content—the latter of which became possible after the release of the CDISC Clinical Data Acquisition Standards Harmonization (CDASH) effort in 2008 [14].

2.2 Data Overload and Quality

Data standards do not necessarily reduce the volume of data that can lead to data overload; however, the CDASH team recognized that they could certainly motivate researchers to avoid collecting unnecessary data [15] and substantially reduce the stress for the sites of dealing with data when data conforms to known structures and familiar conventions. Certainly, most would agree that it's easier to read and rapidly comprehend something that's written in your native language, and CDISC data standards are the common language of clinical research. Data that conforms to known standards simply makes researchers more productive, whether by allowing reuse of common building blocks in setting up studies or in enabling the use of off-the-shelf review tools without the need for excessive configuration, or in creating analysis programs or, finally, in interpreting final results [16]. Just as any post office employee knows that it's easier to deal with the mail once it's been sorted and stacked, so does clinical data become more useful once it's recognizably organized for use according to data standards.

The impact of data standards on data quality has barely been scratched to date in the literature. One of the benefits of the full set of CDISC submission standards was to help FDA reviewers become more productive and minimize misinterpretations of the data [17]. Similarly, having sponsors designing study databases with a clear, consistent end in mind should help to improve operational efficiency by increasing reuse of software components and helping to avoid common errors both by leveraging the learning curve and making it possible to use standard edit checks to identify errors sooner.

But, as the Gartner study realized, an even more fundamental benefit of standards on quality can be achieved when standards are employed at the earliest stages of study planning—in protocol and CRF design [18]. When protocols are defined using the same standardized descriptions of collections of data elements, it should be possible to use these descriptions to set up data collection forms in a clinical data management system, which in turn can generate data listings that conform, in general, to SDTM datasets that provide inputs for analysis.

The FDA is well aware of this. While many of the current FDA guidelines focus on the end product they will receive [19], FDA has long recognized the critical importance of end-to-end traceability of study data, and FDA experts have contributed to efforts to develop structured protocol models. The need for standardized CRF representations was identified as opportunity 45 in the FDA's 2006 Critical Path Opportunities List, [20] which recognized that use of standard CDASH CRF representations can eliminate errors at the site since site personnel are more likely to use familiar CRFs correctly and consistently with fewer misinterpretations.

3. APPLICABLE REGULATIONS

3.1 Standards and Regulatory Authorities

As noted earlier, the ability of CDISC to gain traction among pharmaceutical sponsors was significantly boosted by the FDA's 2004 announcement of their support for SDTM. While the business case for standards should arguably be an adequate carrot alone, it does require significant upfront investment, change, and even some perceived risk to be realized, likely over a multiyear period. As a result, many sponsors likely convinced themselves that they were doing just fine enough using their own internal standards instead of transitioning to CDISC, and either postponed using CDISC or adopted the practice of converting legacy data, which by its very nature only increased costs as an extra step at the end. So, for many, it would take an extra stick wielded by regulators to push them to go all in.

It took some time, but the stick finally began to appear in 2013, which saw the issuance of a clear statement from FDA requiring use of CDISC [21].

Also in 2013, the European Medicines Authority announced a commitment to support data transparency initiatives by requiring that research data be made available publicly, with the apparent goal of eventually requiring conformance to CDISC as well [22]. This was further enforced by statements from the Pharmaceuticals and Medical Devices Agency, Japan (PMDA), announcing a pilot and a plan to require the use of CDISC standards by 2016 [23]. Recognition of the importance of using CDISC standards in all three regions of the International Conference for Harmonization (ICH) offered a compelling case for sponsors to accelerate their internal plans for implementing CDISC standards.

The reason for considering the use of clinical data standards as part of a data transparency initiative like that of the European Medicines Agency (EMA) is directly related to one of the key value propositions—data standards make it possible to pool, compare, and analyze disparate data sources in order to support knowledge discovery. This expectation, in fact, was recognized by Dr. Norman Stockbridge of FDA when proposing the creation of the Janus Data Warehouse in 2002 [24]—a project that had a significant influence on the development of the CDISC SDTM standard. By providing a framework where clinical data could be easily pooled together to support aggregate and comparative analysis, FDA reviewers could conceivably [25] improve their ability to compare the safety and effectiveness of new compounds to current standards of care and more likely be able to continue to build aggregate safety databases that depict how a drug's safety profile evolves over time [26].

Of course, the ability to pool and aggregate data from different drugs or studies in a scientifically sound manner depends on more than structural data standards [27]. Since each clinical study protocol is unique, with different target endpoints, objectives, exposures, populations, and constraints, it's essential to be able to provide context that can guide what data sources can be combined with integrity, which is the purpose of a structured protocol standard. In other words, first you must find which protocols are capable of comparison, and then you combine the data from those protocols before seeking knowledge from the pooled database. Second, while the structures help, it's essential also to have consistent, controlled terminology so that the data values within the database mean the same thing. CDISC has established a controlled terminology initiative in partnership with the National Cancer Institute's Enterprise Vocabulary Services (EVS) [28] toward that end. Third, it's most essential that different individuals develop a common understanding of how to use the standards and how to minimize individual judgments that can lead to inconsistencies in how data is represented—which will likely compromise the integrity of the pooled database. This is an evolving process, involving better standards that close current gaps, better training and accumulated experience, and improved validation tools and techniques to identify inconsistencies and encourage wider adoption among users of data standards.

But clearly, the ability to use standards consistently on the broad reservoir of current and past research data and make it available to a broader research community has the potential to drive dramatic new insights in the use of medical products to improve patient lives—even in some cases to potentially bring back past failed drugs and reapply them for new, safer uses.

3.2 Collaborative Initiatives to Develop Standards

While the major regulatory authorities were still formulating their messages regarding data standards in 2012, other discussions relevant to clinical data standards were also occurring among a group of senior leaders for some of the world's largest pharmaceutical organizations, who were seeking to identify common areas of need where they could work together directly in a precompetitive manner. The benefits of such collaboration initiatives had been previously demonstrated by the Innovative Medicines Initiative in Europe [29], among other public–private partnerships. These discussions resulted in the establishment of TransCelerate Biopharma, Inc. (TCB) in 2012 [30]. TCB's initial portfolio included five major programs [31], one of which was to contribute to the development of therapeutic-area data standards. The importance of applying data standards to specific therapeutic areas of clinical research has long been recognized—since it is those efficacy- and disease-related questions relevant to a particular disease area, patient population, and strategic focus area where the greatest and most impactful benefits can be achieved. But it was the explicit mandate embedded in law through the Food and Drug Administration Amendments Act (FDAAA) of 2012 [32] that encoded this in law that finally caught the attention level of C-level scientific and business executives at major pharmaceutical companies. By mid-2012, TCB announced plans to work with CDISC, FDA, and the Critical Path Institute [33] (a nonprofit public–private partnership) to participate in a therapeutic data standards initiative under the Coalition for Advancing Standards and Therapies (CFAST) [34].

While CDISC had released six earlier documents on therapeutic-area standards [35], the products had generally been limited in scope and often took two or more years to complete. CFAST provided a vehicle for TCB to contribute financial and dedicated in-kind resources to help speed up the development of new standards under an enhanced CDISC process that previously depended largely on the availability of volunteers. The first new standards released under the CFAST initiative were completed in less than a year, with products that addressed a wider scope that was intended to be meaningful to clinical and medical experts, as well as data managers and statistical programmers.

3.3 Realizing the Promise—Putting Standards to Work

While increased regulatory and industry acceptance of data standards has recently opened the door to finally achieving the benefits long promised by data standards, it's clear that the real work has only just begun. As more and more therapeutic-area standards are produced, the burden of ensuring consistency and reusability increases, so the prior paradigm of getting people together to work with spreadsheets and documents over telephone meetings was recognized as no longer sufficient to support the expanding need. It was also clear that standards had to walk a thin tightrope between both ensuring that early adopters don't have to change course midstream as new versions of standards are issued and also being able to more rapidly produce new works—even as science continues to evolve with new methods and areas of interest that require the standards to grow and adapt.

The need to provide a systems infrastructure to develop, house, and deliver standards as electronic metadata led to the development of the CDISC Shared Health and Clinical Research Electronic Library (SHARE) [36]. CDISC SHARE will make it possible to accelerate the development of new therapeutic standards based on reusable high-level research conceptual components, and deliver standard metadata directly to systems for implementation across the full project lifecycle from design through analysis. SHARE will also make it possible to express relationships not just between the various CDISC standards and concepts, but also externally to integrate public ontologies and concepts used in the conduct of healthcare. The potential of reusing healthcare information for research purposes and embedding research concepts more in the conduct of healthcare-related services to many more patients offers a compelling vision for vastly improving the health and care of patients in the future. The Institute of Medicine has explored this intriguing idea in their report on the Learning Healthcare System [37].

But translating the vision of linking healthcare and research through semantic interoperability into reality is an imposing challenge [38,39]. Some points of view contend that research data should uniformly conform to healthcare data standards, such as those produced by Health Level Seven (HL7) [40]. However, HL7 standards are not yet implemented in a consistent manner globally and are largely used to support health delivery transactions and payments rather than research applications [41]. But is research data really the same as healthcare data? [42] Research studies are protocol-driven, and these experimental protocols precisely define how to treat the patient consistent with the experimental design—which may vary considerably from standards of care—as well as how to collect the data. Research data are historically presented in tabular files of rows and columns, which allow aggregation, sorting, and tabulation of results. Healthcare data is captured at a more granular level and does not typically include the detailed CRF questions that accompany a study to measure safety and efficacy. Still, there is overlap between these two data spheres: such as basic demographics, concomitant medications, vital signs, and especially laboratory data. It's also possible to have overlap in medical history, although medical history questionnaires tend to be very diverse and tailored for specific cases (rather than a comprehensive, standardized patient history which should be part of the personal health record that a patient would present to their physician). Thus, reuse of healthcare data is not so easy—protocol-driven research collects data differently than the more reactive world of primary healthcare, the systems are not aligned (having different business, scientific, and especially regional regulatory requirements and attitudes), and very often use different semantic vocabularies for coding information (for example, healthcare typically codes problems and diagnoses in ICD-9 or SNOMED versus adverse events in MedDRA).

But incremental progress is occurring on many fronts. For example, CDISC has collaborated with Integrating the Healthcare Enterprise (IHE) on a set of profiles [43] that enable the use of Electronic Healthcare Record data for multiple research purposes, including patient recruitment and CRF data capture [44]. In Europe, the Innovative Medicines Initiative (IMI) has funded the EHR4CR project [45] to apply such methods, and other efforts are also underway in Japan and other countries. The common thread between these initiatives is a foundation based upon data standards, which are essential to drive the economies of scale necessary to make this vision into reality.

4. SWOT

While the many benefits and opportunities of adopting clinical data standards are compelling, as indicated earlier, progress has been slow due to several perceived weaknesses and threats:

4.1 Strength

Standards make it possible to more rapidly glean knowledge from data and promote data reusability.

4.2 Weakness

Adopting standards requires investment in adapting systems and processes which companies maybe reluctant to commit.

4.3 Opportunity

Data standards can increase productivity in study setup and analysis. Adoption of a common, uniform set of data standards can promote precompetitive cooperation among research participants.

4.4 Threat

Standards are presumed by some researchers to pose constraints on scientific creativity, even though others believe they actually make it possible to advance science.

While many regulatory authorities are now encouraging or requiring the use of data standards, unclear regulatory statements about which standards to have has led some sponsors to delay investing in standards adoption, in the fear that the standards they adopt now may differ from what is ultimately required.

Some sponsors and CROs still fear they may contribute to unintentional disclosure of intellectual property or expose potential product weaknesses to competitors.

5. TAKE HOME MESSAGE

Just as any effective communication between two parties is based on the use of a common language, so do clinical data standards provide the common language for fully realizing the extraordinary opportunity of reengineering clinical research through improved productivity, increased knowledge, more effective dialogue with regulatory authorities, and expanded collaborations throughout the global research community.

REFERENCES

[1] CDISC website: www.cdisc.org. [accessed January 2014].
[2] FDA. Computer assisted new drug application (CANDA) guidance manual. DIANE Publishing Company; 1994.
[3] CDISC 2012 Annual Report. Available at: http://www.cdisc.org/stuff/contentmgr/fil es/0/6497cf2280bc974792a8803e973d1dee/files/cdisc_ar_2012__web_updated_versi onnov.pdf; [accessed January 2014].
[4] CDISC Clinical Research Glossary. Applied clinical trials, vol. 7; December 2011. Available at: http://www.appliedclinicaltrialsonline.com/appliedclinicaltrials/article/a rticleDetail.jsp?id=751876. [accessed January 2014].

[5] Guidance for Industry. Providing regulatory submissions in electronic format – general considerations, IT-2; January 1999. Available at: http://www.fda.gov/downloads/Drugs/DevelopmentApprovalProcess/FormsSubmissionRequirements/ElectronicSubmissions/UCM163187.pdf; [accessed January 2014].

[6] Christiansen D, Kubick W. The CDISC metadata model; November 26, 2001. Available at: http://www.cdisc.org/articles; [accessed January 2014].

[7] http://www.cdisc.org/standards-and-implementations; [accessed January 2014].

[8] FDA Press Release; July 21, 2004. Available at: http://www.fda.gov/newsevents/newsroom/pressann ouncements/2004/ucm108330.htm; [accessed January 2014].

[9] Federal Register, vol. 73, No. 87, Section 129, May 5, 2008.

[10] Kenny Susan J and Litzsinger Michael A. Strategies for implementing SDTM and ADaM standards, PharmaSUG 2005 proceedings. Available at: http://www.lexjansen.com/pharmasug/2005/fdacompliance/fc03.pdf; [accessed January 2014].

[11] Rozwell C, Kush RD, Helton E, Newby F, Mason T. The business case for CDISC standards; March 22, 2006. Gartner https://www.gartner.com/doc/490510; [accessed January 2014].

[12] CDISC Study Data Tabulation Model Implementation Guide. Human clinical trials, version 3.2; December 2013. Available at: www.cdisc.org/sdtm; [accessed January 2014].

[13] Willoughby Cara, Fridsma Doug, Chatterjee Lisa, Speakman John, Evans Julie, Kush Rebecca. A standard computable clinical trial protocol: the role of the BRIDG model. Drug Inf J 2007;41:383–92.

[14] CDISC Clinical Data Acquisition Standards Harmonization (CDASH) version 1.1; January 2011. Available at: www.cdisc.org/sdtm; [accessed January 2014].

[15] Kubick Wayne R. Buckthorn wars and the essence of clinical data; June 2012. Available at http://www.appliedclinicaltrialsonline.com/appliedclinicaltrials/article/articleDetail.jsp.

[16] Kubick W. The elegant machine: applying technology to optimize clinical trials. Drug Inf J 1998;32:861–9.

[17] Kubick Wayne R, Ruberg Stephen, Helton Edward. Toward a comprehensive cdisc submission data standard. Drug Inf J 2007;41:373–82.

[18] Kush RD, Bleicher P, Kubick W, Kush ST, Marks R, Raymond S, et al. eClinical trials: planning and implementation. Boston: Thompson Center Watch; 2003.

[19] FDA study data standards resources. Available at: http://www.fda.gov/ForIndustry/DataStandards/StudyDataStandards/default.htm.

[20] The Critical Path Opportunities List; March 2006, Page 11. Available at: http://www.fda.gov/downloads/ScienceResearch/SpecialTopics/CriticalPathInitiative/CriticalPathOpportunitiesReports/UCM077258.pdf; [accessed August 2014].

[21] CBER/CDER Study data standards for regulatory submissions position statement; September 13, 2013. Available at: http://www.fda.gov/ForIndustry/DataStandards/StudyDataStandards/uc m368613.htm; [accessed January 2014].

[22] European Medicines Agency. Draft policy 70: publication and access to clinical-trial data; June 24, 2013. Available at: http://www.ema.europa.eu/ema/index.jsp?curl=pages/includes/document/document_detail.jsp?webContentId=WC500144730&mid=WC0b01ac058009a3dc; [accessed January 2014].

[23] PMDA Request for electronic clinical study data for pilot project; September 2, 2013. Available at: http:// www.pmda.go.jp/operations/shonin/info/iyaku/jisedai/file/tsuuchi_e.pdf; [accessed January 2014].

[24] 2010 Presentation by Norman Stockbridge at DIA/FDA CDER/CBER computational science annual meeting March 22–23, 2010. Available at: http://www.diahome.org/Tools/Content.aspx?type=eopdf&file=%2fproductfiles%2f21575%2f10014%2Epdf; [accessed January 2014].

[25] Kubick Wayne R. When great ideas meet the real world; February 2010. Available at: http://www.appliedclinicaltrialsonline.com/appliedclinicaltrials/CRO%2FSponsor/When-Great-Ideas-Meet-the-Real-World/ArticleStandard/Article/detail/655353?contextCategoryId=554; [accessed January 2014].

[26] Janus Clinical Trials Repository (CTR) Project. Available at: http://www.fda.gov/forindustry/datastandards/studydatastandards/ucm155327.htm; [accessed January 2014].

[27] Kubick Wayne R. The power and pitfalls of aggregate data; October 2011. Available at: http://www.appliedclinicaltrialsonline.com/appliedclinicaltrials/IT/The-Power-and-Pitfalls-of-Aggregate-Data/ArticleStandard/Article/detail/742590?contextCategoryId=554; [accessed January 2014].

[28] Haber Margaret, Kisler Bron W, Lenzen Mary, Wright Lawrence W. Controlled terminology for clinical research: a collaboration between CDISC and NCI Enterprise vocabulary services. Drug Inf J 2007;41:405–12.

[29] Goldman, M. New frontiers for collaborative research. Sci Transl Med 2013;5:216ed22. Available at: http://dx.doi.org/10.1126/scitranslmed.3007990.

[30] TCB Press Release; September 19, 2012. Available at: http://www.prnewswire.co.uk/news-releases/ten-pharmaceutical-companies-unite-to-accelerate-development-of-new-medicines-170329496.html; [accessed January 2014].

[31] TCB initiatives website: http://www.transceleratebiopharmainc.com/our-initiatives/; [accessed January 2014].

[32] PDUFA 2012. Reauthorization performance goals and procedures fiscal years 2013 through 2017. p. 28. Available at: http://www.fda.gov/downloads/forindustry/userfees/prescriptiondruguserfee/ucm270412.pdf; [accessed January 2014].

[33] C-Path website: http://c-path.org; [accessed January 2014].

[34] CFAST Press Release; November 12, 2012: CDISC, C-Path, FDA, TransCelerate and the global CDISC community launch initiative to accelerate therapies through standards. Available at: http://www.cdisc.org/cfast; [accessed January 2014].

[35] CDISC Therapeutic area standards webpage: http://www.cdisc.org/therapeutic; [accessed January 2014].

[36] CDISC SHARE webpage: http://www.cdisc.org/cdisc-share; [accessed January 2014].

[37] Institute of Medicine. Digital infrastructure for the learning health system: the foundation for continuous improvement in health and health care – workshop series summary; May 2011. Available at: http://www.iom.edu/Reports/2011/Digital-Infrastructure-for-a-Learning-Health-System.aspx; [accessed January 2014].

[38] Mead C. Data interchange standards in healthcare IT – computable semantic interoperability: now possible but still difficult, do we really need a better mousetrap? J Healthc Inf Manag 2006;20:71–8.

[39] Kush RD, Helton E, Rockhold FW, Hardison CD. Electronic health records, medical research and the tower of Babel. N Engl J Med 2008;358:1738–40.

[40] HL7 website: www.hl7.org; [accessed January 2014].

[41] Norman K. Simplifying data standards: CDISC and HL7 Deciphered; June 2010. Available at http://www.appliedclinicaltrialsonline.com/appliedclinicaltrials/article/articleDetail.jsp?id=672337. [last accessed January 2014].

[42] Kush Rebecca Daniels. Data sharing: electronic health records and research interoperability. In: Richesson R, Andrews J, editors. Clinical research informatics. Springer; 2012. pp. 313–34.

[43] Integrating the Healthcare Enterprise (IHE) website: http://www.ihe.net

[44] IHE healthcare link profiles. Available at: http://www.cdisc.org/stuff/contentmgr/files/0/f5a0121d251a348a87466028e156d3c3/misc/cdisc_healthcare_link_profiles.pdf; [accessed January 2014].

[45] EHR4CR website: http://www.ehr4cr.eu; [accessed January 2014].

CHAPTER 22

Data Management 2.0

Johann Proeve

Contents

1. THE NEED

Since the 1980s, the drug development process has become more and more complex. This is reflected not only by more patients being enrolled into clinical trials. In 1983, a case record form (CRF) contained about 8–15 pages capturing patient information. Today, the volume of a CRF easily exceeds the size of 180 pages/forms, with a maximum of 600 pages/forms, which means that many more data are being collected than in the past. In addition to the patient data, the use of EDC (electronic data capture) has introduced an additional approximately fivefold data volume originating from the audit trail of the applications used. Whereas in the past most of the data were generated by the site investigator, this has changed in the past few years. ECG data read results and central lab data results, just to name a few, are provided by specialized third-party companies. Finally, the use of electronic patient-reported outcome data has added to the data volume and the complexity of clinical trials.

All of the above affect the processes, the applications, and the workload in the clinical data management area. On the other hand, not all the data captured are being analyzed and reported via tables, graphs, or listings, i.e., they are not being used.

Compared to the past, many more functions internally as well as externally need an ongoing access to all data from ongoing and from completed clinical trials. This means that all data, patient data, audit trail data, and performance data, and probably in many different formats and cuts, must be

Re-Engineering Clinical Trials
http://dx.doi.org/10.1016/B978-0-12-420246-7.00022-0
245

readily accessible for, e.g., the data managers, medical monitors, programmers, statisticians, clinical project leaders, study managers, project managers, and, to a certain extent, also for the pharmacokineticists, the bioanalytics group, and many more users.

Finally, all the clinical trial data need to be reported to the health authorities as part of a submission, via the so-called integrated summary of safety and integrated summary of efficacy analyses. Currently, the data itself have to be submitted to the U.S. Food and Drug Administration; however, in the future other health authorities, such as the European Medicines Agency and very likely also the Chinese Food and Drug Administration and the Japanese Pharmaceutical and Medical Device Agency, will ask for access to these data.

In essence, pharma companies are faced with a huge volume of patient data and performance data that they need to process, clean, make available to many end users with different requirements, and finally store for many years in a retrievable, human-readable format. How can that process be eased?

2. THE SOLUTION

The overall process of managing the data of clinical trials needs to be simplified and streamlined. There are several aspects to this challenge.

1. *The data capture* component
   a. The volume of data needs to be reduced by simplifying the clinical trial protocols. The focus must be on the most important data to demonstrate safety and efficacy of the test compound in the clinical trial. Secondary and tertiary efficacy criteria must be reduced to an absolute minimum to also reduce the number of data captured [1].
   b. The data items to be collected per study, per project, or even across projects must be standardized as much as possible. The more the items are standardized the easier it will be for all parties involved in the data capture and data processing areas. Studies can be set up faster and more easily and sites will be more familiar with the CRF pages. Preferably, the standards that are common to all clinical trials should even be standardized across sponsor companies. First initiatives have been kicked off (CDISC [2] and TRANSCELERATE [3]). These initiatives will help in streamlining the data capture process, at least with respect to the common items, such as adverse events data, lab analytes, vital signs, medical history, concomitant medication, ECG findings, patient demographics, smoking habits, etc. These data usually already cover more than 50% of the data in a clinical trial.

c. The standardization must cover not only the items themselves but also the code lists used, the edit checks implemented, the formats, and the labels. This will permit an even smoother setup of a trial and the management of the trial data. Site staff will always know what to enter where and which data to make available because they will be familiar with the forms presented, irrespective of whether by pharma company A or B or by a Contract Research Organization.

d. The preferred data capture method for clinical trials has been EDC via applicable hardware and software. This must be the minimum requirement for today's clinical trials operations. Data capture using the paper data documentation approach should happen only in rare cases, i.e., in studies in countries not having the required infrastructure for running an online EDC system. Offline EDC system use must be avoided by all means because of the huge challenges associated with the hardware and software management and maintenance.

e. Very similar to the above, patient-generated data, i.e., data from questionnaires or diaries, should also be captured electronically. The quality of data from paper-based questionnaires and diaries is usually poor and does not withstand health authority scrutiny and acceptance.

f. Nowadays, clinical trial data are frequently being entered into the hospital or general practitioner patient report, whether paper or electronic. These data, for the most part and in a second step, are being transcribed into an EDC system or—even worse—into a paper CRF. A major effort usually has to be undertaken to check the correct transcription from one system to another. This is an extremely labor-intensive task. To reduce or—best case scenario—even avoid these transcription tasks, a direct data capture method should be employed. Tablet applications are available today permitting a direct data capture at the patient bedside or during the patient visit. Such technology helps avoid redundant data capture and the effort of checking consistency with the source data [4], because the data captured via the tablet applications are the source.

g. Long term, and for those cases in which direct data capture using the tablet applications is not possible, the primary data capture at the sites via the electronic health records/electronic medical records must be improved. The better the quality and the structure of the data in the electronic health records (EHR) or electronic medical record (EMR) system the easier to reuse these data for clinical trials, either by academia or by pharma. The data could be used for protocol feasibility, for patient identification, or even for a data transfer from EHR to the sponsor company EDC system [5]. This requires a close cooperation among the EHR/EMR system vendors, the clinics, and the pharma companies.

In conclusion, the main message of the above is that primarily the data capture must be standardized as much as possible. Second, the volume of data must be reduced to the absolutely required data, and data that are "nice to have" should not be captured as part of a clinical development program. Third, long term, the data capture should be moved as much as possible to the source of the data. Finally, manual transcription of data from one system to another should be avoided by all means because it introduces an additional burden for all parties involved in the conduct of clinical trials.

2. *Data access* for review component

    a. Once the data from the various sources have been captured via the different applications, they have to be made available to a broad user community and various systems. This is necessary to facilitate the data review on an ongoing basis or the data reporting by the following.

        – Data managers need access to the entire dataset with all original data entered by the site staff; all external data from, e.g., central labs or bioanalytics units; derived items such as converted local lab data into a standard unit; and coded data, i.e., medical history or concomitant medication data entered in text format and coded to standard glossaries, such as MedDRA or WHO-DD. The data managers also need access to the underlying data structure and the audit trail data to ensure data structure consistency. They usually access the data directly into the EDC system or, for the complete picture of the data, review them in the clinical database management systems. Those systems are either available off the shelf or have been home grown. Off-the-shelf systems are SAS-DD®, Oracle LSH®, and Entimice®, to name just a few.

        – Medical monitors need the data to review individual aspects of the patient data supporting the potential detection of unreported serious adverse events or unexpected safety-related signals in the data. Because they have a different skill set compared to the data managers, and in order not to waste too much time on setting up, e.g., reports or listings in the data review tools, the medical monitors need to have access to the data via simple-to-use and straightforward applications with precanned reports, graphs, and listings. Several applications are available off the shelf, such as jReview®, Spotfire®, or Comprehend®, facilitating the data review (Figure 22.1).

– Project managers are mainly interested in the trial or project status. Data required for this function are mainly available via the audit trail of the studies. A typical example could be how many patients have already been processed completely and are ready for a statistical analysis. A similar question could be which study sites enrolled the most appropriate number of patients for a per-protocol analysis. These data can be made available by home-grown systems and derived from the clinical trial database or directly from the EDC system.

– Pharmaco-vigilance case managers need access to a particular subset of the data mainly related to the serious adverse events. Those data could be, for example, the adverse event data themselves, the demographic data, data on medical history, applicable laboratory analytes data, risk factors, etc. These data need to be made available to pharmaco-vigilance in a timely fashion, i.e., usually within 24 h after gaining knowledge of a serious adverse event. The pharmaco-vigilance data are usually stored again in a separate system supporting appropriate reporting of the data to the health authorities. Those systems are, e.g., Clintrace®, Argus®, and Aris G®. Pharma needs to ensure that the data in the clinical database and those in

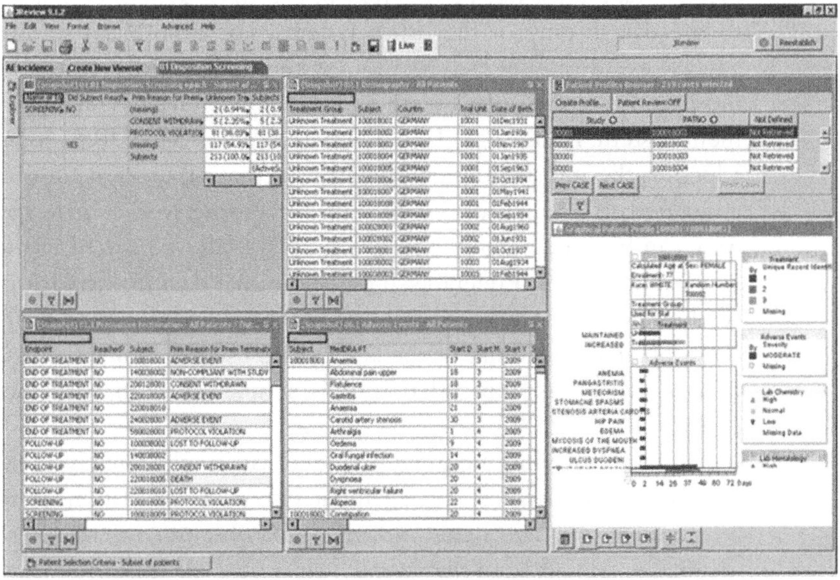

Figure 22.1 jReview® output for data review by medical monitors using tabulations and graphs in combination for easy data review and assessment.

the pharmaco-vigilance database are in sync, i.e., no discrepancies between the data in the two systems are acceptable.

— Statistical programmers and statisticians require an ongoing access to the data permitting them to start working on the statistical analyses and reporting programs while the study is still running. They have requirements for the data structure that may be different from the structure used by the other functions above. The analyses are run in SAS® because SAS® is the standard analysis tool used by the health authorities as well.

b. The requirement to deliver the clinical trial data (e.g., entered by the site staff) and the underlying meta data (i.e., the database structure in EDC, the structure in Oracle LSH®) and the performance data (i.e., site performance data from the audit trails, e.g., which field has been changed how many times in the EDC system) to so many different systems as described above without losing consistency of the data results in some basic requirements for the storage of the data.

— The data need to be up to date at any point in time. This means, once the data have been captured in the EDC system, they also need to be available in any other system shortly thereafter.

— The data need to be consistent across the systems. This means, original data must not be different in the EDC system compared to the data in any of the other systems. For example, a serious adverse event captured in the EDC system must be the same as in the pharmaco-vigilance system and the clinical database management system. Additional data, however, such as MedDRA codes added to the investigator adverse event verbatim, or local lab data converted to a common set of units, or the derived relative day data, can be added at any point in time and also be stored in the applicable systems. Preferably, these additional data in the various systems are also consistent with one another. This requires a thorough up-front planning of the algorithms used to generate these derived data, something that sounds simple, but can be rather complex.

— It must be clear who modified or added data to the already existing data in the database management system. These data need to be stored in separate fields and must not obscure/overwrite the original entries. A time stamp and a clear user identification must be available. In essence all the data manipulations and modifications must be transparent.

- The data audit trail data must be available in a human-readable format. The audit trail data are required by several functions, and the data on who made which change to the data when and—in the EDC system—for what reason need to be retrievable. In addition, the audit trail may also be accessed by health authority inspectors and thus requires making the information available in a legible way instantaneously.

In essence, data management must ensure that the clinical trial data can be accessed by anybody internally or externally required to see and work with the data. Effort must be made to ensure the data are not being copied into too many different databases to ensure continuous consistency of the data. Preferably, the data should be maintained in one clinical trial database management system and all applications should access this database for data review purposes. This may not always be manageable; however, the fewer database copies exist the easier for the maintenance of the data.

3. *The reporting* of the data, the metadata, and the performance data in many different systems and versions is another major burden to the organization, potentially resulting in slight differences in the tables, graphs, or listings. Different users may have different reporting requirements, requiring different data structures and slices of the very same data.

   a. Investigational New Drug Application and Development Safety Update Report annual reports are predefined reports by health authorities with specific data cut requirements [6].

   b. Data monitoring boards may require a data cut on a particular date, irrespective of the data available to the sponsor company beyond this specific predefined date. This may mean data to be excluded for this snap-shot.

   c. Pharmaco-vigilance requires reports on patients with serious adverse events in the clinical database. These data must be reconciled against the data in the pharmaco-vigilance database to ensure full consistency between the two databases, the clinical trial database and the pharmaco-vigilance database.

   d. Project management needs to know the status of a program or the trials of the program, but on a high level. Those metric reports are usually required on a monthly or quarterly basis and cover aspects such as number of patients treated, number of patients available for an interim analysis, expected duration for reaching a specific milestone of a trial, number of outstanding queries, number of patients that finished the study, and many metrics related to the study status, the

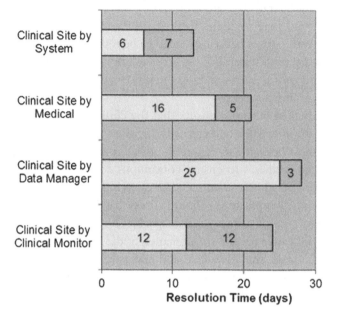

Query Resolution Time (days) by Query Type

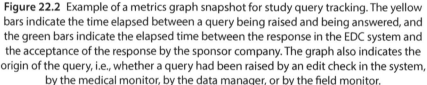

Figure 22.2 Example of a metrics graph snapshot for study query tracking. The yellow bars indicate the time elapsed between a query being raised and being answered, and the green bars indicate the elapsed time between the response in the EDC system and the acceptance of the response by the sponsor company. The graph also indicates the origin of the query, i.e., whether a query had been raised by an edit check in the system, by the medical monitor, by the data manager, or by the field monitor.

site status, the patient status, and even the visit status. The data used are mainly performance data rather than patient data and can be derived from the metrics data or the audit trail. Those metrics are important for managing the trials [7]; however, one always needs to keep in mind that the analyses do not come for free, either (Figure 22.2).

e. Clinical project management, study managers, and several other functions working jointly on a study may require slightly different reports on a more frequent basis. Those could be reports driven by patient data or by performance data, such as patients violating in- and exclusion criteria, patients with acceptable compliance with respect to tablet intake, visit dates entered into EDC, or sites with queries outstanding for more than two weeks. Toward interim analyses and the end of a trial those reports will be required to be run more frequently (Figure 22.3).

Country	Unit	Number	Run-in	Screening	End of Screening	Visit 1 (Base line) (Day 1)	Visit 2 (Day 7 + - 2)	Visit 3 (Day 30 + - 2)	Visit 4 (Day 60 + - 2)	Visit 5 (Day 90 + - 2)	Study Medication	Premature Discontinua-tion	Follow -Up Visit	Last Visit
AUS	40002	400020001	2013-08-14	2013-10-31	2013-11-13	2013-11-13	2013-11-13	2013-11-21	2013-12-12	2014-01-13	2013-11-13			
AUS	40002	400020002	2013-08-28	2013-10-03	2013-10-16	2013-10-16	2013-10-24	2013-11-12	2013-12-12		2013-10-16			
AUS	40002	400020003	2013-10-29	2013-12-04	2013-12-11	2013-12-11	2013-12-18	2014-01-09			2013-12-11			
AUS	40003	400030001	2013-07-31	2013-07-31										2013-07-31
AUS	40003	400030002	2013-08-21	2013-08-21										2013-08-21
AUS	40003	400030003	2013-08-16	2013-09-09										2013-09-09
AUS	40003	400030004	2013-08-01	2013-09-05	2013-09-12	2013-09-12	2013-09-19	2013-10-11	2013-11-08	2013-12-12	2013-09-12			
AUS	40003	400030005	2013-08-12	2013-08-12										2013-08-12
AUS	40003	400030006	2013-08-14	2013-08-14										2013-08-14
AUS	40003	400030007	2013-08-19	2013-08-19	2013-08-26	2013-08-26	2013-09-03	2013-09-24	2013-10-24	2013-11-25	2013-08-26		2013-12-23	2013-12-23
AUS	40003	400030008	2013-08-19	2013-08-19	2013-08-28	2013-08-28	2013-09-04	2013-09-26	2013-10-28	2013-11-25	2013-08-28		2013-12-23	2013-12-23
AUS	40003	400030009	2013-08-22	2013-08-22	2013-08-29	2013-08-29	2013-09-04	2013-09-27	2013-10-28	2013-11-29	2013-08-29		2013-12-23	2013-12-23

Figure 22.3 Patient tracking system output showing the status of the visits in the EDC system for the first couple of patients of a trial.

Reviewing the above requirements clearly demonstrates that the many customers and the various systems can be kept "under control" only by reducing the volume of data, by trimming the number of systems employed, and in particular by ensuring a consistent definition of the reports required. The last is a main resource consumer and the more consistent the definitions are the easier to manage the various requests. Personal preferences on layout or definition of data cuts must be avoided by all means because they are not likely to add value but rather increase complexity.

3. SWOT

Strengths	Weaknesses
Focus on main efficacy and main safety data	Lower customer acceptance
More consistency in the data	Fewer options on customization
Fewer data errors	Potential for missing development opportunities by lack of introduction of new data items
Easier for site staff and investigators	
Less burden for patients due to fewer exams	
Better acceptance by health authorities	

Opportunities	Threats
Reduction in cost and resource requirements	Potential failure of main efficacy criterion resulting in—worst case—nonapprovability of a compound
Faster study setup and closure	
Better company-wide understanding of the content of the data captured	

4. APPLICABLE REGULATIONS

1. Guidance for Industry: Electronic Source Data in Clinical Investigations, U.S. Department of Health and Human Services Food and Drug Administration, Sept. 2013
2. www.FDA.gov/Drugs
3. ICH (International Conference on Harmonisation of Technical Requirements for Registration of Pharmaceuticals for Human Use) Development Safety Update Report, E2F, Aug. 17, 2010

5. TAKE HOME MESSAGE

The main messages from this chapter are:

1. Standardize the data collection, data storage, and data checking as much as possible, preferably across projects or even companies. The majority of data items are being collected across all clinical trials irrespective of the indication or therapeutic area. The data collected usually do not make a difference with respect to whether a drug works. This can be achieved by joining the CDISC organization and working with consortia such as TRANSCELERATE. Internally, senior management needs to be convinced of the benefits of standardization. The benefits can be demonstrated, for example, by using a time-tracking system to show the effort it takes to create an electronic case report form or a set of tables from scratch compared to taking existing standards and delivering the same case report form or table based on those standards more quickly. The numbers should convince every manager in the organization.
2. Reduce the number of data points collected to the absolute minimum and stop collecting data that are of secondary or tertiary interest. Those data frequently only increase the burden for the investigative site, the patients, the sponsor organization, and finally also the health authorities. Once marketing authorization has been granted, those additional data can easily be captured in simple, straightforward phase IV trials or via registries.
3. Ensure that the data for review, data cleaning, serious adverse event reporting, assessment for central monitoring boards, and also the statistical analyses are in sync. This can be achieved by keeping the data—preferably—in one and only one location and granting access to all functions with a vested interest in the data.
4. The definitions of reports, graphs, and listings—whether for patient data or underlying performance metrics—must be streamlined as much as possible. This will help the entire organization to arrive at a consistent

conclusion with respect to the efficacy and safety of the compound in development. The best way of getting to a sound set of commonly applicable tables, graphs, or listings is the setup of an interdisciplinary team with members from various functions in the drug development organization. Those team members need to agree upon the definitions of the deliverables, including but not limited to the algorithm to be applied to the data, and simple aspects such as the headers and footers, the labels, the format, the date, and the location where the report had been generated. Finally, they also need to agree upon the frequency of the metric reports to be run. All of the above will help automate the report generation to the maximum extent.

5. Metrics based on the audit trail of the EDC system and also the other systems applied by data management can be used to support and steer the entire study conduct process. The metrics can clearly point to the bottlenecks during the conduct of a clinical trial. For example, metrics can highlight the sites with a delay in data entry into the EDC system, a delayed response to queries raised by the sponsor company, or the enrollment of an undesired patient population. Similar metrics can be used to follow up on the timely monitoring activities by clinical research associates or monitors. The number of cleaned patients versus those entered can easily be retrieved from the clinical database and appropriate actions be initiated as applicable. All of the above thresholds can be agreed upon by either a top-down approach or having the study team agree upon those thresholds. In turn, this will permit anybody in charge to see whether a trial is on track, slightly off track, or already completely off track. This does require, however, that those reports are looked at by sponsor staff, completely understood, and eventually also acted upon.

REFERENCES

[1] Eisenstein EL, Lemons 2nd PW, Tardiff BE, Schulman KA, Jolly MK, Califf RM. Reducing the costs of phase III cardiovascular clinical trials. Am Heart J March 2005;149(3):482–8.
[2] www.CDISC.org.
[3] www.transceleratebiopharmainc.com/our-initiatives/.
[4] Guidance for Industry. Electronic source data in clinical investigations. U.S. Department of Health and Human Services Food and Drug Administration; September 2013.
[5] Coorevits P, Sundgren M, Klein GO, Bahr A, Claerhout B, Daniel C, et al. Electronic health records: new opportunities for clinical research. J Intern Med December 2013;274(6):547–60.
[6] Furlan G, Douglas S. The developmental safety update report. The new way to drug safety or a born-again old report? DIA Glob Forum August 2011;3(4):37–42.
[7] Djali S, Janssens S, Van Yper S, Van Parijs J. How a data-driven quality management system can manage compliance risk in clinical trials. Drug Inf J 2010;44:359–73.

CHAPTER 23

What Do the Sites Want? The Trial Master File

Andrew Mitchell, Jochen Tannemann, Kevin McNulty

Contents

1. THE NEED

In today's clinical development environment, it has become increasingly difficult to find sites that can successfully meet patient enrollment guidelines and adhere to complex study protocols. Data from Tufts Center for the Study of Drug Development underscores this trend, finding that between 1995 and 2005, there were 21% fewer volunteers being admitted into trials and a 30% increase in patient dropouts.[1] This same research also found that the number of routine tasks per trial increased by 65% and the average clinical trial staff work burden increased by 67%.[2]

Top-performing sites are well-sought after and are often working on multiple studies with multiple sponsors simultaneously. Approximately a third of sites are working on more than 20 studies in a year (Figure 23.1).

Given these facts, finding these top-performing sites and then maintaining a strong and collaborative relationship is a high priority for sponsors and contract research organizations. Yet, the complexity of clinical research and the increasingly stringent regulatory oversight can make this difficult to accomplish. Sponsors often throw technology at challenges (Figure 23.2) to improve efficiency without carefully thinking through all the business processes from the site perspective, and sites are often reluctant to embrace change and tend to adhere to paper-based solutions (Figure 23.3).

---

[1] Tufts CSDD Impact Report.
[2] Ibid.

Re-Engineering Clinical Trials
http://dx.doi.org/10.1016/B978-0-12-420246-7.00023-2

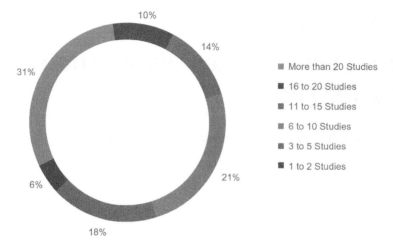

10%

14%

31%

■ More than 20 Studies

■ 16 to 20 Studies

■ 11 to 15 Studies

■ 6 to 10 Studies

■ 3 to 5 Studies

■ 1 to 2 Studies

21%

6%

18%

Figure 23.1 Number of clinical studies sites conducted on an annual basis.[3]

[3] CenterWatch-Intralinks 2013 Site Survey.

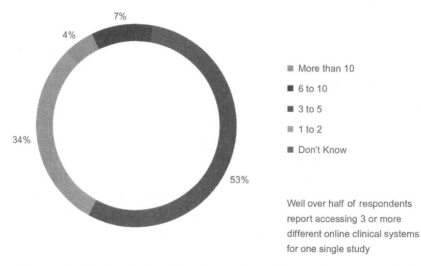

7%

4%

34%

■ More than 10

■ 6 to 10

■ 3 to 5

■ 1 to 2

■ Don't Know

53%

Well over half of respondents report accessing 3 or more different online clinical systems for one single study

Figure 23.2 Number of online clinical systems typically accesses during a study.[4]

[4] Ibid.

2. THE SOLUTION

Technology applied correctly, however, does offer a means to streamline procedures, reduce workloads, improve collaboration, and increase audit readiness, while still maintaining regulatory compliance. Considering the

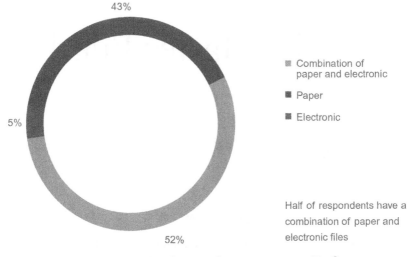

Figure 23.3 Type of storage for investigator site files.[5]

⁵ Ibid.

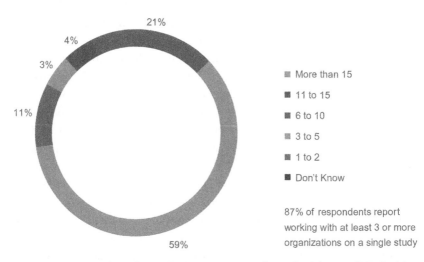

Figure 23.4 Number of organizations sites typically work with on a clinical trial.

number of parties (Figure 23.4) involved in a trial, automating complete business processes through technology offers the ideal solution.

There has been a large industry focus on the trial master file (TMF), and yet almost all commercial solutions do not address the full scope of the TMF. Most electronic (e)TMF solutions focus on the interaction between the

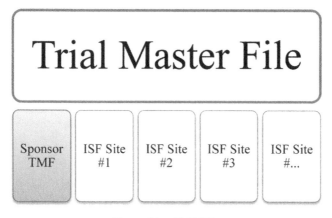

Figure 23.5 TMF, ISFs.

TMF and the sponsor, but neglect the interaction with the sites. Yet, international regulation define the full scope of the TMF as both the sponsor file and the investigator site file (ISF) (Figure 23.5):

The TMF is normally composed of a sponsor file, held by the sponsor organization and an investigator site file, held by the investigator. These files together are regarded as comprising the entire TMF for the trial and should be established at the beginning of the trial.[6]

The challenges in implementing this specific solution are driven by privacy and data ownership requirements. Both areas of the TMF (sponsor and ISF) include records that are private to the respective organizations.

By using private data rooms for the sponsor TMF and ISF, and additionally controlling the interaction of documents originating from the sponsor (such as protocol and investigator brochure) and those originating from the investigator (such as financial disclosure, medical license), information can be protected at each area that is not to be disclosed to the respective other party.

The sponsor and investigator should also be able to grant access to private files to relevant parties in relation to specific tasks and surveillance activities. These tasks include inspections by health authorities and remote monitoring activities through the clinical research associate (CRA).

During the past few years, a wide consensus in the commercial community has been reached to organize TMFs in accordance to the Drug Information Association TMF reference model (Figure 23.6). The TMF should reflect this structure. The TMF reference model organizes artifacts in zones and sections. Additionally, for each document a level (study, country, site) and the ownership (sponsor, investigator) can be defined.

[6] MHRA, *The Gray Book*, p. 330.

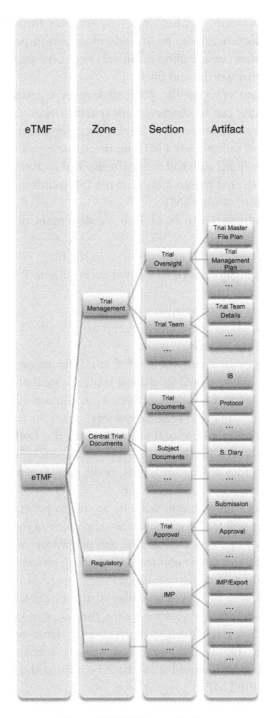

Figure 23.6 TMF organization.

The full TMF will be the final and only resource for study documents. The source of documents can be an individual person providing a document (the originator) or a feeding eClinical system. An artifact stored in the TMF has to be trustworthy and final.

Each document entering the TMF undergoes a default filing process. This default process can be shortened for specific document related workflows if the different roles are taken by the same person.

Differing from the sponsor TMF, the investigator will usually not have specialist staff for filing and will maintain the ISF in avocation. Therefore, there are some essential requirements for the ISF solution:

- Clear integration with eTMF
- Temporary permission to be able to see document or download for a short term
- Sponsor sees metadata to know what is in the file
- Principle investigators need to see and access files in ISF all the time
- Should be a repository
- Hide tasks that are not pertinent or timely
- Table of contents to know where things are
- Improved user experience

Artifacts may be pushed into the TMF from different originating feeding systems. Because systems used in clinical trials are validated, the respective interfaces also need to be validated. Systems without a validated interface are classified as "nonqualified feeding systems."

A qualified feeding system will push data into the TMF, and document metadata from the feeding system are persistent throughout the feeding process: This includes eSignature status, revision and version history, and document ownership.

Nonqualified feeding systems will not be able to push data directly into the TMF, but they will feed documents into the inbox of the TMF. They will trigger the review process and act as the originator of a new artifact. Depending on the risk assessment the default filing process might be shortened for nonqualified feeding systems.

The eTMF defines the documentation status of a clinical trial. At different time points, different requirements for the status of documents apply. Study phases such as preparation, start-up, conduct, close-out, and reporting define a different volume and amount of artifacts stored in the TMF. The TMF responsible person should at any time be informed on the quality and completeness of the TMF.

The TMF receives external information to measure the completeness of a TMF at a given time point. Usually, this information is kept in a clinical trial management system of the sponsor. However, this information is not standardized. The eTMF should not take over trial management functionality but can provide an interface to receive the required information either manually or as an automatic upload.

Focusing on the entire business process and then applying technology offers the most complete and efficient solution for the TMF. Implementing a solution that focuses solely on sponsor–TMF interaction is incomplete and does little to improve sponsor relationships with sites.

3. SWOT

Strengths:
- Improved compliance and efficiency at site—all documents in one place while ensuring that control is always retained by the site
- Improved compliance and efficiency at sponsor—enablement of remote monitoring visits
  - Allows for more efficient use of monitor time to focus on protocol-related issues versus documentation
- Reduce risk to the sponsor:
  - Increased visibility into the site
  - Reduce reliance on individual CRAs
  - Improve consistency across sites
  - Site inspection readiness
- Reduce use and storage of paper

Weaknesses:
- More complicated to implement than paper systems
- More initial training needed
- Internet access needed
- Higher up-front investment and system costs

Opportunities:
- Remote source data verification for paper-based studies
- Reduced distribution costs versus manual processes
- Improve eTMF filing by categorizing and prioritized assignment of content received from the sites
- Higher quality of documents from sites in sponsor TMF
  - Eliminate manual reconciliation of the ISF and TMF (always in synch)

- Real-time access to documents as appropriate

Threats:

- Site may not make full use of the system due to lack of training
- Understanding or interest and potentially higher workaround at the site level

4. TAKE HOME MESSAGE

Information at each area that is not to be disclosed to the respective other party can dramatically improve document management efficiency and quality.

An independent, site-controlled electronic investigator site file would

1. Support ISF filing at each site
2. Manage distribution and collection of content between ISF and sponsor TMF systems
3. Enable remote monitoring and review of a sites paperwork as part of sponsor risk-based monitoring strategy
4. Enable archiving ISF information at end of trial, with ongoing access for authorized personnel

5. APPLICABLE REGULATIONS

21 CFR 11; European data privacy laws.

CHAPTER 24

From Data to Information and Decision: ICONIK

Malcolm Neil Burgess, Nicholas J. Alp, Gareth Milborrow

Contents

1. THE NEED

The fundamental motivation for clinical data analytics is to improve quality in clinical trials. We define quality as "the absence of errors that matter in decision making for patients." How do we move from processing and analyzing data to a place where we can make rational and consistent decisions to improve quality? First, we have to eliminate the data that does not matter in order to start to make sense of the data that does matter. Traditionally, attempts to reduce the collection of extraneous data were aimed at achieving this goal. Although this did enrich the data, it did not come close to achieving the critical mass necessary to ignite a chain reaction to convert the data into useful information (let alone knowledge). Much of the data does matter but only when aligned and compared in context and in such a manner as to transverse the divide so that information can then be extracted (or visualized). When visualization is then coupled with effective and timely decision making, you have a situation where the power of the data is fully

Re-Engineering Clinical Trials
http://dx.doi.org/10.1016/B978-0-12-420246-7.00024-4
265

harnessed, and the decision-making process becomes almost intuit for those able to "read" the knowledge stream. The ICONIK platform developed by ICON allows these three stages to be achieved in close to real time; the fact that intelligent decisions can be made in very close to real time on data that is placed in various appropriate contexts (knowledge packages) means that for maybe the first time, our clinical studies can be effectively managed during their execution based on what is actually happening at our sites—rather than what we think is happening at our sites. By defining what constitutes the right context and data that will enable effective decision making and how to produce appropriate visualizations to enable the information to be interpreted, close to real-time decisions can then be routinely made. By wrapping the right people and processes around the technology and analytical models, and by subjecting our systems to a continual cycle of evaluation, validation, and refinement, we have made this complex transition and interpretation a routine part of the ICON-process landscape. ICON patient-centered monitoring combines real-time, centralized data analysis with on-site and off-site contact and interventions to dynamically identify, mitigate, and manage risk to quality in a study. We define risk as the probability of errors or noncompliance with ethical principles, GCP, regulations, or protocol in any clinical trial process, leading to concerns with subject rights and safety or reliability of data. How we visualize these risks is a key part of our process and systems. The ICON patient-centered monitoring approach is designed to increase the quality and efficiency of monitoring activities, with resources targeted to support sites with any identified risk indicators.

2. THE SOLUTION: ICONIK INTEGRATED CLINICAL DATA PLATFORM

ICON has developed and implemented the proprietary ICONIK (ICON Immediate Knowledge) integrated information platform to provide transparency throughout the management, reporting, and analysis of data relating to drug development. At the core of the system is the Oracle Life Science Hub (LSH) which acts as our main clinical data repository—providing security and full traceability of the data from point of entry to point of exit. ICONIK provides enhanced quality in scientific management and trial oversight through streamlined data-driven decisions, and provides the foundation to increase efficiencies and substantially improve quality by giving transparent and shared access to a "single source of the truth" to ICON and sponsors.

Figure 24.1 illustrates the flow of operational and clinical data (in near real time) from the individual primary source systems into the ICONIK data repositories and how these data are presented in a visual and interactive way to the study and sponsor team members, including key functional groups such as the centralized monitoring team, medical monitors, and clinical trial managers.

Data is loaded using a proprietary software system we have designated as the Study Data Mapper. Once the programming enhancements have been made for a specific study, the loading of the data becomes an automated process that can be set to run as often as once a day. The periodicity of how frequently we run the data load depends on the critical nature of the study itself and also how frequently data is being generated. But daily data loading is our routine processing time frame, with the visualizations being updated dynamically once the data changes. So ICONIK provides a single and integrated view of all study information, refreshed in near real time (nightly is

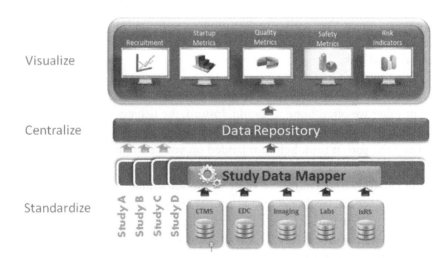

Figure 24.1 Architecture and function of ICONIK. There are multiple independent primary data sources in a typical clinical trial, for example, clinical trial management systems (CTMS), electronic data capture (EDC) systems, medical imaging data, laboratory data, and interactive voice/web response systems (IxRS). These primary sources often have independent data structures and formats. The ICONIK study data mapper transforms these data structures into a unified format, enabling these discrete data streams to be aggregated and integrated into repositories, not only at a study level but also across multiple studies in the program. From these repositories, data can be surfaced and analyzed in near real time, in any location, through a range of web-based reporting and analytical tools.

the normal routine), from study startup to database lock. Using these data, a trial can be evaluated efficiently from a scientific, safety, and quality perspective across a single study, or indeed an entire portfolio of studies on a compound. Analytical operations, from the detection of a safety signal to the data quality analysis of a site, can be performed dynamically, consistently, and efficiently.

3. THE SOLUTION: DATA, INFORMATION, AND KNOWLEDGE: QUALITY AS IT RELATES TO RISK

Staring at a spreadsheet of uniformly gray digits on your computer screen, you would be forgiven for being under the impression that the data represents a uniformly objective truth that is static in nature and closely, if not absolutely, tied to the site. On the surface, there is very little to distinguish the history of the data on one tab from another, giving the illusion that all data has a common history and that all data came to appear on your screen through a uniform process that affected one data set no more than any other; an impression that leads you to believe that all data holds more or less equal value (or information) in the detection of risk.

This could not be further from the truth.

Not all data is what it seems, and not all data holds the unbiased, transparent value we often hope it should. Instead, the detection of risk through the analysis of data requires a detailed understanding of the origin of the data and the path it took before it landed on your computer screen. Failure to fully appreciate the dynamic nature of the data, its life, and its purity, will almost certainly undermine the value of the subsequent analysis.

In this section, we hope to convey the dynamic, complex, and sometimes deceptive nature of the data with the aim that you will be able to identify these features in your study and, by association, the ability of that data to consistently reflect risk.

Let's start with an apparently simple example: vital sign data. Typically, we are presented with three core columns containing the systolic measurement, the diastolic measurement, and the heart rate measurement, all taken simultaneously at some point in history. On the surface, this is a relatively simple data set; a patient identifier followed by a series of numbers (the vital sign data) alongside the metadata describing the time and date the data was taken (and possibly some other clinical parameters, for example, the patient's position).

But, in reality, this data set is far from straight-forward. For a start, some of those measurements were taken on digital blood pressure meters and some were performed manually. Furthermore, the percentage of readings taken on digital meters varies from site to site, country to country, and study to study based on therapeutic indication (cardiology studies have a particularly high percentage of readings taken on digital meters), regional wealth (Western countries tend to have more digital readings than third world or emerging markets due the expense of the meters), and personal preference of the site staff. This is important. Analysis of the data derived from digital meters reflects the accuracy of the meter, not the integrity of the site. However, data obtained from a manual measurement, in contrast to a digital measurement, is permanently and very closely linked to the site's integrity for several reasons listed in the following text.

First, it is difficult for anybody to retrospectively influence the data. To better understand this point, let's briefly examine another data set— concomitant medication (conmeds). In the author's experience, it is not unusual for a site to omit a number of conmeds from the patient's case report form (CRF), probably due to the burden on the site and because of a perceived lack of value of the data. However, even if the site does not document all of the conmeds, a vigilant clinical research associate (CRA) will detect the omissions and request that the conmeds are added to the CRF. It is vitally important that you, the reader, understand this subtle event: Initially, the site did not perform to the standards required, but following the actions of the CRA, the site added the missing data. If a risk analysis was performed on the conmed data prior to the CRA visit, there was a good chance we would have detected the site's inappropriate behavior, but once the CRA took corrective action, analysis of the conmed data would [probably] no longer detect the noncompliance. This transition reflects the subtle but important difference between quality and risk. Following the CRA's corrective action, the quality of the data improved (particularly its accuracy and completeness) but the risks may not have changed—risk is a trait, not a data point. Critically, our subsequent ability to detect that risk trait has been masked by the corrective action. As a result, the subsequent value of the conmed data as an indicator of risk is greatly reduced because we are no longer analyzing the activities of the site but, instead, the collective actions of the site, the CRA, and the site's compliance with the corrective actions—statistically referred to as confounding variables. Trace evidence tends to remain, but it can be heavily masked. We will return to conmeds later in this section, but for now, let's get back to the vitals data.

Unlike conmeds, it is very difficult, if not impossible, for the CRA to retrospectively influence the vitals data. Source document verification (SDV) merely serves to confirm that the data in the CRF is consistent with the data in the source documents. Even if the CRA became suspicious that a specific blood pressure reading of 120/80 mm Hg appeared improbable, considering the sea of blood pressure data with identical values, it is very difficult for the CRA to retrospectively argue the point. After all, the CRA was not there on the day of the measurement, and who is to say the reading was not 120/80? Or so the investigator will argue. Also, the CRA does not have a global, statistically supported view of the data. Instead, they are embedded in the details of the data, reviewing each individual data point and compiling a limited impression of the site. Therefore, aside from making corrections to transcription errors, vital sign data goes largely unaltered throughout the life cycle of study. To be clear, this is not to say that the views and actions of the CRA are irrelevant, but the message is that the CRA can only operate within the confines of human capability and the process.

A second valuable feature of vital sign data derived from manual measurements is that the manual blood pressure readings are strongly influenced by the operator (digital readings are not of course). This may seem obvious, but the implications are profound, and the ability to detect these influences are not always immediately obvious to an analyst without a medical background. For example, a typical approach to the analysis of blood pressure data when in pursuit of risk (or fraud) detection is to calculate the standard deviation (or variance) of the systolic or diastolic measurements and to compare the result on a per site basis with the other sites collectively. If the standard deviation is unusually high or low at any one site, the conclusion is that there maybe a problem, and a CRA should be dispatched. This approach is fraught with problems, not least of which is the question "What do we expect the CRA to do about it?" But, let's look at some characteristics of the data first.

Systolic and diastolic measurements are highly correlated and are not independently variable. As the systolic reading increases, so does the diastolic reading (typically by about half of the systolic increase). This correlation is ingrained in the clinician over the years of his or her practice but, importantly, the correlation is by no means universal or absolute. In some diseases, for example, aortic regurgitation, the exact opposite may occur, and the diastolic reading may, in fact, decrease as the systolic increases, albeit it a rarity by comparison.

Number preference is widely used: clinicians often round off the blood pressure readings to the nearest five or zero, for example, 120/80 or 135/85, and this is generally considered acceptable in routine clinical practice. Digital blood pressure meters do not do this.

Last, the range of available readings is often surprisingly narrow. In a study requiring normotensive patients, the acceptable range of systolic measurements might be between 100 and 140 mm Hg. But if the clinician is rounding off to the nearest 5, this is a mere nine systolic values at baseline (100, 105, 110, 115, 120, 125, 130, 135, and 140 mm Hg systolic) and far less if there are only one or two patients who will each remain within a biologically narrow systolic range over time.

With this in mind, the use of standard deviation as a tool for detection of risk using blood pressure data becomes challenging. Standard deviation can only be used on either systolic or diastolic measurements independently (there are exceptions, but they have their own limitations), does not take into account the difference between manual and electronic blood pressure readings, and is a measure of data spread in a data range which is often inherently narrower than anticipated. That is not to say it does not work. In fact, it does work, but only to a degree. In the author's experience, standard deviation worked well to detect those sites that had unrelentingly repeated the measurement 120/80 over and over, but it did not work well when the investigator deliberately attempted to deceive—arguably a site of even greater concern. In cases where there is an attempt to deceive, the investigator may deliberately spread the data over a few systolic and diastolic readings, for example 140/90, 120/80, and possibly 110/70. However, because there are only nine possible systolic values available to the investigator (presuming he/she rounds off to 5 mm Hg), as compared to the 41 possible values available to a digital meter, it is very easy for him/her to create the illusion of adequate data spread and avoid detection, often deflecting our attention to smaller sites with few patients and, thus, a very limited range of systolic data, albeit completely genuine data.

Instead of standard deviation, what is needed is an algorithm(s) which takes into account the existence of digital blood pressure meters, the correlation of systolic and diastolic data, the intra- and inter-patient variability, the presence of number preference, and the interoperator variability—ideally presented to the user in a simple to understand format. The key to the algorithm(s) is to capitalize on the [fraudulent] investigator's ingrained sense of correlation and staccato data spread, neither of which replicate real data. When this is achieved and combined with a well-defined stepwise approach to the analysis, the blood pressure readings, unlike conmeds, provide a persistently valuable window into the site's risk profile that is largely untainted by repeated monitoring and that is continuously updated throughout the life cycle of the site as new readings are taken (the high frequency of vital sign measurements is another valuable benefit of this data set).

Like blood pressure data, the heart rate data is also more complicated than initially meets the eye because heart rate data is often extrapolated, not actual. As a result, it is our experience that standard deviation does not work as well as we hope and, like blood pressure, we need to create an algorithm(s) which is specifically suited to heart rate data to detect those sites that are deliberately and systematically fabricating data. In our experience, heart rate data does have one small but significant advantage over blood pressure data: using a good deal of clinical acumen, it is possible to use simple algorithms to instantly demonstrate that the data is fabricated. When combined with evidence of suspicious blood pressure data, the verdict is almost conclusive, and we are able to direct the CRA to conduct very specific, well-defined procedures to prove it. This is the advantage of a well thought out, carefully executed risk detection and management plan.

As you read through the earlier paragraphs, I hope you have started to build an idea of how subtle and complex the vital sign data can be despite the apparently simple nature of the systolic and diastolic values as they neatly line up on your screen. Of course, this subtleness is not restricted to blood pressure data, heart rate data, or conmeds but extends across all data sets. Each data set has its own unique characteristics which you can better understand if you ask the following questions of it: when in the study life cycle is the data collected, who collects the data (the source), who can influence the data, is it causally related to risk? Let's look at some of those questions a bit closer.

The timing of collection within the study life cycle is important because it allows us to understand when the analysis is relevant and where the gaps in our risk coverage may exist. For example, almost all companies analyze randomization (or screen failure) rates in order to detect issues with protocol compliance. We do too. Indeed, we have causally mapped randomization rates to the risk "protocol (study) compliance," and with some subtle tweaks, it works well. But it is only effective during the period of recruitment, and we need to find at least one other indicator of protocol compliance to cover the maintenance period of the study if we are to provide end-to-end risk monitoring.

Sometimes it is not simply that the data is no longer collected but, instead, that the site's compliance changes over time, based on the perceived value of the data. For example, conmeds are often poorly collected at Visit 1 (V1) because it is a considerable effort, and there is no guarantee that the patient will be randomized. However, there is an improvement in the collection once the patient is randomized because the same data is now closely associated with safety events (adverse events), and the volume of data is reduced (fewer patients). Therefore, postrandomization conmed data can be a more valuable indicator of risk than the prerandomization data. Note that we are referring to risk, not quality, and in our opinion, risk is a trait. We are looking for indicators which are sensitive and specific to those traits we consider to be risk prone. Sometimes risk and quality are synonymous, sometimes not.

Next let's consider the source of the data. Sites are a collection of people with a variety of qualifications and responsibilities. These various people interact with the patients and each other at different points in time, and each has a specific role, some of which are data related. The data we collect is, therefore, a composite of those roles. for example, in larger commercialized sites, the principle investigator is simply a figurehead. He/she does not actually see patients or collect data on most days. His/her clinical duties are largely delegated to one of possibly many subinvestigators, who in turn delegate some of the more routine tasks to the nursing staff. This is a fairly standard model in larger sites. As a consequence, the blood pressure measurements in larger sites are likely to have been delegated to the nursing team, and the use of the blood pressure data as a risk metric is reflecting the activity of the nursing team, not the doctors at these sites. This complex mosaic affects our risk assessment because we must ensure that the risk analysts identify at least some data which can only come from the medical doctors. This data can then be supplemented with information from the broader team. By doing this, we can provide very detailed guidance to the CRA: whom to interview, what questions to ask, which files to review. It is important to also realize that the roles are not static. For example, conmeds are often collected by the nursing staff in mass screening programs, but after randomization, the conmed data is collected as part of the medical doctor's consultation with the patient. In these cases, we sometimes notice a completely inverse pattern to the one described earlier: the V1 conmed data is very high quality and drops off dramatically after randomization. The data completeness then gradually improves as the CRA conducts the SDV and makes inquiries related to new adverse events and medication documented in the patient's health records.

A well-constructed risk detection platform is one which provides sensitive and specific risk-detection algorithms that cover the study over its whole life cycle, cover all the roles in the site, are unaffected by monitoring (or at least partially immune to monitoring), and correlate with all the risks traits we are trying to detect. Ideally there should be no point in the study during which a particular risk is not being monitored or could be masked beyond our detection capabilities. We hope these musings will give you insight to what are the relevant markers for your studies to ensure you are adequately monitoring and managing the relevant risks.

4. THE SOLUTION: USING THE INFORMATION/KNOWLEDGE TO MANAGE THE RISK IN REAL TIME

The ICON patient-centered monitoring strategy is defined by the following principles:

- It is designed to meet regulatory and quality requirements for GCP and is consistent with guidance documents published by the FDA [1] and EMA [2] on risk-based quality management and monitoring.
- It uses scientific analysis of emergent data, together with clinical research associate (CRA) site knowledge, to direct central, off-site and on-site monitoring activities.
- It is an adaptive strategy that uses site milestones, data volume metrics, and risk-indicator-based triggers to identify variances in site performance and to target appropriate interventions.
- It optimizes resource utilization, reduces SDV of noncritical subject data, and aims to deliver higher quality and cost-effective clinical trial management.

Specifically, the ICON patient-centered monitoring process is aligned with the recently-published TransCelerate Biopharma position paper on risk-based monitoring [3], and encompasses:

- A formal protocol risk assessment, data category review, and the development of a study-specific monitoring plan, in consultation with relevant stakeholders in different functions.
- A definition of critical data categories that impact key GCP requirements for subject rights and safety, investigational product efficacy and safety, and data integrity.
- Reduced on-site source data verification (SDV) appropriate to study risk, focusing on SDV and source data review (SDR) of critical data, defined in discussion with the sponsor, supported by comprehensive, centralized, clinical data review by the clinical data analysts (CDAs).
- Prespecified milestones and site activity metrics that trigger site contact.
- Use of real-time risk indicators by the centralized monitoring team to evaluate site performance and to guide and trigger specific monitoring

actions. These analyses are communicated to the study team at a regular frequency (for example, monthly).

- Flexible use of additional targeted monitoring activities, including additional SDV and SDR and other interventions directed to sites, based on site performance analysis, according to defined rules, and with traceable actions.

- Flexible use of off-site visits and on-site visits to support sites, perform root cause analysis of detected errors or noncompliance, and mitigate performance and compliance issues.

On-site activities continue to play a key role in quality management. These activities include confirmation of subject-informed consent; investigational product accountability; site file review; site relationship management; source data review; and source data verification (particularly of critical data). However, on-site monitoring alone is not well suited to the detection of comparative performance signals, trends, and patterns across multiple subjects, sites, and countries, or the monitoring of uncommon events to identify sites that may need corrective action. These activities are best performed by centralized monitoring of aggregated data using technology specifically designed for these purposes.

Figure 24.2 provides an overview of the ICON risk-based monitoring process. This is driven by a cross-functional approach that involves particular attention to communication and documentation of information and decisions.

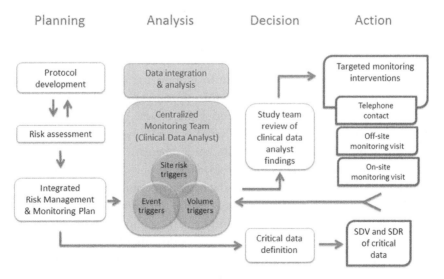

Figure 24.2 Overview of ICON patient-centered monitoring process.

5. THE SOLUTION: RISK ASSESSMENT

The first stage of the ICON patient-centered monitoring process is to determine the specific risks and global risk-level associated with the clinical trial and protocol, in line with quality by design principles. Optimally, this process begins during early development of the protocol, in collaboration with the sponsor, and prior to protocol finalization. The project team meets with the relevant stakeholders to discuss and define these risks using the risk assessment tool. Multiple criteria relating to the trial protocol, patient population, investigational product, data management, and geographic criteria are evaluated (see example in Table 24.1). Each risk criterion is assigned a weighted score, and risk indicators and potential mitigating actions are assigned. In addition, a composite study risk score is calculated based on the weighted scoring system for each criterion. The risk score informs the cross-functional team's discussion of the integrated cross-functional risk management strategy (for example, including medical monitoring, data management, and site monitoring), and detailed monitoring plan specifications.

6. THE SOLUTION: INTEGRATED RISK MANAGEMENT PLAN

An integrated risk management plan is developed using the outputs of the risk assessment process. This document defines plans for a range of activities, including communication, governance, quality assurance, medical monitoring, data management, study start up, vendor management, documentation control, and site monitoring.

The study specific monitoring plan (SSMP) forms one component of the integrated risk management plan. The core document provides guidance and specific instructions relating to monitoring of the investigational sites, including the minimum criteria for monitoring and site management tasks that will be conducted throughout the course of the study. Specific sections are included in the SSMP, clarifying the study-specific monitoring and SDV schedule, together with the comprehensive clinical subject data review activities performed by the centralized monitoring study team and the triggers that may lead to potential additional monitoring activities.

The team completes a template to describe the monitoring visit schedule and SDV/SDR strategy, which outlines the baseline or minimal on-site monitoring visit schedule for the study. This document also establishes the minimal number of off-site monitoring visits and minimal number of telephone contacts the monitor will have with the investigational sites, and

Table 24.1 Example of risk assessment

Number	Criteria	Level	Study score	Study-related information and comments	Suggested risk indicator trigger
1	Study phase	High	5	Early phase II	Vital sign values
2	End point	Low	1	Objective end point in lab data	
3	Study design	Medium	3	Interventional study with simple design	Number of AE
4	Risk of procedures	Low	1	Few invasive procedures, close to standard of care	
17	Geographic score	High	5	Two participating countries with high risk	Number and type of protocol deviation
Overall study score			45		
Study monitoring risk level			Medium		

The project leader and a cross-functional team of relevant subject matter experts review the categories and level of risks (in up to 17 categories), in order to design a risk management strategy to address these risks. The example in the table records the risks in study phase, study design, study procedures, and geography with their level, score, and description. Each study criterion is scored in order to design the risk management strategy and associated risk indicators with their specific thresholds. The study monitoring risk level score provides a high-level indication of the intensity of monitoring recommended.

defines targeted minimum categories of data for SDV and SDR, and includes the specific data points, subjects, and visits where 100% SDV is mandated.

In the "Guidelines for Additional Monitoring" document, the team defines the risk indicators that are analyzed by the centralized monitoring team to identify variant or outlier site performance and the thresholds that will define outlier sites and trigger an intervention. This document is completed by the study team with centralized monitoring team support. The choice of risk indicators and trigger thresholds for each risk indicator can be adapted (i.e., made more or less stringent) by the study team in collaboration with the sponsor, depending on the needs of the study.

The study team defines the three categories of triggers in the following hierarchy (risk indicator triggers override data volume triggers, which override milestone triggers):

- *Risk indicator triggers*—Comparative evaluation of site activity across the study, according to objective risk indicators, indicates the need for the site contact to perform investigative or corrective action. Risk triggers are considered in three domains: "recruitment" (e.g., screening to randomized ratios, withdrawal rates), "reporting diligence" (e.g., adverse events reported per randomized subject per month exposure; concomitant medication per randomized subject), and "data quality" (e.g., variability index of vital sign data, to identify digit preference, data rounding tendencies, or biologically implausible data).
- *Data volume triggers*—For example, a site contact is recommended when the volume of data or subjects at a site is above a defined threshold to justify a full day on-site visit to perform SDV, SDR, and other on-site activities.
- *Milestone triggers*—These are triggers relating to defined milestones at a site that initiate an on-site monitoring visit, for example, the first subject randomized at a site.

The Guidelines for Additional Monitoring document also defines the recommended monitoring interventions based on the significance or severity of the finding, risk level involved, and the current monitoring visit plan. The CRA, together with other key members of the study project management team, determines the specific course of action to best investigate, clarify, or resolve each finding at each specific site.

The central monitoring team analysis of the risk indicators and triggers defined by the SSMP document is conducted through the use of the ICONIK data integration platform, described in the following text.

During site management and monitoring activities, the CRA may also make observations whereby specific risks, data trends, or triggers may be identified. All such CRA observations are documented in the monitoring visit report and action item module within ICON's clinical trial management system (CTMS). CRA observations are formally discussed in the monthly combined project study team meetings, so that comprehensive risk and mitigation information is shared between the centralized monitoring team and the site-facing team. In addition to these scheduled meetings, high-risk CRA observations are immediately escalated and brought to the attention of the entire study team.

The clinical data analyst (CDA) assigned to each study prepares the Centralized Monitoring Plan using a template to define the centralized monitoring analysis process, the analysis frequency of risk indicators and triggers, and any other associated project-specific activities.

The core SSMP document is updated when required by the project management team and CDA, in consultation with the sponsor, and updated versions are distributed to the study team members.

The following examples from the ICONIK analytics tools and visualizations are presented in the following text; these examples relate to risk indicators for recruitment, reporting diligence, and data quality, which the CDA can review along with other prebuilt listing data reports, distribution analyses, or graphical charts to evaluate site performance. Using a suite of dynamic filters and drill-down functions, the CDA can interact with the data to generate immediate analytical outputs. Because the primary data sources are fully aggregated and integrated, multiple domains of data can be evaluated simultaneously at subject, site, and study level (Figures 24.3–24.5).

7. THE SOLUTION: CENTRALIZED MONITORING ACTIVITIES

Using the ICONIK data reports, the clinical trial study data is analyzed by the CDA for each risk indicator defined in the SSMP (screen failure rate, randomization rate, AE underreporting, etc.) to detect a potential site risk—termed a "finding"—which may result in the need for additional monitoring activity at the investigational site. These CDA findings are not in themselves considered definitive evidence of a quality problem, but rather as an observation or hypothesis that requires further investigation.

All CDA findings are entered by the CDA into a specific module within ICON's clinical trial management system (CTMS) by category or domain type: reporting diligence, data quality, recruitment, and others. Each finding

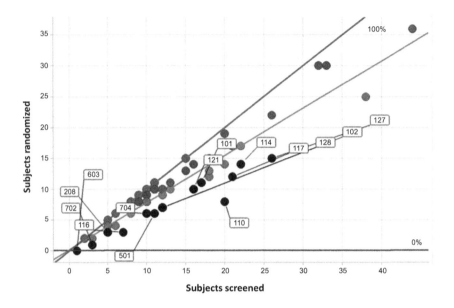

Figure 24.3 Risk Indicators—recruitment domain; subject randomization to screening ratios by site. This figure shows a screen shot from ICONIK clinical data analysis. The scatterplot shows the distribution of sites in a Phase 3 study: comparing the number of subjects screened (X-axis) versus the number of subjects randomized (Y-axis) per site. The red line indicates a 1:1 (maximum) randomization to screening ratio. The green line indicates the mean randomization ration for this population of sites. Dynamic algorithms enable the CDA to select the lower quartile (25%) of sites with low randomization to screening ratios—these sites are automatically highlighted with site number labels. This trigger threshold can be changed according to the risk assessment and SSMP documents. For example, the analyst can choose to identify the sites in the lowest or highest 5%, 10%, or any other proportion of this distribution. The study team would focus on the recruitment activities of these sites to investigate and mitigate this performance issue. *(For interpretation of the references to color in this figure legend, the reader is referred to the online version of this book.)*

is also assigned a priority score of low, medium, or high based on the centralized monitoring team's predefined scoring system of analyzed triggers.

For any high-priority finding entered into CTMS, the site CRA and project management team receive an immediate alert email triggered by the system. After each risk indicator or trigger finding is analyzed, scored, and entered into CTMS by the CDA, an overall site score is calculated by the CDA and assigned to each site. Sites with no findings receive no score; however, each site with any findings is assigned a composite risk score of low, medium, or high, according to the number and severity of findings.

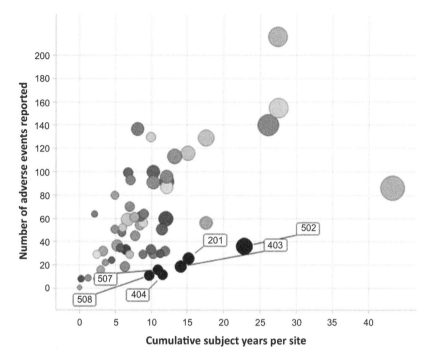

Figure 24.4 Risk indicators—reporting diligence domain; adverse event reporting by site. This figure shows a screen shot from ICONIK clinical data analysis. The scatterplot shows the distribution of sites in a Phase 3 study, comparing cumulative randomized subject years (X-axis) versus the total number of adverse events (AE) reported by each site. The area of each dot in the scatterplot is proportional to the numbers of random- ized patients at each site. Highlighted and labeled sites are in the lowest 10% of the distribution—these thresholds can be changed by the CDA using dynamic algorithms and tools within the ICONIK system, as determined by the SSMP. In the interactive visu- alization, hovering or clicking on elements in the scatterplot provides comprehensive data listings on the selected site. These sites will be highlighted as CDA findings to the study team for further investigation.

The composite site risk score is also entered into the CTMS system for tracking within ICON's clinical trial site performance reporting tool, visu- alized as a dashboard.

The study team holds regular study cross-functional meetings to present the CDA findings, review the highest priority sites, and address any issues or questions regarding CDA analysis information. During this time, action plans to address the identified issues may also be discussed and prepared among the clinical study team members. In addition, information from the CRA experience with sites is fed back to the centralized monitoring team.

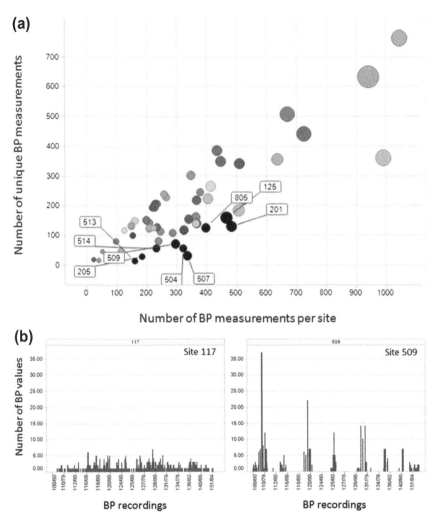

Figure 24.5 A: Risk indicators—data quality domain; vital sign variability by site. This figure shows a screen shot from ICONIK clinical data analysis. (a) The scatterplot shows the distribution of sites in a Phase 3 study, comparing the total number of reported blood pressure (BP) measurements (X-axis) versus the total number of *unique* blood pressure data points reported by each site (Y-axis). The size of each dot is proportional to the number of patients randomized at each site. A low number of unique BP measurements indicates that certain BP values are reported multiple times. Highlighted sites (black) indicate the sites in the lowest 15% of the distribution—these thresholds can be changed by the CDA as determined by the SSMP. In the interactive visualization, hovering or clicking on data from any site in the scatterplot provides comprehensive patient-level data on this site. (b) The figure shows data distribution histograms from two sites in this distribution. Site 117 is a typical site from the mean of this population, reporting 366 individual blood pressure (BP) measurements from 13 subjects. The BP

All decisions, interventions, and outcomes are documented by the CRA in the CTMS system. It is the responsibility of each site CRA to check the CTMS on a regular basis (at a minimum weekly) to identify new CDA findings that have been raised following the CDA analysis.

After discussion within the clinical team, the CDA findings addressed by the CRA with the site are entered into the CTMS and the responses are reviewed by the CDA for appropriateness to the issue. The CDA marks the finding as closed upon review of the additional monitoring intervention and outcome.

Figure 24.6 shows an overview of the centralized monitoring activities and the interactions with the study clinical operations team.

8. THE SOLUTION: ADAPTIVE SITE MONITORING ACTIVITIES

Site monitoring activities are conducted according to the SSMP, ICON standard operating procedures, GCP, international and local regulations. The CRA ensures that activities are executed according to the study requirements and specifications.

The ICON patient-centered monitoring strategy employs the following additional site monitoring activities to ensure all site performance and compliance issues, including CDA findings, are addressed: on-site monitoring visit, off-site monitoring visit, and telephone contact.

- The on-site monitoring visit is conducted by the site CRA to conduct SDV, review source data, study documentation (SDR), and to verify appropriate conduct of the study by the investigator. After each visit, the CRA issues a monitoring visit report using the CTMS system. This type of visit is triggered in addition to the baseline on-site monitoring visit.
- Off-site monitoring visits are formal telephone conferences performed by the CRA to assess the performance of the investigational site, support

---

values are distributed across a wide range, with 218 unique recordings, and BP values reported to the nearest 1–2 mm Hg. In comparison, site 509 (one of the outlier sites) has reported 288 BP values from 11 patients. The BP values are distributed in distinct groups, with only 70 unique recordings, many recordings reported to the nearest 5 or 10 mm Hg, and many values such as 110/80 mm Hg reported on more than 10 occasions. The analysis suggests the site is rounding BP data to the nearest 10 mm Hg and failing to perform this procedure per protocol. Site 509 and the other outlier sites would be highlighted as CDA findings to the study team for further investigation and site training and support. *(For interpretation of the references to color in this figure legend, the reader is referred to the online version of this book.)*

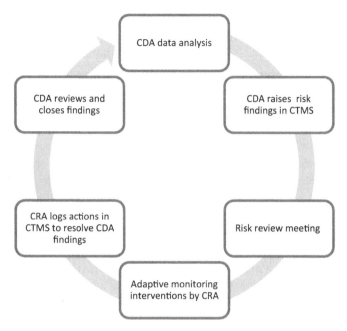

Figure 24.6 Integrated monitoring cycle. The CDA undertakes site quality and performance analysis on a scheduled basis (for example, monthly), communicating individual findings to the CRAs responsible for each site. High-priority sites are discussed at the study team risk review meeting, at which feedback from the CRAs is also shared with the central monitoring team. The CRAs undertake targeted monitoring interventions, integrating information from the CDA with their own direct knowledge of their sites. The CRA logs specific actions in response to each CDA finding, and these are reviewed by the CDA before each finding is closed.

staff with data queries, train, or update staff on new study information, and may be used as per the additional monitoring guidelines as a method to address CDA findings with the site. Off-site monitoring visits follow a formal appointment and agenda with the site study coordinator and investigator, have a structured agenda, and a follow-up letter is issued to the site. A report is generated in CTMS to document the information.

- Telephone contact is a focused means of communication with the site and is typically shorter than a formal off-site monitoring visit. This form of contact is designed to maintain communication, provide updates, and drive quality at the site.

The use of additional monitoring interventions is discussed during the clinical study team meetings, and the CRA and clinical team determines the most effective method to address the CDA finding and site performance issue.

Other specific interventions may be required in the case of major or repeated findings, including, but not limited to:

- Site re-training
- Co-monitoring/QC visit
- For cause audit
- Clinical Trial Manager (CTM)/sponsor/affiliate/national coordinating investigator contact to site
- Site closure.

Any additional monitoring interventions that are decided and performed to address CDA findings by the CRA are documented either in CTMS, or if through telephone contact, by use of a telephone contact record form that is filed as part of the trial master file (TMF).

9. SWOT

Strength	Weakness
The process and systems described are in use for multiple active projects and have been tried and tested for their ability to perform as expected.	Focus on a holistic solution using existing technology and concepts—future developments in technologies and concepts might make this approach outdated relatively quickly. As with any holistic solution, this is one way to tackle the problem. There may be other alternate approaches that achieve the same goal to effectively managing clinical studies.
Covers all core aspects necessary to perform interactive monitoring of your clinical sites and their performance.	

10. APPLICABLE REGULATIONS

International Conference on Harmonization (ICH), Good Clinical Practice (GCP) and all applicable Food and Drug Administration (FDA), European Medicines Agency (EMA), and Pharmaceuticals and Medical Devices Agency (PMDA) regulations.

11. TAKE HOME MESSAGE

ICONIK allows data to be placed in context and in a timely fashion—typically within 24 hours of data collection. ICON has developed many algorithms that allow ICONIK data to be interpreted in context to extract and visualize potential risks to the patient and the successful conduct of clinical studies. ICON has developed various process and procedures that allow these identified risks to be ameliorated or avoided, and these systems, processes, and procedures together enable ICONIK patient-centered monitoring to provide more effective, efficient monitoring of clinical studies. The result is to improve the safety of the patient and increase the likelihood of a definitive outcome to the study itself by improving the overall quality of the study execution and the data itself.

REFERENCES

[1] Guidance for Industry: oversight of clinical investigations — a risk-based approach to monitoring; 2013. www.fda.gov/downloads/drugs/guidancecomplianceregulatoryinfor mation/guidances/ucm269919.pdf.
[2] Reflection paper on risk based quality management in clinical trials; 2013. http://www .ema.europa.eu/docs/en_GB/document_library/Scientific_guideline/2013/11/WC50 0155491.pdf.
[3] Position paper: risk-based monitoring methodology; 2013. http://www.transcelera-tebiopharmainc.com/content/risk-based-monitoring-methodology-position-paper/.

CHAPTER 25

Knowledge Management
Looking after the Know-How

Nick Milton

Contents

1. THE NEED

The pharmaceutical industry is a very unusual type.

It is unlike almost every other industry, in that the vast majority of projects fail. Less than 5% of drug development projects lead to a commercial product. This means that in more than 95% of the cases, the only product from a drug development project is knowledge. The company has learned a little bit more about this molecule, this receptor, this therapy area, and the sum total of the company knowledge has increased by a significant amount.

But, if knowledge is the only product, how well is that product managed? In any other industry, the deliverables from a project are managed. If a project creates a new product, it is handled by a product manager. If a sales project delivers a new client, this is handled by a client manager. The project results in a new office opening in a new country, then this is handled by an office manager. So who manages the knowledge created from drug development projects? Who makes sure it is compiled, collated, and made available to future projects?

Note that here we are talking about knowledge rather than information or data. We are talking about the development of insights and understanding,

Re-Engineering Clinical Trials
http://dx.doi.org/10.1016/B978-0-12-420246-7.00025-6

rather than filing the results of clinical trials. We are talking about what those trials mean, rather than the raw data itself.

And there is another side to knowledge in pharmaceutical organizations, which is a knowledge of how drug development projects operate. Development projects face huge challenges. They are often staffed by people from multiple functions, in multiple countries, often working on multiple projects at once, and they face increasingly strict and complex regulatory challenges. It is not an easy business, developing a new drug, and the major pharmaceutical organizations make it even more difficult for themselves as a result of their team structure. Where a small independent company, made up of a handful of people working at the same office, can share and build their collective knowledge through day-to-day conversation, a large, multinational company does not have this luxury. If a large multinational company is to continuously learn about drug development and a constantly changing marketplace, this has to be done deliberately.

When it comes to the details of medical research, we have a third challenge. Even as I write this, I realize that many people will see it as a huge and sweeping generalization, but researchers are not always the most extroverted of people. Research is a task that requires high levels of individual dedication and intellectual focus, information gathering, and problem solving, and (say, compared to being a sales manager) suits introverts better than extroverts. When it comes to sharing knowledge in a world of introverts, there needs to be a degree of structure to ensure this happens on a regular and timely basis. Knowledge doesn't just flow, it needs to be requested. And when knowledge does not flow, it accumulates in the brain of the researcher. We end up with an organization of learners, rather than a learning organization—an organization of experts rather than an expert organization.

The risk to the pharmaceutical industry is clear. Ninety-five percent or more of projects create a potentially valuable product which could be a huge asset to future growth, but this product is not managed, it is locked away in organizational silos and carried in the memories of (potentially introverted) individuals. Therefore, it is at risk of loss through retirement, redundancy, poaching by small startups, and just ordinary forgetting.

2. THE SOLUTION

The solution to this problem is to start to treat knowledge as a real asset that has to be managed and to introduce a system of knowledge management (KM).

Knowledge management can be considered as a management approach focused on maximizing the benefits and strategic and tactical value of organizational knowledge. Knowledge, in this context, is defined as the organizational capability or know-how by which individuals, teams, and projects make the most effective decisions and take the most effective actions for business delivery.

If we think of knowledge as "know-how" and as a decision support tool, then we can see how it is different from information and data. In the pharmaceutical world, there are two forms of know-how:

1. Knowing how molecules and receptors interact in various species, and how these interactions affect bodily and mental functions.
2. Knowing how to work together as an integrated multidisciplinary global team to rapidly and effectively develop, test, and either reject or pass a new drug through the approval process.

So how do we manage something as intangible as know-how? First let's look at knowledge management as a discipline and how it has developed over the years.

Recognizing the importance of knowledge at the beginning of the knowledge age, in the 1990s, the initial concept was to capture an organization's knowledge in documents and place them in repositories so that those needing the knowledge could easily access it. However, over time it became evident that employees could not search for knowledge that they did not know they needed. As knowledge repositories grew ever larger, searching took more time than employees had. To be useful, organizational knowledge needed to be validated, categorized, and synthesized. The idea developed of "knowledge owners" who would take accountability for these processes.

It also became apparent that only a small portion of the knowledge gained during work activities could be written down. Researchers have found that 80% of an organization's knowledge is in the heads of knowledge workers and cannot be documented. To gain access to this knowledge, referred to as tacit knowledge, a new way of transferring the knowledge was developed. Several structures have emerged, such as the "communities of practice" which provide the opportunity for conversation among workers that are geographical separated. At the same time, project-based knowledge management approaches were introduced.

Through the history described above, it became recognized that individual knowledge management tools and processes will not, on their own, deliver value, and that an integrated knowledge management framework is necessary. The elements of such a framework are explained in the following sections.

2.1 The "Learning Before, During, and After" Model

This model describes how knowledge management activities can fit within the cycle of business activity.

The management of knowledge, like the management of quality or resources, needs to be systematic rather than ad hoc and needs to be tied into the business cycle. In drug development projects where multiple activities take place, knowledge can be addressed at three points. The project team can learn at the start of an activity, so that the project begins from a state of complete knowledge (learning before). They can learn during the activity, so that plans can be changed and adapted as new knowledge becomes available (learning during). Finally, they can learn at the end of the activity, so that knowledge is captured for future use (learning after). The people and teams who manage the projects can use knowledge to improve their results and reach their goals. This model of "learn before, during, and after" was developed in BP during the 1990s (see Ref. [1]) and also appears to have been developed independently in several other organizations. Shell refers to this as "ask, learn, share."

However, there is more to the model than the learning before, during, and after cycle. The knowledge generated from the project needs to be collated, synthesized, and stored as knowledge assets (guidance documents, or wikis which track the development of understanding of a molecule) in order that knowledge deposited in the "knowledge bank" at the end of the project becomes more useful when accessed at the start of the next project.

Communities of practice need to be established to manage and share the tacit knowledge assets so that researchers and scientists around the world can discuss the development of knowledge in any one therapy area.

This five-component model (learning before, learning during, learning after, synthesis of knowledge into knowledge assets, and building communities of practice) is a robust model that creates value wherever it is applied. The model is illustrated in Figure 25.1.

2.2 People, Process, Technology, and Governance

The four aspects of roles, processes, technology, and governance are key enablers for any management system, as shown in Figure 25.2. A knowledge management framework needs people to be assigned roles and accountabilities; it needs processes embedded into the project framework for knowledge identification, capture, access, and sharing; it needs technology for the

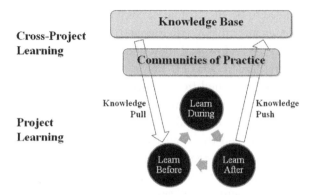

Figure 25.1 The "learning before, during, and after" model for knowledge management.

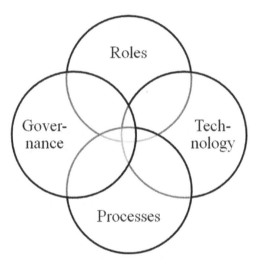

Figure 25.2 The four main enablers of knowledge management.

storage, organization, and retrieval of knowledge, and it needs governance of the knowledge management system to ensure that it is being applied.

2.3 A Knowledge Management Model for Pharma

Every organization will need to tailor a knowledge management framework to their own circumstance, but each of the frameworks is likely to contain some or all of the elements listed below. Already, many of the major multi-nationals such as Astra Zeneca, Merck, Pfizer, and Glaxo SmithKline are building and deploying their own knowledge management systems using many of these elements, as described in Goodman and Riddell [2].

1. There will need to be effective processes within the projects for capturing new knowledge after major activities and after project phases. The classic process here is the "retrospect," described in Milton [3], which is a team meeting where all members of the project team spend up to a day discussing what has been learned from the activity or project phase. They will discuss the medical learning, any new knowledge that has been gathered relating to the therapy area, and also learning about the way they worked together as a team and the way that the project itself was handled and managed. These meetings require an external objective facilitator and very detailed notes will be taken. The conversation will cover what was expected, what was actually delivered, the root cause between the two, and the lessons for the organization and for future projects.

2. There will need to be a mechanism for handling these lessons. New lessons about the therapy area need to be forwarded to the community of practice or the knowledge owner for the therapy area, so that the knowledge base may be updated. New lessons about the project process need to be forwarded to whoever is in charge of the project process, so the project guidelines can be updated as required.

3. There will need to be a knowledge owner for major areas of knowledge, such as project management, regulatory approvals, clinical trials, and the main therapy areas. That person will be accountable for making sure that a body of knowledge is created, maintained, and kept updated, and that any old knowledge is removed. Technologies such as wikis can be very useful here for hosting a continuously updated body of knowledge. An example of this is Pfizer's internal wiki, known as Pfizerpedia (see Ref. [4]).

4. There will need to be a community of practice for major areas of knowledge to make sure that people have an avenue for discussion about new problems, new questions, new lessons, and new insights. Often the community of practice is led by the knowledge owner, and the community often acts as both the contributors to, and the users of, the body of knowledge on the wiki.

5. There will need to be a process for making sure that new projects access and learn from the lessons of the past. One or two companies have experimented with the idea of a "learning plan" for projects, which allows them to plan out and monitor the effectiveness of their learning from the experience of others.

6. Within the projects, there may need to be simple processes for regular review of learning so that the projects themselves can take action if things

change. The standard process is the "after action review" (also described in Ref. [3]), a brief and regular learning activity typically applied within the military and the emergency services for rapid and effective learning.

7. There will need to be enough governance to ensure that all of this happens. This will require a knowledge management team somewhere in the organization to set the expectation for knowledge management, to define the processes and roles that will be needed, to acquire any necessary technology, to train people in the application of knowledge management, and to monitor how well knowledge management is being applied.

3. SWOT

There are several strengths, weaknesses, opportunities, and threats to the introduction of effective knowledge management within pharmaceutical organizations. These are listed below.

3.1 Strengths

Knowledge management is a relatively cheap intervention that delivers a lot of value. It focuses on an asset that the organization already has—its knowledge—and connects up that knowledge across the organizational silos. Knowledge management is a simple concept, and there are a wealth of proven practices and technologies to enable knowledge management. There is a relatively strong history of the concept within the pharmaceutical industry, so it is not like you are trying to introduce something new.

3.2 Weaknesses

Although knowledge management is a simple concept, that does not make it easy to do. It is at its heart a change initiative, and it represents a significant and distinctive cultural change. Knowledge that was once seen as a personal asset, the property of the researcher, needs to be treated as a corporate asset from which others can learn (and who in return will share their own learning). In some companies, there may be several cultural barriers that will need to be overcome: rivalry, internal competition, "knowledge is power" and "not invented here," for example. Knowledge management needs to be introduced as a change program, and change programs take a long time and need strong support from senior management. Through all of this change, the value of knowledge management may not initially be easy to see. Knowledge is an invisible and intangible asset, and it is not until the change is completed and knowledge is reused and combined into new insights that the value can be seen.

3.3 Opportunities

Introducing knowledge management provides many opportunities. It can speed up processes, through continual learning, it can exchange practices across diverse departments, it can improve communication within global teams, and it can radically improve the understanding of treatments and therapies.

3.4 Threats

Knowledge management is something which it is easy to "half do." The temptation is to go for a quick fix and to introduce one of the many technologies which the vendors ensure you will deliver knowledge management, as if by magic. This way lies disaster. Knowledge management can easily be derailed by cultural elements such as internal competition, organizational silos, over-strong hierarchies, knowledge hoarding for prestige or power, or a blame culture.

4. APPLICABLE REGULATIONS

There are no regulations applicable to knowledge management.

5. TAKE HOME MESSAGE

- Knowledge is usually the only deliverable from a failed drug development project, and yet, that knowledge (the know-how, the experience and the insights, rather than the data) is seldom managed.
- To manage knowledge requires a framework of roles, processes, technologies, and governance.
- Knowledge management is a relatively simple, though not easy, intervention that delivers value from an asset you already own.

REFERENCES

[1] Gorelick C, Milton N, April K. Performance through learning: knowledge management in practice. San Diego: Elsevier; 2004.
[2] Goodman E, Riddell J. Knowledge management in the pharmaceutical Industry – enhancing research, development and manufacturing performance. London: Gower; 2014.
[3] Milton N. Knowledge management for teams and projects. Oxford, UK: Chandos Publishing; 2005.
[4] Mullin R. Seeing the forest at Pfizer; a radical knowledge-sharing initiative takes hold at the world's largest drugmaker. Chem Eng News 2005;85(36).

CHAPTER 26

Taking Control of Ever-Increasing Volumes of Unstructured Data

Henrik Nakskov

Contents

1. THE NEED

Today data is the fastest growing element in human history. Unlike a century ago, when economic growth was dependent on factors such as good supply chain management, the industrial assembly line, and exchange of physical goods, today's modern economic growth is dependent on the ability to

Re-Engineering Clinical Trials
http://dx.doi.org/10.1016/B978-0-12-420246-7.00026-8

handle and manage large volumes of unstructured information. The competitive advantages of good production methodology, craftsmanship, and well-trained staff have been replaced by the ability to structure information and react fast.

This chapter will look at ways to help you navigate through complex clinical trial data and information structures without drowning in complexity and technology. In particular, we will look at:

- Using the growing wave of data to your advantage.
- How managing data complexity is not just about technology.
- How processes, organizational psychology, and people need to learn to use technology and data to their best advantage.
- How to use past and real-time data to improve and develop.
- Combined, all of these points will lead to the foundation of future decision making, knowledge leadership, and knowledge management.

1.1 The Myth of Predictable Data

Modern organizations rely on structured information and data intelligence to make decisions. However, all the various forms of data intelligence structures, such as reports, visuals, listings, and other indicators have one fundamental flaw that is often overlooked: Human nature can never be expected to react predictably. Although the data might be neatly arranged in a predefined structure indicating predictability and certainty, when humans are involved, so too are discrepancies.

When we consider that the data shown in these various structures is the result of human activity, it becomes clear that regardless of the sophisticated technology involved, blind reliance on data is not the way forward. Critical thought and the ability to question data still remain highly relevant. In the field of clinical drug development, this is even truer as problems with data quality can have far-reaching consequences that can ultimately affect patient safety and an organization's very existence.

The movement of data through the clinical trial process can in many ways be compared to the shipping of valuable content. The ship in itself is not important; what is important is that it has the required stability to transport the goods, is able to dock at the harbor, and that it can unload and load its valuable content safely and efficiently. In the same way, we have to maintain focus on the data that is being transported and moved. It is just an enabler.

2. THE SOLUTION

2.1 Understand Your Business, Your Processes, and Your People

Taking control over the seemingly uncontrollable world of data is actually very straightforward and can be described in seven stages. By mastering all the seven stages, you will be on the way to mastering data quality. However, before we look at the seven stages, it is necessary to understand the competencies that are needed.

The ability to be successful as an information supply chain unit requires business context and process knowledge. Ideally, you should possess a high degree of both in-depth specialized knowledge and an understanding of all the interconnected processes—the "Big T" skill set. These skills involve being able to talk to people, investigate connections, draw process diagrams, handle data exchange connections, evaluate the impact of influences, know the system's data conversion, create communication channels, and finally, have the ability to "sell" your information.

Although you may not consider yourself to be a sales person, being able to create buy-in and acceptance from the business owners and stakeholders you work with will decrease reluctance to accept change and hasten the progress toward the goal of better data quality. By getting to know the human element of your business, you also have a better chance of predicting the unpredictability of your customers and preempting their needs in the future.

2.2 Seven Stages on the Journey to Data and Information Control

2.2.1 Understand Context

Data management is the development, execution, and supervision of plans, policies, programs, and practices that control, protect, deliver, and enhance the value of data and information assets. In short, it is about handling the fastest growing part of our world. In the clinical process, data comes from two main sources: clinical trial data from patients and clinical trial conduct data related to the actual execution of the trial.

The potential and competitive advantage of data comes from the ability to control the flow of changes that originate from the data-information-knowledge growth. This is not just about technology. It is about understanding data and interpreting data in the context of its origin. Good information management is about *data causality*. In other words, it is about the ability to understand the connections that come from nonlinear volumes of information. By being able to understand the business context and the clinical process and then applying this understanding to the data, you can see cause and effect and react appropriately.

There are people who would argue that the craftsmanship of data management on its own is enough, but it is not. Basic data management skills will only open the gateway to data handling. Once the gate has opened, you have to know which methodology to apply and which tools to use depending on the business context.

If your background is pure data management, it would be advisable to spend three to five years in clinical drug development to get a foundational background. If you come from a clinical background, you should start reading, programming, and learning about how data is used.

If you do not have either of these skill sets, you should prepare for a long learning curve or change careers. Without having a foot in each camp, you will never be able to successfully manage data management. Data cannot lie, and you will ultimately be held accountable.

2.2.2 Ensure Data Quality

Data quality is the foundation for reliable decision making. However, information management is never static. This means ensuring data quality is an ongoing process achieved by managing the data and those processes that create the data. While it may sound simple, it is complicated by the fact that any research and development process looks for answers to questions that have been asked by humans in order to gain answers from other humans. All information transition carries the potential for misinterpretation and translation. To secure data quality, you need to be sure that the meaning of the message has not changed.

IT compensates for the increase in data volumes, and it can be tempting to be seduced by its orderly graphs and reports. But you should never forget your critical sense and common sense. You need to continuously question the data. Is this data a true reflection of the processes and conditions under which it was captured? Is this what was meant by the message of the data?

The sources of quality lie within understanding the specific business process and being able to make associations from the business to the data. Simple techniques like data triangulation, visualization, outliers detection, and medical conditional analysis can help you validate the data and ensure no significant discrepancies are included. This type of validation takes time and effort, but there is no way around it if you are serious about ensuring data quality.

2.2.3 Track Data

As discussed earlier, total predictability in the clinical trial process is simply not possible, and therefore, data cannot just be taken at face level. Your organization's competitive advantage lies in the ability to handle data and convert it into information.

One solution is to start thinking of the data tracking process as a separate process. This means that the tracking in itself is the goal, not data management or data quality. Data tracking can easily be compared to traditional logistics. Just as logistics might include air, sea, road, or rail transport of goods, information can be submitted in the form of a paper entry, ePRO, remote data entry, device specific (e.g., spirometry), or a hematology parameter in acute care ambulance, and many other sources.

That is why it is important to stay focused upon where the data is in the chain. You should be able to explain where each data element is in the supply chain, where it came from, where it will go next, and the different time stages each data element will go through.

The next step is to actively use this information to make decisions related to the two previously described steps. Data always tells a story, so if it is delayed, the reason for the delay may impact other data elements. Remember that when a data element is transported from one system to another, the probability of the data element remaining unchanged is only 50%. Either it is correct or it is not correct. That is why during data management activities, it is necessary to secure data quality via systems validation and verification in order to increase the probability of data elements being correct, close to 100%.

For this reason, data tracking is not only a good service for your information customers, but also a good data risk indicator. During my career as information manager, I have seen some obscene systems and application landscapes handling clinical data, where data is exchanged 5–10 times though independent systems/applications, often by independent departments. The results of these complex systems were distorted data, which was used to make bad decisions that ended up costing money, time, and trust.

System landscapes need to reflect business needs and incorporate tracking at every stage. Decisions are continuously being made at many different points in the information chain. By understanding and continuously reevaluating data, you minimize risk and increase your chance of clinical trial success.

2.2.4 Develop the Right Metrics

Metrics are more than just monitoring of an algorithm. When developing metrics that can have a significant influence on an organization, you need to take into account human behavior and the dynamic nature of your organization. This is summed up neatly in the principle of Le Chatelier, which states that any change in a system at equilibrium results in a shift of the equilibrium in the direction that minimizes the change.

A seesaw is the easiest way to illustrate this principle. As any child can tell you, when the person at the lower end of the seesaw gets off, the equilibrium changes, and the other person comes down. Or if we apply it to information management, what was true before your own deliverable of information to the business created a reaction may no longer be true as the reaction changes reality.

Any given metric will influence the behavior and decisions being taken—for better and for worse. So, consider carefully before firing off a lot of lists, numbers, and visualization of the past activities and estimates of the future, maybe enriched with real-time analysis. Remember that what you are showing is an extract of reality, based upon your judgment and selective skills. Each metric draws on a limited amount of information originating from a gigantic pool of data. While what you show is perfectly true, it is not representative of all data and can easily mislead.

On the other hand, it is just as important that you do not drown your customers in information as you try to show all the good data you can get out of the system. The true master of information management is revealed though what you have not included.

If your customers own more than three metrics for each evaluation scheme, the data owns them. Three metrics is the cutoff point where the customer stops thinking. Instead of using the information as a guide, people let the information be the cause of reaction and stop thinking. Faced with too many metrics, they will stop being critical and instead become addicted to data.

The market of information you are offering should not be there to replace good, solid knowledge and common sense; it should be a service. Customers should not be blindly following your offerings as their guiding star. Metrics should only ever be a supporting service.

Before you start creating metrics, consider the following questions:
• Will the consequences of the metrics be changes in the organization that are wanted?
• Do the people in question like to be monitored?
• Will the metrics undermine the practice of good cooperation?
• Is the assumption of causality (cause and effect) correct?

- How will the metrics be implemented?
- Who will have insight into the metrics' output?
- Will the metrics be linked to employee's goals?
- Should any external stakeholders be involved?
- Where is the ownership placed for the metrics?
- Will the metric give additional insights which lead to a broader understanding of how the company reacts?
- How can we capture feedback?
- What is the frequency of need changes?
- How do we handle any dysfunctions that are caused by a metric?
- How do we capture learning and establish operational development? This final question is covered in more detail in the next step.

2.2.5 Operational Development: Use Your Knowledge

If you have been through the first four stages, you should now understand the business context around your data; be aware of the need for quality data, the benefits of tracking, and you should have the right metrics to support decision making. The next stage is to use the knowledge you have gained in a knowledge management (KM) system.

This is where technology that can leverage the development of knowledge comes in. To create an optimal knowledge management system, you need to consider all the previously outlined parameters and be highly systematic in the actions you take so you can use the knowledge you have gained during other stages. Within the system, you need to implement procedures for how to capture the evaluation of metrics, learning, feedback, organization reaction, and operational causality.

The capture of ideas that come from interpretation of the metrics is of particular benefit. The following categories are examples of categories that could be used:

- Human reaction
- Operational parameters
- Logistical perspectives
- Decisions support
- Organizational level
- Data sources identification
- SQL source code
- Visuals
- Your own support unit structures

2.2.5.1 Sharing What with Whom?

Once you have got the information into the system, you need to decide who can get the information out. If your KM system does not enable knowledge sharing, it can easily end up being just another database that nobody uses. Consider if it is relevant for knowledge to be shared between departments, between functions, between companies in the same field, or between all companies?

If you allow too many people to share information, it could backfire, resulting in data overload. Alternatively, you might find yourself in a situation where people are reluctant to let their activities be monitored. The recipient of your information must be competent and willing to receive your information. A clear structure on information exchange with information submitted to the right people in the right format will save you considerable time and frustration farther down the line.

2.2.6 Information Supply Chain Management (ISCM)

ISCM is built on the foundation of the first five stages. It ensures you get the right information to the right recipient at the right time.

- The right information has to be the right data in the right context, quality, and form.
- The right time is exactly when you or your customers need it, not too early, not too late.
- The right recipient is identified though your content and operational knowledge.

To measure the effect of the information, you need to create feedback procedures. This is not only for feedback, such as what do people think of it, but feedback on a more basic level: Did your customer receive the information or not? Did it get there at the right time or not? Did the package meet expectations? Remember, you are not measuring whether the effect is good or bad (i.e., wanted or unwanted) but effect and reaction. In essence, you are measuring if steps one through five were efficient and effective.

There is a full toolbox to help you with ISCM: the established theory of supply chain management. This contains a number of feedback procedures and communications tools, like the bullwhip effect, nonlinear feedback, parallel processing, JIT theory, supplier–buyer psychology, and more.

Note that ISCM (Information Supply Chain Management) is not the same as tracking described in step three. Tracking focuses on pure information logistics (IL) and does not include any information about data quality nor any information content evaluation.

ISCM is taking all perspectives into consideration, like technology, time, service, people, reaction, effect, development, and summing up all the preceding steps to a deliverable to your information customers.

2.2.7 Integration of External Service Suppliers

One of the big changes the Internet has brought is the ability to exchange complex information fast and make it easy and intuitively understandable. This has enabled suppliers to specialize in different stages of the production process.

For example, in the manufacturing industry, this has facilitated the physical replacement of production facilities. Car generators are now produced in one country for almost all automobile brands; windshields are produced in a specialized factory in all different shapes and forms. The catalyst for all of this happening is not the location of the production facility but the ability to exchange and understand the blueprint for the activity.

The same changes are also taking place in R&D teams in the pharmaceutical industry—but with extra communication challenges. Pharmaceutical R&D is like one big dish of spaghetti with lots of interconnected processes. Some are executed in parallel and some serially. With the growth in cross-functionality, processes are no longer linear, and communication lines can easily get tangled. This is compounded by the fact that when you outsource tasks, functions, or processes, you add an extra layer of communications. But the effect is not just an extra layer of communication. It is more likely that it is x^2, where x is the number of information transactions taking place between the CRO and business owner.

So a prerequisite for ensuring successful cooperation is expectation management and measurement, taking all the previous phases into account. Building up a strong relationship with your suppliers with clearly defined metrics will allow you to build a knowledge base that you can use for any future projects.

This expectation management also applies to the incitements that drive you and your suppliers. Be aware of any changes in incitements during the project. An incitement analysis carried out with your supplier can align your goals and cement the working relationship.

A reliable activity which can save you from a lot of problems in connections with outsourcing is the development of an information management strategy.

3. SWOT

3.1 Strengths: Why Is the New Concept Better?

The degree of growth in information and its uncontrolled nature will not be reduced in the future. This approach gives you control without losing vital information. Although it may seem like an unmanageable task, following the seven steps will achieve data quality. The steps are interconnected and contribute to each other, but they can also be executed independently. As the saying goes, the best way to eat an elephant is bit by bit.

3.2 Weaknesses

Nothing comes without a cost. This approach is considerable both in time, complexity, and cost. If taken lightly, you can quickly spend a lot of time and money without obtaining any benefits. This makes it necessary to spend extra time on the structuring of this approach. This can be done through a COP (clinical operation plan).

3.3 Opportunities

Ones you have gone through the seven steps, you will have a solid decisions foundation. It can be reused in other areas in business and can be incorporated as part of the company's culture.

3.4 Threats

It takes time. And many companies do not have the ability or money to wait.

4. COP

The table of content in a COP can vary greatly between companies and between trials, reflecting the indications for which the clinical trials are conducted.

An example of a general COP could contain the elements below:
- Communication plan
- Data flow identification
- IL (information logistics)
- ISCM (information supply chain management)
- DI (data intelligences)
- Data handling plan (DHP)
  - Data exchange plan
  - Cross-check activities
  - Metrics identification
  - SQL development
  - Data sources
- Data quality review committee plan
- Stakeholder identification

- Recruitment plan/strategy
- Training plan
- Risk analysis plan (including risk grid)
- Site management strategy
- Lessons learned
- Potential in- or out-sourcing plan

5. A LITTLE WARNING

5.1 There Is No Free Lunch When It Comes to Data Quality and Information Management

You may see systems advertised that offer full data quality and peace of mind so you can sleep easy at night, safe in the knowledge that your data quality is assured. But these magic solutions do not exist and never will because this sort of software would require total predictability in all processes. With the data growth and the increased frequency of changes we see throughout the industry, the predictability they would require will never be available. The bottom line is that there is no way around hard work, in-depth, well-established knowledge about the business and good relationships with your customers.

5.2 Turning Quality Data into Sound Decisions

What you have been reading is a description of what to supply for your customers and how to do it.

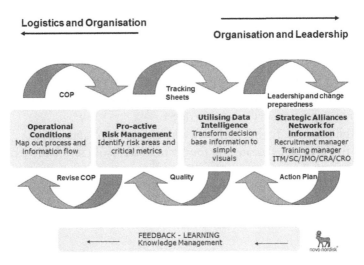

The following chapter looks at the next step of how the data is used in organization and leadership. These two areas are the powerhouses that propel your business. Ensuring good data quality is the engine room. It provides the power but cannot steer. Above deck, steering takes place on the bridge—the organization and leadership. When these two elements work together to make decisions based on quality data, your ship can be steered safely into the harbor of clinical trial success.

6. APPLICABLE REGULATIONS

1. Guideline for Good Clinical Practice. http://www.ich.org/fileadmin/Public_Web_Site/ICH_Products/Guidelines/Efficacy/E6/E6_R1_Guidlines.pdf
2. European Union law on clinical trials of medicinal products for humans.http://eur-lex.europa.eu/legal-content/en/ALL/;jsessionid=SCHnTxGRS2NsnncLqrvWd1rq2jxgpLDnqQC2TYx0J244FP9F5CRL!746316659?uri=CELEX:32001L0020.
3. US regulations for the conduct of clinical trials. http://www.fda.gov/ScienceResearch/SpecialTopics/RunningClinicalTrials/default.htm.
4. EU Guideline on good pharmacovigilance practices (GVP).http://www.ema.europa.eu/docs/en_GB/document_library/Scientific_guideline/2012/06/WC500129138.pdf.
5. US FDA Guidance on Quality Risk Management. http://www.fda.gov/downloads/Drugs/GuidanceComplianceRegulatoryInformation/Guidances/UCM073511.pdf.

7. TAKE HOME MESSAGE

Obtaining control over an ever-increasing amount of unstructured data and using this to your advantage is possible. It requires an in-depth knowledge and understanding of the clinical and the technological world, spiced up with some degree of service-mindedness.

The prerequisite for success is to take a structured approach.

The first five steps create the foundation; step six creates the exchanges and step seven the integration.

CHAPTER 27

Share the Knowledge Based on Quality Data

Liselotte Hyveled

Contents

1. THE NEED

Over the last 20–30 years, the level of information available for processing has increased dramatically. Unlike the 1970s, when we were exposed to 500 consumer messages daily, today we are exposed to up to 5000 [1]. Of these 5000 messages, we engage in 76, recall 12, and act on 5—the equivalent of 0.1%. In the pharmaceutical world, there has been a similar increase in data generation. For example, a regulatory file has grown from a mere 7 pages in 1952 to 930,000 pages in 2008 and 14 million pages in 2013 [2], most of which are generated from clinical trials.

This makes the ability to work with and manage all aspects of data a hugely important skill, not least in the pharmaceutical industry. As a result, companies that are able to combine strong data management skills with organizational knowledge are in the best position to increase productivity and the overall quality of regulatory documentation, such as that from clinical trials. This chapter examines how managing, visualizing, and communicating data

Re-Engineering Clinical Trials
http://dx.doi.org/10.1016/B978-0-12-420246-7.00027-X

effectively throughout a trial can enable swift action, which can help a company gain and maintain a competitive edge.

Most pharmaceutical companies have already understood the need to generate data that can provide content. However, if not managed efficiently, it can often result in large data dumps, which then easily become just another task vying for a person's often already compromised attention span.

This is why there is a clear need to give your data *context*. This can be achieved by deciding which data are most important for ensuring a successful clinical trial and then clearly communicating these data. Visual reports are an ideal medium for achieving communication. Unlike written reports, data that have been turned into visuals are often clearer to understand and more easily digestible. However, being able to clearly communicate the right data is just one part of better knowledge sharing and data management; data also need to be shared in a well-defined knowledge structure.

2. THE SOLUTION

This chapter examines how better knowledge sharing and data management throughout a trial can enable swift action to be taken when needed. It describes an optimal knowledge structure for monitoring, sharing, and acting efficiently on data during a clinical trial. The structure has four components: tools, process, organization, and people, as shown in Figure 27.1.

The process and tools are usually predictable assets, whereas the people and the organizations are more unpredictable. Hence, we try to control the predictable assets and understand the unpredictable.

There are three main groups that work together to share relevant knowledge: data team, knowledge team, and action team. These groups work together to continuously collect process and act on the data. Using their combined knowledge and skills, they can accurately highlight any areas of concern, and then act swiftly to minimize trial errors, increase changes of success in the clinical trials, and avoid potential audit findings. This cycle of data and knowledge sharing in the knowledge-sharing infrastructure creates continuous improvement throughout the life cycle of the clinical trial.

To facilitate knowledge sharing, the team works using a "boiler room" concept. The boiler room is a place where concise, highly focused meetings for the exchange of knowledge among people with different skill sets in the organization. It ensures a common understanding and transparency, with a view to improving solutions for current and future tasks.

Knowledge Infrastructure

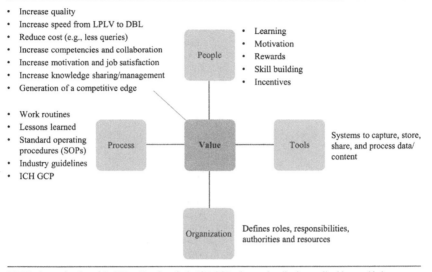

- Increase quality
- Increase speed from LPLV to DBL
- Reduce cost (e.g., less queries)
- Increase competencies and collaboration
- Increase motivation and job satisfaction
- Increase knowledge sharing/management
- Generation of a competitive edge

- Work routines
- Lessons learned
- Standard operating procedures (SOPs)
- Industry guidelines
- ICH GCP

People
- Learning
- Motivation
- Rewards
- Skill building
- Incentives

Process   Value   Tools   Systems to capture, store, share, and process data/content

Organization   Defines roles, responsibilities, authorities and resources

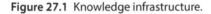

LPLV = last patient last visit. DBL = Data base lock. ICH GCP = internationalised centralised harmonidation good clinical practice.

Figure 27.1 Knowledge infrastructure.

3. IDENTIFYING CRITICAL DATA

Once you have identified the elements of your knowledge structure, you need to map out and prioritize your knowledge assets. This means creating an inventory list that describes the business needs and the key value drivers in the trial. What needs to be known in order to accomplish the trial's organizational goals with the optimal speed and quality? In other words, you have to find out which core knowledge/data need to be captured, and the difference between what is known and what needs to be known or generated. Here, it is used to remember that data quality is not only defined by volume.

The following questions may help to guide you through this process:
Which data define the primary or secondary endpoints in the trial?
Which data indicate a process flow?
Are any pieces of data interdependent?
What is the time frame for collecting the data?
What are the data volume, velocity, variety, and veracity? (see Figure 27.2)

4. THE KNOWLEDGE STRUCTURE IN PRACTICE

Having identified the data you want to capture and generate, you need to involve the right stakeholders and teams with the relevant organizational

Quality Data – Not Only Data Volume

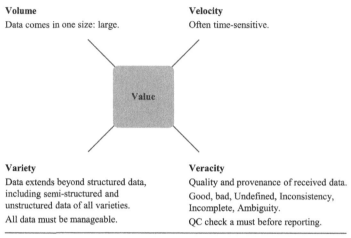

Volume
Data comes in one size: large.

Velocity
Often time-sensitive.

Value

Variety
Data extends beyond structured data, including semi-structured and unstructured data of all varieties.
All data must be manageable.

Veracity
Quality and provenance of received data.
Good, bad, Undefined, Inconsistency, Incomplete, Ambiguity.
QC check a must before reporting.

Figure 27.2 Quality data—not only data volume.

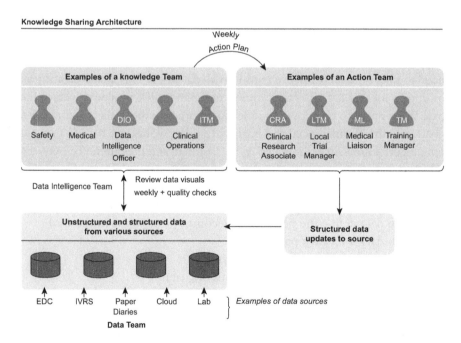

Figure 28.3 Knowledge sharing architecture.

knowledge. As seen in Figure 27.3, there are three main groups: data team, knowledge team, and action team. These teams work together to continuously collect process and act on the data. Using their combined knowledge and skills, they can accurately highlight any areas of concern, and then act swiftly to minimize trial errors and potential audit findings. This cycle of data and knowledge sharing creates continuous improvement throughout the life cycle of the clinical trial. Let us take a closer look at the different groups involved.

5. THE DATA TEAM

The data team works closely with the knowledge team to identify the specific trial data required. Once identified, the data team determines the source and nature of the input and transforms these data into digestible visuals. Here, it is important to keep all visuals simple, clear, and easy to understand, as a good visual should be intuitive to understand with minimal explanation needed. Visuals can be consistent throughout the trial or special visuals can be requested if necessary. Be prepared for several review rounds with the knowledge team when creating the visuals. Even when the visuals have been finalized, it is recommended that the data team continue to review the format and content regularly to avoid data report blindness.

6. THE KNOWLEDGE TEAM

This group of critical stakeholders represents different aspects of the business with their own spheres of strategic knowledge and experience. Their role is to meet regularly, ideally weekly in the boiler room, to review data. They use the visual reports to identify gaps, errors, and breakdowns that have occurred in data collection. At the end of each meeting, they draw up a plan detailing the corrective action needed. In this way, the knowledge officers are able to highlight any areas of concern that can impact the trial before they have adverse effects further downstream.

7. THE BOILER ROOM

This is a room where the knowledge team meetings are held. It should be designed for short, effective face-to-face meetings lasting approximately 30 min. At these meetings, each knowledge officer in the knowledge team presents selected data visuals for immediate feedback from the other knowledge officers. This results in a plan of corrective actions. To encourage speed of thought, focus, and engagement in the discussions, it is recommended that the room is kept deliberately sparse with no chairs.

During these meetings, a model for problem solving can be applied as a support for generating the action plan:

1. **Problem:** What is the root cause of the problem?
2. **Cause:** Why has the process broken down?
3. **Temporary solution:** What can we do straight away to prevent the problem from escalating?
4. **Permanent solution:** What can we do to permanently fix the issue and prevent it from happening again?

8. THE ACTION TEAM

Unlike the knowledge team, which has a more strategic mindset and is typically based in headquarters, the action team is typically the operational team based "in the field." The action team is responsible for executing the action plan. It is in close contact with all other key stakeholders and provides feedback to the knowledge team on an ongoing basis for use in the review meetings.

An example of the knowledge structure is seen in Figure 27.3.

9. AN EXAMPLE FROM REAL LIFE

The following example comes from a recent diabetes trial designed to ensure that the patients have optimal glycemic control, as indicated, for instance, by HbA1c or Glycomark.

During the trial, the knowledge infrastructure described earlier consisting of data team, knowledge team, and action team was set up. These three groups worked closely to ensure that the investigators were following the trial-specific process and guidelines, so that there was timely interaction with the local trial staff if any corrective action was necessary.

Because the trials were executed globally using varying information technology standards, the patients entered information about their glucose levels and insulin doses, food items, and similar in a paper diary. These data items were subsequently transferred manually to electronic data capture (EDC). Lab data were stored in the lab database, and other information was generated via an interactive voice web response system.

The knowledge officers in the project started out by deciding which key data from the trial needed to be transformed into data visuals. These visuals, along with other selected data items (e.g., standard tracking on recruitment, etc., and nonstandard, for example, on time from diary collection to EDC entry), were presented weekly to the rest of the team in the project boiler room. This allowed them to identify breakdowns in any of the data flows before a major breakdown in a process occurred. For example, patients may have completed the information inaccurately in the diary data entry process, the data entry process might have been wrong or delayed, or samples may have been missing.

When the selected data did not follow the expected path toward improved glycemic control, the knowledge officers in the knowledge team defined the corrective action to be taken on their weekly action plan. This plan was passed on to the action team for operational implementation and subsequently followed up the week after.

All these actions support ensuring timely intervention and global standards.

At this point, one could ask why this kind of corrective action is not just carried out by the clinical research associate (CRA) as a routine check. The answer to this lies in the fact that the CRA often suffers from information overload, due to the increasing demand for data surveillance, data entry, reporting, and similar. Often, CRAs are unable to see the connection between missing data and a breakdown in an entire process or a consequence of this further down the data stream.

The action team used the plan to take local action (sometimes via the CRA) and then provided feedback to the team in the boiler room. This created an ongoing basis for review at the next weekly knowledge sharing meeting—in effect, it created a continuous cycle of improvement throughout the life cycle of the clinical trial.

10. ORGANIZATIONAL PSYCHOLOGY

So far, we have looked at why knowledge infrastructure of this kind in a clinical trial is important; provided some tangible questions to consider when identifying your data report need; and looked at a real-world example. Now we need to focus on the human aspect of this process and consider how to get the teams engaged in sharing, understanding, and acting on the data.

Of course, there are the classic incentives such as compliance and motivation in the form of some kind of reward. But the true value of sharing knowledge based on quality data comes when the teams are committed to the project and *data are the connecting factor* for the network. This culture creates a sense of community around the trial. Once this is established, involvement, commitment, creativity, and ownership evolve, leading to greater self-esteem in team members. Knowledge sharing is no longer an autonomic process on a fixed schedule, but a master class—*a mindset*. This takes both time and effort and requires continuous, clear, and transparent goals. In other words, this is organizational psychology put into practice.

Looking back at the example described earlier from the diabetes clinical trial, one of the most effective ways of creating this commitment came from the boiler room meetings. Commitment to these meetings did not happen instantly. It had to be established. In fact, it took approximately 3 months before the meetings were prioritized and valued by most team members, and even longer before the various groups began to work efficiently as a team. This has to be expected: The team has to go through a period of adaptation and experience first-hand the results of this way of working.

It should also be remembered that the knowledge of the team is tacit as well as explicit. Transferring tacit knowledge is more effective through human interaction, which is why the boiler room framework is so much more effective than e-mailing reports to other stakeholders. Moreover, this practice also adds to the valuable social side of sharing knowledge.

Due to the speed of the data and knowledge exchange, a network of people with broad tacit and explicit knowledge is needed to keep up with the changes in the processes or procedures at the investigational sites. As a collaborative team, the impact of their knowledge is highly effective. However, this requires that each individual recognizes the other members as being of equal importance. All team members bring their own set of skills and experience to the meeting and need to be able to translate their knowledge into something everyone present can relate to and understand. Egos and self-importance need to be left outside the boiler room door, as they will hinder this collaborative approach.

This is why, when knowledge is to be shared, it is not enough to ensure two-way communication where you exchange "data and services." The optimal knowledge ecosystem requires personal engagement, face-to-face interactions, and recognition of the importance of each team member.

When a knowledge infrastructure has been implemented as described earlier, the value that it can generate for a business includes:
- Early identification of issues in a clinical trial to allow corrective actions to be implemented and changes made
- Fast and effective insight into the process and identification of potential gaps

- Minimization of errors and audit findings and a reduction in queries
- Better quality of pivotal clinical trial data generated for regulatory approvals
- Identification of new optimized ways of working
- Reduction in the time spent on drug development
- An increased competitive edge

These are the tangible benefits of knowledge sharing through quality data. On the intangible side, you may also see increased people skills, an increased sense of trust, more openness, and a greater curiosity on the part of your team. Instead of blindly following standard operating procedures, they are forced to consider what action should be taken. All of these factors will ultimately increase your company's capacity to innovate.

11. SWOT

We summarize using a SWOT (Strength, Weakness, Opportunity, and Threat) model:

S: Collaborative approach allows early identification of issues and corrective action that can reduce time spent on drug development and increase competitive advantage

W: New way of working requires commitment and change in mindset from those in the various teams

O: Fast and effective insight into the process and identification of potential gaps

Minimization of errors and audit findings and a reduction in queries

Better quality of pivotal clinical trial data generated for regulatory approvals

T: It takes time and commitment for the process to be effective and bring value.

12. TAKE HOME MESSAGE

- Identify the data that are critical for trial success
- Understand the data and its sources
- Choose the right visualization
- Keep it simple and consistent
- Avoid data overload

- Create a personal network and a face-to-face data sharing process and space, the boiler room
- Execute action plan and follow up frequently
- Never assume
- Remember, it takes time, every time, for this process to be effective
- It takes time for people to connect via data
- Once established, this approach brings great value on many levels

REFERENCES

[1] Hyveled L, Nakskov H, Karpour P. 2347 DIA. Knowl Inn Clin Oper Excellence June 2008:2347.
[2] Internal Novo Nordisk A/S data.

You Need Processes, Systems, and People

CHAPTER 28

You Need Processes, Systems, and People—It's All about the People (and Their Competences)

Mike Hardman, Martin Robinson

Contents

1. THE NEED

Clinical research is a rapidly developing and dynamic environment. The sector is undergoing a range of significant changes. In the commercial field, pharma companies are increasingly outsourcing clinical trials to Contract Research Organisations (CROs). The search for new markets, treatment-naïve patient populations, and the need to drive down costs has seen increasing number of studies in nontraditional geographical areas such as China and India. Pharma companies are attempting to maximize the data they collect from each study by having an increasing number of trial objectives. Therefore, studies are becoming ever more complex, making them challenging from both an investigator's and monitor's perspective. Furthermore, the growing use of adaptive trial design has added new levels of intricacy in the way that research is conducted.

Re-Engineering Clinical Trials
http://dx.doi.org/10.1016/B978-0-12-420246-7.00028-1
319

Regulatory changes have also had an impact on the clinical trial process. There has been an attempt to harmonize trial approvals and the methods by which Ethics Committees function in the European Union, and directives have been transposed into local laws, introducing legal consequences for serious incidents of noncompliance. Information is much more readily exchanged between regulatory authorities, and there is growing pressure for sponsors and other researchers to publish all trial results irrespective of their conclusions about the efficacy and safety of new treatments. The European Medicines Agency is working toward modifying the EudraCT database so that all trials registered will have a summary of their results, made publicly available through the EU Clinical Trials Register (EU-CTR).

The regulators have also issued several guidance documents regarding risk-based monitoring. The European Medicine Agency's reflection paper on risk-based quality management in clinical trials [1] addresses the problem that practices are not proportionate or well adapted to specific trials. In 2013, the FDA finalized its guidance for a risk-based approach to monitoring [2]. This document was produced in response to the growth in the number and complexity of trials. The FDA's position is that a risk-based approach is dynamic, flexible, and focused on mitigating risks to patients, data quality, and trial integrity.

All of these changes have required the clinical research sector to rethink its practices, particularly with respect to reengineering processes to enable sponsors to initiate and execute trials more rapidly and cost-effectively. There has also been added pressure on the workforce to adapt to these changes. The roles of clinical research monitors and data managers in particular are changing. There still appears to be a lack of talent and shortage of skilled people in some areas. The merging of some CROs and the increased use of outsourcing by pharma companies has created additional demands for competent Clinical Research Associates (CRAs) to work in this dynamic and changing environment. The solution of some CROs is to try and poach staff from each other and a general reluctance to grow their own talent. Pharma companies contribute to the problem by requesting CRAs of a certain number of years' experience to work on their trials rather than demanding proof of competence of their project team members [3] This desire for experience over competence is particularly dangerous in an environment which is very dynamic. With such a volatile background, it is vital that individuals maintain their professional competence, as the number of years' experience is a decreasingly valid measure of performance.

2. THE SOLUTION

All stakeholders, pharma, and CROs need to be able to demonstrate that their staff are competent, no matter where in the world the study is being conducted. In addition, they need to be able to manage turnover in the project team by not only keeping it under control, but also knowing that when they need to replace a team member, the new person joining the team is as competent as the individual leaving it. The use of competency profiles is also a more robust basis for mutual recognition of competence and supports the mobility of staff.

Using competence as a performance measure allows more objective appraisals to be conducted, and training and personal development needs can be identified more accurately and specifically. Staff recruitment and selection is a more precise science when competency frameworks are used. Employers have a much greater chance of selecting people for the right job roles. Consequently, staff turnover, which is a constant problem for pharma companies and CROs alike, is reduced.

Many employers still have the bad habit of promoting people based solely on the number of years' experience without regard to whether or not the individual is suited to their new position. The result is that these people struggle in their new position which may carry significant responsibility. The organization is damaged; teamwork and morale may suffer, and incompetent managers can have a significant effect on employee turnover. A survey conducted by the Chartered Management Institute revealed that 47% of people felt they were in a badly managed workplace, leading them to leave their job [4]. Replacing staff is costly as the accountancy firm PricewaterhouseCoopers reported when it revealed that the cost of hiring a new person to replace an existing employee who is performing optimally is equal to that person's annual salary [5].

Finally, having competent clinical researchers benefits all parties in the clinical research sector. Sponsors have a greater chance of reduced inspection findings; protocol design and compliance has the potential to be improved, and most importantly, the rights and well-being of clinical trial subjects are increasingly protected.

2.1 How Can a Competence-based System Be Introduced?

Clinical research is a truly global enterprise. Many trials are multinational spanning several continents simultaneously. There are increasing numbers of trials being conducted in the so-called developing world. Any competence-based system should work universally so that the appropriate standards of performance are maintained no matter where the trial is being conducted. Both the Declaration of Helsinki (October 2008 version) and the *WHO Handbook for Good Clinical Research Practice (Guidance for Implementation, 2005)* describe the need to have competent investigators. However, both documents neglect to mention the competence of any of the other key roles in clinical research.

Because of the increasing globalization of clinical research, there is an increasing pressure for standardization so that quality systems are applied consistently and that patients' rights and well-being are upheld universally. Both sponsor organizations and investigator sites have a responsibility to make sure that their staff are competent and have access to the appropriate learning and development resources. Organizations must invest in developing their staff so that a learning culture permeates throughout the system.

What should be the components of such a framework? First, each person should have a well-defined job role that specifies the key responsibilities and areas of work that the job covers. Second, each job role should have an accompanying competency framework. This is a document that describes the specific core competences required for the job role. These competences are expressed as the essential knowledge, skills, and behaviors to perform the job to the required level of performance. Third, each person should have an individual learning and development plan that enables them to become competent in their respective role.

Having these three components in place allows learning and development needs to be targeted specifically and efficiently and gives managers and staff alike a set of objective standards that facilitate mutually constructive performance reviews. The result is that training and other learning interventions can be carried out in an efficient and streamlined way that allows for the maximum potential return on investment in terms of time and cost.

Some job roles in clinical research lend themselves more easily to definition, and thereby standardization, than others. The roles and responsibilities of investigators and monitors are outlined reasonably comprehensively in The International Conference on Harmonisation (ICH) Harmonized Tripartite Guideline, for Good Clinical Practice (GCP) E6 (R1) in Sections 4 and 5.18, respectively. Competency frameworks for investigators and monitors can be developed using the information in the guideline as a starting point.

An Internet search reveals that some initiatives are already underway in an attempt to provide a competency framework for clinical investigators.

The Multi-Regional Clinical Trials (MRCT) Center at Harvard University in the United States is proposing a set of minimum training standards for principal investigators and clinical staff [6]. The International Academy of Clinical Research has facilitated the setting up of an international and multidisciplinary task force to develop a competency framework for clinical investigators [7]. The Innovative Medicines Initiative (IMI) project Pharma-Train has developed a set of core competences for pharmaceutical physicians and nonphysician scientists [8] and has developed a European approach to clinical investigator training [9]. Furthermore, in the United Kingdom, Vitae has developed a researcher development framework [10], and the IMI Education and Training projects have developed LifeTrain, a European framework for continuing professional development in the biomedical sciences [11] For a competency framework to be a valuable and helpful tool, it must be concise yet comprehensive, universally applicable both internationally and across the complete spectrum of types of clinical trial, and be an incentive for clinical researcher to strive for excellence. Clinical researchers, particularly investigators, are understandably averse to anything which appears to add to their bureaucratic load. However, because so much is at stake regarding the health, well-being, and rights of clinical trial subjects, it is vital that there is some system for verifying competence. Other industries where there are significant hazards to health and welfare or where there is the potential for substantial financial risk have systems in place to certify practitioners. The Gas Safe Register in the United Kingdom is a system for the certification of gas engineers that verifies they are competent to work safely and legally on boilers, cookers, and other gas appliances. The International Institute of Business Analysis (IIBA) has a system of accreditation for business analysts. For the operation of pleasure craft, there is an International Certificate of Competence (ICC), which may be issued to anyone who has successfully completed certain national boating licenses. These are just some of the many diverse examples of schemes in other fields.

3. SWOT ANALYSIS

3.1 Strengths: What Are the Benefits of Having a Competence-based System of Verification?

Having a competence-based system of verification can only raise clinical research standards. Having an international system that recognizes competence allows greater mobility and flexibility within the global workforce. This enables a resource to be transferred where it is needed and enables an international and consistent standard of performance to be achieved. A recent example of mutual recognition of GCP training for investigators has been developed by TransCelerate [12]. Developing and verifying competence allows new talent to be developed efficiently and effectively with the result of new intake of hires being fully and rapidly productive. It is vital that the clinical research sector has a steady stream of new talents as this brings new ideas and innovation by their ability to challenge the status quo through fresh eyes. Using competence as a performance measure enables a much more specific and targeted approach to identifying and meeting training needs. Sponsor organizations can employ staff, either permanently or on contract, with greater confidence that their new hires are competent to fill their respective roles.

Career progression and succession planning is a much more precise science using a competence-based system. It is vital that a good fit is found between a person's ability to do their current job and their capacity to fulfill a higher role with more responsibility. The result is a thriving organization, staffed with people who have both the confidence and competence to carry out their work to a consistently high standard.

3.2 Weaknesses: If a Competence-based System Is so Good, What's Stopping Us from Implementing It?

Unfortunately, competence is not well understood as a fundamental concept. For example, when selecting CRO staff to work on their projects, pharma companies inevitably opt for the number of years' experience rather than proof of competence. Because clinical research is such a dynamic environment, years of experience can rapidly become a devalued currency. Sometimes experience can equate to complacency and apathy to learning new skills.

Another challenge is that verifying competence requires more effort and thought than counting the number of years' experience. There is a general lack of expertise in developing competency frameworks and using them appropriately. Most training organizations or training functions within organizations focus on inputs rather than outputs. There is an overreliance on the documentation of attendance of training courses rather than measuring what these learning interventions achieve in terms of their participants learning new skills. Attending a training course can be a very passive activity if the learning environment is unstimulating and the "participants" are not motivated to learn. Training is often overused as a compliance tool in reaction to an internal quality assurance audit or regulatory inspection.

Naturally, training may be a vital part of the corrective and preventive action (CAPA), but there is clearly a systemic flaw in an organization if this is regarded as a standard solution to noncompliance.

The regulatory authorities must also shoulder some of the responsibility for the current state of affairs by their overzealous attention to the documentation of training. This reinforces a box-ticking mentality which values having up-to-date GCP training records more than having people who are competent to ensure the protection of the rights and well-being of clinical trial subjects and the integrity of the trial and its resultant data. Unfortunately, the adage of "what gets inspected gets done" often rings true.

Line managers often have a poor understanding of competence. The result is that training and development needs are not satisfactorily identified, and unnecessary training is carried out or, conversely, vital learning needs remain unmet. Even when an employee attends a training course, there is often no debrief with their manager to reflect on what was learned in the training course and how that can be applied back in the workplace to embed the learning, practice the newly acquired skills, and develop competence.

3.3 Opportunities: Action Is Needed Rather than Reaction

The history of clinical research has not always been particularly savory. The sector is frequently reactive to incidents such as unintentional disasters or deliberate misconduct. The Nuremberg Code, the forerunner of the Declaration of Helsinki, was formulated in 1946 and specifies 10 key principles under which medical research must be carried out.

The thalidomide tragedy in the early 1960s occurred when large numbers of pregnant women were prescribed the drug for morning sickness. Thousands of children were born with deformities of their limbs. The authorities reacted by the passing of the Kefauver-Harris Drug Amendments Act in the United States in 1962, which tightened restrictions surrounding the surveillance and approval process for drugs to be sold in the United States. Manufacturers were required to prove that new treatments were both safe and effective before they were marketed. Further legislation saw the Investigational New Drug (IND) process introduced in 1962. This addition to the regulations required that all new drug research had to be approved by the FDA before it could commence. Equivalent legislation soon followed in Europe. Universal harmonization of GCP took a major step in 1997 when the ICH GCP guidelines were finalized between the regulatory bodies of the European Union, Japan, and the United States.

In contrast to the reactive, but rightly necessary, legislation introduced as a result of these catastrophes, this is a great opportunity for the clinical research sector to demonstrate a willingness to be proactive and introduce an accreditation system based on competence verification. The result would be a clear signal that the sector values its workforce and also demonstrates a commitment to patient safety and data integrity. The public, who are sometimes provided with a jaundiced view of medical research by the press and media, would be given increased confidence that people involved in medical research were competent to manage trials and that people who volunteered were treated with care and dignity and not regarded as "human guinea pigs."

The clinical research sector cannot afford to be complacent and convince itself that all is well. The evidence suggests that there is plenty of room for improvement.

According to the UK's regulatory agency, the MHRA, in their latest report [13], 81.3% of commercial sponsors that the MHRA inspected had at least one major and/or critical finding. For noncommercial sponsors, the figure was even higher at 96.4%, and over one-fifth had at least one critical finding. Bearing in mind that a critical finding is one when the safety or well-being of trial subjects have either been or have significant potential to be jeopardized, and/or the clinical trial data are unreliable, then these statistics do not provide much confidence. The most common types of findings in the noncommercial sector were Investigational Medicinal Product (IMP) management, pharmacovigilance, and organizational oversight. These are worrying trends, as shortcomings in all of these activities can have a potentially serious impact on subject well-being.

On an international scale, data from the European Medicine's Agency (EMA) [14] makes equally disturbing reading. In that year, the EMA surveyed inspection information from their EudraCT database. This database contains summary information about all clinical trials of investigational medicinal products with at least one site in the European Union. The EMA collected data from 366 inspections worldwide, mostly at investigator sites, and discovered that nearly 70% of the organizations had at least one critical or major finding.

The clinical research sector needs to take a significant step to raise its standards and improve this profile of findings. It needs to do this in a climate of new challenges such as rapidly evolving technology, new geographical territories, and novel processes in the way that research is conducted, such as using a risk-based approach. By focusing on competence rather than experience, a fresh and novel approach can be developed to create a workforce that is motivated, hungry to learn, and flexible and dynamic to meet these new opportunities and challenges. This is a chance to make a significant step forward to develop new talent, contribute to the full employment of gifted young people, help longer serving employees maintain their professional competence, and to raise standards globally.

3.4 Threats: What Are the Consequences of Not Adopting Competence Verification to Develop Talent?

Some of the biggest obstacles of developing talent based on assessing competence are complacency, resistance to change, a dearth of expertise in assessing competence, and a lack of willingness to invest in the development of people.

If we do nothing, quality will inevitably deteriorate with the consequential risks to patients and the increased costs associated with rectifying errors and trials where no conclusions can be drawn because of poor execution and quality control. Analysis of clinical trial data queries [15] reveals approximately one CRF page in every five requires a data query. According to a white paper *Improving Clinical Trials Speed and Cost through Query Reduction* by David S. Zuckerman [16], the average cost of resolving a data query is about \$130. Imagine a clinical trial where patient enrollment stands at 300 and the CRF contains 70 pages. Based on the conclusions from the research above, we can reasonably estimate $300 \times 70 \times 0.2 = 4200$ data queries. At an average cost of \$130 to resolve each query this would equate to a total budget of \$546,000 to complete data query resolution for this fairly modest trial. There would appear to be ample opportunities for cost reduction by having competent monitors based just on reducing the number of data queries alone.

Unfortunately, many organizations, particularly when in a financial recession or when under extreme pressure to reduce costs, will sacrifice investment in the training and development of their staff. Increasing time and price pressure on CROs from their clients means less outlay in budget and availability for training. The result is a vicious circle where there is a danger that trials will overrun and go over budget because of a lack of competence. CROs are very wary of losing their best staff to their competitors resulting in the bizarre situation that they will hold back from developing their own people for fear of supplying a steady stream of competent staff to their rivals, expertise that they have developed and nurtured themselves. This, combined with a lack of management expertise in verifying competence and an overreliance on using the number of years' experience as a yardstick for ability, are the factors which are holding back the best opportunities for developing staff and raising standards.

Applicable Regulations.

None.

4. TAKE HOME MESSAGE

Using competence verification to develop and assess talent in the clinical research sector would make a significant contribution to improving the way that clinical trials are planned and executed. The value of developing new processes and new technology cannot be fully maximized unless there are competent people to exploit these advances. At worst, progress in improvements in the way that trials are conducted will stagnate and may even decline if peoples' competence profiles are not fit for this rapidly changing and dynamic work environment.

Employers have a responsibility to provide a framework for developing competent staff which includes the appropriate investment in competence-based learning and development as well as ensuring that managers have the skills to nurture talent. Each individual working in clinical research should have an obligation to develop themselves against performance standards and to gain recognition (accreditation or certification) of competence wherever possible. The regulatory authorities must move to inspecting methods of how sponsors and investigator sites ensure their staff are competent rather than reviewing attendance of training and, if necessary, they should introduce the need for accreditation. This is a great opportunity for the clinical research sector to make a major step forward in developing a talented, flexible global workforce that is equipped to meet the challenges of conducting top-quality clinical trials globally while protecting the rights and well-being of clinical trial subjects worldwide.

REFERENCES

[1] http://www.ema.europa.eu/docs/en_GB/document_library/Scientific_guideline /2013/11/WC500155491.pdf.
[2] http://www.fda.gov/downloads/Drugs/Guidances/UCM269919.pdf.
[3] Robinson Martin. What will it take for the industry to accept proof of competence over experience? Appl Clin Trials Online July 8, 2013.
[4] Half of workers quit jobs due to bad management. Chartered Management Institute. http://www.managers.org.uk/news/half-workers-quit-jobs-due-bad-management.

[5] Failure to retain competent employees costing UK businesses £42bn a year. Price WaterhouseCoopers. http://www.ukmediacentre.pwc.com/News-Releases/Failure-to -retain-competent-employees-costing-UK-businesses-42bn-a-year-f27.aspx.

[6] http://mrct.globalhealth.harvard.edu/pages/investigator-competence.

[7] IAoCR Task Force Develops Global Clinical Research Competencies. http:// iaocr.com/.

[8] Silva Honorio, Stonier Peter, Buhler Fritz, Deslypere Jean-Paul, Criscuolo Domenico, Nell Gerfried, et al. Core competencies for pharmaceutical physicians and drug development scientists. Front Pharmacol 2013;4:105.

[9] Boeynaems Jean-Marie, Canivet Cindy, Chan Anthony, Clarke Mary J, Cornu Catherine, Daemen Esther, et al. A European approach to clinical investigator training. Front Pharmacol 2013;4:112.

[10] http://www.vitae.ac.uk/researchers/428241/Researcher-Development-Framework .html.

[11] Hardman Mike, Brooksbank Cath, Johnson Claire, Janko Christa, See Wolf, Lafolie Pierre, et al. LifeTrain: towards a European framework for continuing professional development in biomedical sciences. Nat Rev Drug Discov 2013;12:407–8.

[12] http://www.transceleratebiopharmainc.comV.

[13] GCP Inspection Metrics 1st April 2009–31st March 2010 (Version 04/03/13).

[14] Annual report of the good clinical practice inspectors working group 2012.

[15] Desai Pankaj B, Anderson Christopher, Sietsema William K. A comparison of the quality of data, assessed using query rates, from clinical trials conducted across developed versus emerging global regions. Drug Inf J 2012;46:455.

[16] David S Zuckerman, Improving Clinical Trials Speed and Cost Through Query Reduction. Customized Improvement Strategies LLC. http://www.rx-business.com/pdf/ data%20analysis%20and%20reports/CIS%20Query%20Reduction%20White%20 Paper.pdf.

CHAPTER 29

Managing the Change—You Need Processes, Systems, and People

Heather Fraser

Contents

1. THE NEED

Pharma organizations have a choice to make. Their business model is broken, and the surrounding health system is changing. So, do they carry on their current approach of cutting costs while investing research dollars in searching for new medicines in already congested therapeutic areas such as oncology? The alternative is to completely rethink their role within the wider healthcare ecosystem, where traditional boundaries are currently being redefined, and a full range of stakeholders are converging with the patient and consumer at the center (Figure 29.1) [1,2].

The latter option requires a substantial adjustment, but brings with it the opportunity to thrive, becoming a very different entity from today. This choice of path will need careful management with change programs potentially spanning both within and outside traditional enterprise boundaries. Governance and strategies for the new business model will need to be defined and include organization and people as well as technology and processes.

Re-Engineering Clinical Trials
http://dx.doi.org/10.1016/B978-0-12-420246-7.00029-3

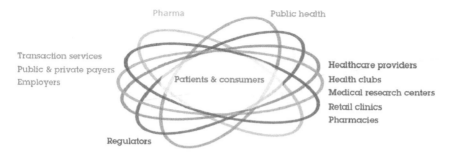

Figure 29.1 Healthcare stakeholders, including pharma, are converging to provide better patient-centered care and empowering consumers to take greater responsibility for their health.

2. SWOT

The change process recommended in this chapter benefits from looking outside the traditional boundaries for pharma. But, this brings with it potential pitfalls such as working across different organizational cultures as well as financial and regulatory tensions. The opportunity offered is one of enhanced value with rewards for the organization as well as others in the healthcare ecosystem and, ultimately, the patient. The biggest threats come, perhaps, from the regulatory authorities (Table 29.1).

3. THE SOLUTION

This chapter will describe how the change outlined earlier will be managed across five dimensions, with examples of the impact on the clinical development process:

- Governance and strategy—How do you govern change across borders; what metrics system needs to be in place to measure the success of the change?
- Organization and people—What new skills will be required; how do you instill a collaborative culture?
- Processes—How do you change business process?
- Tools and technology—How do you incorporate new tools such as social media and analytics in the development process; what standards need to be in place?
- Regulatory—What are the trade-offs between the different approaches and any associated risks?

Table 29.1 What is the impact the changes involved in healthcare convergence on the business?

Strength	Weakness
• Rethink the business beyond the pill and instead focus on the health and wellness of patients and consumers	• Requires individual organizations to leave behind business models based solely on the product and convene their thinking around the consumers and patients
Opportunity	**Threat**
• Improved quality and lowering costs of healthcare • Provides innovative ways of providing patient-centered care	• Regulations may inhibit the change • Standards need to be implemented across both geographical and ecosystem borders

3.1 Governance and Strategy

A comprehensive plan for governance is a basic requirement with high-level sponsorship as an important success factor. The structure may be permanent or a temporary entity and connected by virtual or physical means. For example, do you have an integrated clinical trials governance plan with all involved parties both inside and outside your enterprise—the clinical supply management function; the hospital pharmacy, investigators; clinical research organizations? In addition are metrics and incentives aligned both across and outside the business? Are you using analytics and other tools to better match patients with clinical trials and track the performance and leading indicators?

3.2 Organization and People

Organizations are facing major decisions relating to business structure and their strategic place in the new ecosystem (Figure 29.2) [3]. In parallel, they must decide on how they change their existing organization to meet their vision. Will you keep the traditional hierarchical organization and leadership model with expertise and management systems aligned to business domains? Alternatively, will you build an innovative organization that is open, transparent, and collaborative, and shares resources beyond the enterprise to rapidly address new opportunities? Do you have the right skill balance internally? Indeed, should innovation be embedded into all roles within R&D-intensive industries, such as pharma? What further capabilities do you need to cultivate in house or partner externally to

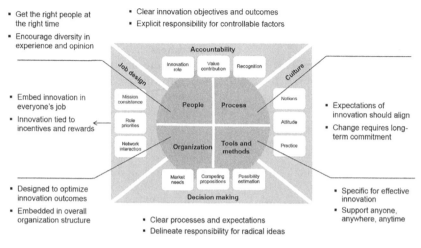

Figure 29.2 Innovation should sit within the organization—dedicated innovation roles, functions, and processes must be nimble.

acquire—from biotech, academia, hospitals, or elsewhere? Finally, how do you build a strong learning culture drawing from expertise from inside and outside and using dynamically formed teams to help the organizations to meet their vision?

3.3 Processes

Having defined their new business structure, pharma executive's next need to look at adjusting existing systems and processes. Will you optimize processes and systems vertically across business domains, functions or therapeutic area or integrate horizontally using a component-based approach? The industry leaders of tomorrow will make a strategic decisions on which processes to retain internally; which to outsource or which services to share. In addition, how do you ensure your processes are dynamic and any changes, such as analytics insights, are integrated on an on-going basis across the enterprise?

3.4 Tools and Technology

Emerging technologies such as mobile, social, analytics, and cloud are expanding dynamic possibilities for all types of innovation as well as lowering barriers to imitation.

While analytics tools can potentially benefit individual organizations, the realization of optimum benefits requires analytics to be applied across the entire healthcare ecosystem. Clinical development can benefit from using these new tools. For example, analytics can help better match patients with clinical trials, and mobile tools can help tracking performance in real time, whether they are in the clinic or being remotely monitored at home. In addition, how do development organizations use social business tools and capacities to actively listen to patients and consumers to discern their needs for future trials?

3.5 Regulatory

Regulations governing healthcare and medicines continue to become more onerous and are likely to impede convergence. A full understanding of the trade-offs from different regulatory approaches is essential. The leaders of tomorrow—who will work with the regulatory authorities to balance the desire to spur innovation and change with the need for structure, safety, quality, and compliance?

4. APPLICABLE REGULATIONS

All ICH GCP; FDA, EMA, and PMDA regulations relating to development and various industry and ecosystem standards such as HL7, CDISC, and HIPAA.

5. TAKE HOME MESSAGE

Change to the business models of pharma organizations is inevitable if they are to flourish in the future. How they go about managing this change, both inside and outside their organizational boundaries, will determine their level of success. Change in governance, strategy, technology, business processes, and regulations will also need careful handling. Successful innovation today needs to be more collaborative, open, and continuous if it is to meet the needs of the pharma company of the future.

REFERENCES

[1] Lefever G, Pesanello M, Fraser H, Taurman L. Fade or flourish – Rethinking the role of life sciences companies in the healthcare ecosystem. IBM Institute for Business Value; 2011.
[2] Mason B, Bacher G, Reynolds H, Fraser H. Collaborating beyond traditional boundaries – What convergence means for our health care systems. IBM Institute for Business Value and AHIP Foundation's Institute for Health Systems Solutions; 2013.
[3] Marshall A, de Rooij M, Biscotti M. Insatiable innovation – from sporadic to systemic. IBM Institute for Business Value; 2013.

CHAPTER 30

How Quality Performance Metrics Enable Successful Change

Linda B. Sullivan

Contents

1. THE NEED

As many companies in the pharmaceutical industry focus on improvements—whether in terms of cost, production, personnel, quality, or other areas—they often find themselves changing at a rate inconsistent with their expectations, and sometimes in ways they had not originally planned for. A focus on minimizing turnaround time may result in a decrease in the quality of data, or there may be significant cost overruns due to extra resources needed to complete the task in a timely manner. Often, single-minded attempts to cut costs can be shortsighted, causing more harm than good at a company. With all this in mind, organizations are encouraging policies and practices that support assessing risk during the planning stages of a project. By proactively managing risk factors, surprises during execution can be avoided. In order to successfully manage any changes and risks in how organizations execute clinical trials, quality performance metrics are useful—even necessary.

Re-Engineering Clinical Trials
http://dx.doi.org/10.1016/B978-0-12-420246-7.00030-X
337

2. THE SOLUTION

2.1 Quality Performance Metrics: An Introduction

The mantra "What gets measured gets fixed" lies at the heart of quality performance metrics [1]. All the performance areas mentioned earlier certainly can be quantified and measured: costs, cycle times, quality of data collected, efficiency, and so on. The real question is how to measure these areas of focus in a way that is helpful to companies and consistent through various scenarios. We can do this by using agreed-upon standards of measure—also known as metrics. Quality performance metrics, in particular, measure the number of errors or percentage of errors relative to a specified set of requirements. Quality performance metrics can assess the number of protocol amendments, errors per information transmission, protocol quality score, frequency of database errors after lock, percentage of subjects with inadequate informed consent, and so on. Using metrics to measure the quality of performance in each of these areas makes it easy to highlight both successes and shortcomings that can be improved on, and to make meaningful comparisons.

Quality performance metrics can be used to drive change in how individuals, departments, companies, or even the industry design, execute, and manage clinical trial processes. Having these measurements allows us to determine the areas in which change has successfully occurred, and better examine the areas in which changes have been suboptimal. Also, proactively using quality performance metrics encourages a culture of risk management (or even risk prevention) that reduces problems in the long run.

Quality performance metrics are a critical component of a larger process of continual improvement, characterized as the "plan–do–check–act" (PDCA) cycle [2] (Figure 30.1). For instance, instituting amendments to

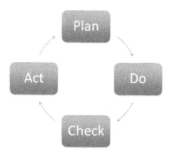

Figure 30.1 The plan–do–check–act cycle.

a protocol (i.e., changes at the "act" step) results in cost overruns and time delays; thus a retroactive focus on quality comes at a financial cost to the company—a study by the Tufts Center for Drug Development showed that more than 40% of clinical-trials protocols were amended before the first patient visit had even occurred [3]. Amended protocols averaged 2.3 amendments and four months of incremental time for implementation, and amendments that included cost data showed an average cost of almost half a million dollars per amendment. Using these numbers means that an average protocol has cost overruns of just over a million dollars, and time overruns of a third of a year! The goal of using quality metrics is to advance to a proactive level of managed change, i.e., introducing the quality metrics at the "plan" and "check" steps of the PDCA cycle in Figure 30.1. When used at those points, protocols will be evaluated by these metrics and revised *before* implementation, resulting in fewer amendments after implementation, fewer cost and time overruns, and increased performance quality [4]. As usage of metrics permeates a company's culture, use of these metrics will be proactive at increasingly higher levels of management, thus allowing more processes to be carried out with less rework, and fewer overruns and other complications.

The ultimate goal of quality performance metrics is to improve, as the name suggests, quality of performance within processes. The end result can include increased training, improved communications, and better data management, among other prospects [5]. Quite often, this goal includes reducing the amount of costly rework.

2.2 Using the Right Metrics

In order to make the best use of quality performance metrics, a company's key metrics have to be selected for their value [6]. Four questions help in selecting the most useful or valuable metrics (Figure 30.2):

1. What are you measuring? What is the question you are trying to answer with the metric?
2. How and when will it be measured? Can it be measured?
3. Who will track and report the metric?
4. Whose performance is being measured?

Above all, the metrics chosen should focus on measuring "quality that matters" or quality that is "fit for purpose." This means that companies should select metrics that will let them assess aspects directly impacting patient safety or data quality. Today's IT systems can aggregate and report an overwhelming number of metrics, but a recent survey showed that less

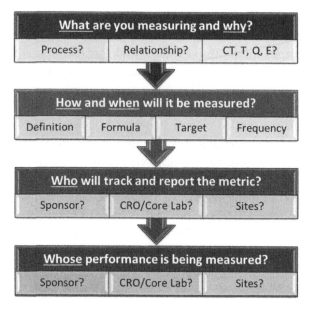

Figure 30.2 Key metric selection questions.

than one-fifth of companies collected, reviewed, and effectively used quality performance metrics [7]. When organizations focus on "quality that matters," they should be selective about which metrics they utilize. Specifically, they should select metrics that target critical-to-quality processes [8]. For example, including metrics that assess the quality of a protocol before final approval—thus avoiding costly protocol amendments later in the study—brings a quality focus to the design of a clinical trial. Unfortunately, many organizations focus their efforts on achieving a time-related metric—"time to enroll first patient," for example—which is not the most useful, effective, or performance-quality-focused metric to measure. As these organizations strive to achieve the "time to enroll first patient" metric, they lose sight of the importance of developing and approving a scientifically sound, executable protocol, and selecting high-quality sites that can enroll the right patients and provide quality data (Figure 30.3). A focus on getting the first patient enrolled often means approving a protocol that needs to be amended shortly after the team has enrolled the first patient. These organizations have achieved their first-patient targets, only to have protocol amendment(s) slow down the rest of the enrollment process. Thus, achieving the first-patient target does not mean that the rest of the enrollment performance expectations will be

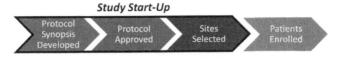

Figure 30.3 Steps in a study start-up.

Metrics that measure performance of related tasks
should be reviewed together to understand the
combined performance ...

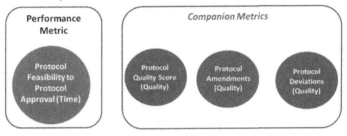

Figure 30.4 Some performance metrics should be reviewed together as companion metrics.

achieved. Rather, the goal should be to select, measure, and monitor metrics that are directly relevant and useful for improving a protocol, which in turn leads to faster overall enrollment even if the first patient enrolls a bit later than expected.

In addition to selecting the right metrics to measure, it is important to realize that these metrics should not be assessed in isolation. There are multiple perspectives that must be taken into account (e.g., the quality of the protocol *and* the quality of the sites relative to that protocol). Only by looking at multiple metrics simultaneously can overall performance quality be increased. Thus, when instituting change based on information from a specific metric, it is necessary to take into account related metrics as well. Often, several metrics tend to cluster together (Figure 30.4), and a change that affects one metric is likely to have a similar (or perhaps inverse) effect on those "companion" metrics. Examining those companion metrics allows change to be targeted more narrowly and carefully. Many times, the various companion metrics may have inverse relationships to one another. This is best visualized with the image of a balloon (Figure 30.5): If the goal is to compress the balloon, pushing in on one side causes the other side to expand, but does not result in any change in the overall size of the balloon. However, pushing on all sides of the

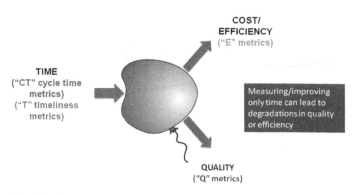

Figure 30.5 Performance metrics are paired to ensure performance improvement.

balloon simultaneously will indeed compress the balloon. Similarly, measuring only one type of metric (say timeliness) may improve that metric while degrading others (e.g., cost). Measuring companion metrics of multiple types (timeliness, quality, cycle time, and efficiency/cost), however, will usually result in overall performance improvements. To return to the previous example, "time to first enrolled patient" may come at the expense of a well-designed protocol and a thorough approval process. Similarly, sites may be selected in haste and may not be well matched to the protocol requirements. If (and when) problems result from these decisions made in haste, the solution will mean cost increases and a decline in efficiency. Often, improvement is made a goal with the implicit assumption that costs should remain fixed. By including cost as a specific metric to be balanced with the others targeted for improvement, it becomes more likely that costs will be contained or even reduced through the actions taken to improve the other chosen metrics. The quality of data collected, for example, can sometimes be improved by automating both data collection and transmittal—for example, having a machine automatically transmit ECGs right away rather than having a researcher potentially introduce human error by manually fixing them the next day. That researcher could instead assist in other procedures, resulting in a more efficient and speedy operation. Successful change for multiple metrics can only be achieved through an organized plan that targets all relevant metrics simultaneously.

2.3 Evaluating and Visualizing Metrics Data

In recent decades, exponential improvements in technology, as well as its proliferation in nearly all aspects of the pharmaceutical industry, has made it far easier to measure and track nearly anything that can be quantified. Similarly, the availability and raw power of data-analytics software means that calculations that once took days to complete can now be performed in a few keystrokes. As database systems become increasingly interconnected, the criteria for success within a specific metric can now be measured across multiple companies, and data can be compared across the industry at large. This visible opportunity for competition can galvanize companies or departments that need an additional spur to begin improvements in quality performance of processes.

A potential challenge in using and evaluating metrics is that they may not be interpreted correctly. Different forms of visual presentation are useful for different types of analysis and for highlighting different trends or patterns [9]. Although it is often tempting to select data and chart types that are eye-catching (such as a pie chart), the primary goal in creating charts should be making useful information available for interpretation and extrapolation (such as using a line or bar chart to compare variations over time) (Figure 30.6) [10]. People should be trained to understand these different forms of data visualization and to make informed, logical decisions (to take action, to target a specific problem, etc.) that are rooted in this same data. It is not enough to simply measure and report metrics; those measurements have to be an effective catalyst for improvement and change.

2.4 Using Metrics for Successful Change

As companies begin to consistently use quality performance metrics to better manage changes and improvements in their processes and general operations, they should closely monitor all aspects of the system being changed to make sure that improvements in one sector do not come at the expense of another sector. Often, using standardized quality performance metrics throughout a company results in increased and improved communication between disparate departments, and streamlines redundant or unnecessary operations. Consequently, it is important to move toward industry-wide standardized performance metrics, so that organizations can compare results across their own studies and compare their company's performance with that of other companies.

In order to integrate metrics within a workplace or a full company, individuals should be trained in the uses and advantages of metrics. This education can occur in many different formats, such as full-day seminars and workshops, or through sequences of short videos and webinars. Exposure is

Status: Yellow

Owner: John Doe

Metric Definition:
Total queries generated during the month for all clinical trials divided by total CRF pages entered by data management for all trials during the same month.

Included/Excluded Data:
Phase II, III, and IV queries included.
Phase I queries excluded.

Type I queries included. Type II queries excluded.
Paper CRF queries only.

Data Sources:
All data from Data Management.

Data Integrity Issues:
None

Reporting Frequency:
Monthly

Goal:
.05 queries per CRF page on a monthly basis by December.

Comparison:
Best paper CRF query rate found in the literature is .06

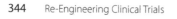

Monthly Queries Per CRF Page

Trends: Improving

Probability of Achieving Goal: Low

Improvement Strategies:
√ Instituted new site training method last December.
√ Began measuring CRAs on their site query rates in March.
√ Began sending query rate data to sites in August.
  Will begin following up with sites on query reports next month.

Variances:
February and March data were worse due to launch of a trial in a new therapeutic area where we were using new sites.

Corrective Actions for Variances:
None

Figure 30.6 A run chart compares variations over time.

frequently the first step in the process of teaching people about quality performance metrics, followed by basic categorization of different metrics types, and then exercises in practical application of these metrics. Only through proper training and education will individuals be able to successfully contextualize and utilize quality performance metrics within their action plans for process improvement.

Another challenge in implementing a successful metrics system is that people may worry that they will be punished. Above all, quality metrics must be used within a culture that actively supports quality performance improvement, not punishment of people. As such, the application and analysis of these metrics needs to be designed specifically to reward people for measuring and improving quality performance—not just time and cost. For example, clinical study staff that demonstrate success in improving specific metrics, such as "percentage of final reports issued to sites within agreed turnaround time" and "number of protocol amendments" might be granted larger research budgets or priority usage of shared equipment. With top-down management support, a culture supportive of improvement through quality performance metrics is entirely possible.

An emphasis on top-down management support also forestalls the other potential challenge to effective use of metrics: silos within companies. Occasionally, different departments, working groups, or other collectives may be so deeply partitioned from one another that they have little to no communication. When this happens, these "silos" will rapidly diverge from one another in their needs, goals, expectations, and workplace cultures. This concern can be minimized by proactive management—if silos are held accountable for the impact that their output has on the ability of other departments to do their work, the "silo effect" will be reduced dramatically. Using a common set of quality performance metrics—which, again, are standards of measurement—will prevent this lack of communication from balkanizing a company's many divisions.

Ultimately, quality performance metrics are crucial to successful change in how organizations plan, execute, and manage clinical trials (Figure 30.7). With quality metrics, protocols can be designed that better meet stated goals of cost, efficiency, quality, and more. And with quality metrics, companies and the pharmaceutical industry as a whole can more successfully meet current and future challenges.

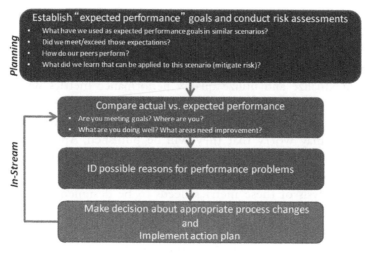

Figure 30.7 Why do you need performance metrics?

3. SWOT

3.1 Strengths

- Enables companies to identify and target problems in quality and performance
- Results in specific problems being resolved without increases in cost or other issues

3.2 Weaknesses

- Requires senior management support and culture change
- Requires training to use metrics effectively

3.3 Opportunities

- Regulatory agencies support quality risk management approaches
- Advancements in IT systems and data-analytic platforms improve access to the data needed to create and report metrics

3.4 Threats

- Nonalignment of regulatory agencies' quality management expectations
- Data to create metrics may not be available and/or may be difficult to access
- Silos within companies make it difficult to align needs and expectations
- Aversity to change

4. APPLICABLE REGULATIONS

- N/A

5. TAKE HOME MESSAGE

- "What gets measured gets fixed": Using quality performance metrics sends a message that quality is a priority and allows management to identify and quantify specific issues.
- Metrics should be selected for usefulness and predictiveness.
- Analyzing multiple metrics enables improvement without cost overruns and other issues.
- Top-down support for proactive use of quality performance metrics results in successful change.

REFERENCES

[1] Zuckerman DS. What gets measured gets fixed: using metrics to make continuous progress in R&D efficiency. Monit 2012:23–8.

[2] Sprenger K, Nickerson D, Meeker-O'Connell A, Morrison BW. Quality by design in clinical trials a collaborative pilot with FDA. Ther Innovation Regul Sci 2013;47(2):161–6.

[3] Getz K, Zuckerman R, Cropp AB, Hindle AL, Krauss R, Kaitin KI. Measuring the incidence, causes, and repercussions of protocol amendments. Drug Inf J 2011:265–75.

[4] Wool L. Intertwining quality management systems with metrics to improve trial quality. Monit 2012:29–35.

[5] Kleppinger CF, Ball LK. Building quality in clinical trials with use of a quality systems approach. Clin Infect Dis 2010;51(Suppl. 1):S111–6.

[6] Dorricott K. Using metrics to direct performance improvement efforts in clinical trial management. Monit 2012:9–13.

[7] Sullivan LB, Wool L. Performance metrics in clinical trials: putting the promise into practice. Monit 2012:7–8.

[8] Sullivan LB. Defining "Quality that matters" in clinical trial study startup activities. Monit 2011:22–6.

[9] Hake P. Clinical metrics 102: best practices for the visualization of clinical performance metrics. Monit 2012:15–21.

[10] Zuckerman DS. Pharmaceutical metrics. Gower Press; 2006.

CHAPTER 31

Conclusion

Brendan M. Buckley, Peter Schüler

Contents

1. TAKE HOME MESSAGE

Even though the pharmaceutical industry depends heavily on the discovery of innovative products, it is intensely conservative in the manner in which it conducts clinical trials.

For example, it could reasonably be argued that the most important technical development in the conduct of clinical trials occurred in the fifteenth century when printing with moveable type was invented. It took over a decade before electronic data capture (EDC) largely replaced paper-based case record forms. Even with EDC there is an unacceptable delay in the flow of information. The verification of data is highly labor intensive and costly. Despite the encouragement of the major regulatory agencies, embodied in guidance on matters such as adaptive trial designs and risk-based monitoring, industry moves with reluctance, fearing that change from conventional ways of working is too risky. However, the realities of economics and the ongoing division of diseases into ever less common therapeutic sub-types now mean that the pharmaceutical industry cannot afford to hope to improve the drug development process by small incremental steps. The previous chapters have described a wide variety of options for an overdue change. Ultimately, progress needs to come from the implementation of many of these together, championed by companies that manage the risks of change by realigning their internal processes to mitigate them. Those that embrace this because they realize the imperative to evolve quickly will succeed into the future. The dramatic manner in which digital photography swept away a giant and long-established film-based industry illustrates how those who stagnate may lose.

Re-Engineering Clinical Trials
http://dx.doi.org/10.1016/B978-0-12-420246-7.00031-1

INDEX

Note: Page numbers followed by "b", "f" and "t" indicate boxes, figures and tables, respectively.

CPSIA information can be obtained at www.ICGtesting.com
Printed in the USA
BVOW10*0400060215

386359BV00001B/1/P

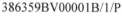